AF774251

Dental Age Assessment

Aman Chowdhry • Priyanka Kapoor
Editors

Dental Age Assessment

A Global Perspective

Springer

Editors
Aman Chowdhry
Faculty of Dentistry
Jamia Millia Islamia
New Delhi, India

Priyanka Kapoor
Faculty of Dentistry
Jamia Millia Islamia
New Delhi, India

ISBN 978-3-032-08787-4 ISBN 978-3-032-08788-1 (eBook)
https://doi.org/10.1007/978-3-032-08788-1

© The Editor(s) (if applicable) and The Author(s), under exclusive license to Springer Nature Switzerland AG 2026

This work is subject to copyright. All rights are solely and exclusively licensed by the Publisher, whether the whole or part of the material is concerned, specifically the rights of translation, reprinting, reuse of illustrations, recitation, broadcasting, reproduction on microfilms or in any other physical way, and transmission or information storage and retrieval, electronic adaptation, computer software, or by similar or dissimilar methodology now known or hereafter developed.
The use of general descriptive names, registered names, trademarks, service marks, etc. in this publication does not imply, even in the absence of a specific statement, that such names are exempt from the relevant protective laws and regulations and therefore free for general use.
The publisher, the authors and the editors are safe to assume that the advice and information in this book are believed to be true and accurate at the date of publication. Neither the publisher nor the authors or the editors give a warranty, expressed or implied, with respect to the material contained herein or for any errors or omissions that may have been made. The publisher remains neutral with regard to jurisdictional claims in published maps and institutional affiliations.

This Springer imprint is published by the registered company Springer Nature Switzerland AG
The registered company address is: Gewerbestrasse 11, 6330 Cham, Switzerland

If disposing of this product, please recycle the paper.

Preface

The lack of an extensive, internationally applicable reference on dental age assessment in the field of forensic odontology was identified as a gap in the literature, which gave rise to the concept for this book. It was becoming more and more obvious that a special volume on dental age estimation was necessary following the success of our earlier work, *Handbook of Forensic Odontology: A Global Perspective* (2018). With collaboration from leading scientists across the globe, we provide *Essentials of Dental Age Assessment: A Global Perspective*—a work influenced by multidisciplinary insights and international expertise.

We would like to sincerely thank the Springer Nature production team for their dedication, professional support, and direction in making this book a reality. Their work has been crucial in shaping this book into a polished and accessible academic resource.

This book covers a wide range of age estimation methodologies, from prenatal to adult stages, while integrating classical and contemporary approaches. It is intended to be both academically rigorous and easily readable. In order to enhance student learning, each chapter includes multiple-choice questions (MCQs), mind maps, and well-illustrated graphics. In-depth discussions are held on cutting-edge subjects including DNA methylation, artificial intelligence, and radiocarbon dating, as well as conventional methods like the London Atlas and Camariere techniques.

In an effort to put knowledge into practice, the book also highlights the usefulness of age assessment through report writing that is supported by literature. With contributions from all around the world and an approachable structure, this book hopes to become a fundamental resource for forensic odontology researchers, practitioners, educators, and students everywhere.

In addition to being a trustworthy companion in forensic and academic contexts, we hope that this volume makes a significant contribution to practice and learning.

New Delhi, India

Aman Chowdhry
Priyanka Kapoor

Contents

Introduction to Dental Age Assessment

1

Aman Chowdhry and Priyanka Kapoor

Abbreviations

CA	chronological age
CBCT	cone beam computed tomography
CT	computed tomography
DAE	dental age estimation
DNA	deoxyribonucleic acid
IOPA	intra oral periapical radiograph
IUL	intra-uterine life
OPG	orthopantomogram

1.1 Concepts and Definitions

- Forensic age estimation:

  "Expertise in forensic medicine that aims to define, in the most accurate way, the chronological age of a person of unknown age involved in judicial or legal proceedings" [1].
- Chronologic age:

  The difference between the individual's date of birth and the date on which the age is being calculated [2].

A. Chowdhry (✉)
Oral Pathology & Microbiology, Faculty of Dentistry, Jamia Millia Islamia, New Delhi, India
e-mail: achowdhry@jmi.ac.in

P. Kapoor
Orthodontics, Faculty of Dentistry, Jamia Millia Islamia, New Delhi, India
e-mail: pkapoor@jmi.ac.in

© The Author(s), under exclusive license to Springer Nature Switzerland AG 2026

A. Chowdhry, P. Kapoor (eds.), *Dental Age Assessment*,
https://doi.org/10.1007/978-3-032-08788-1_1

- Dental age:
  It is the assessment of the stage of dental maturity based on various factors including calcification, mineralization, eruption, and/or post-eruption morphologic changes seen in teeth. Dental age can be an indication of chronological age for an individual.
- Skeletal age:
  It is an interpretation of skeletal maturity, primarily assessed on radiographs (hand-wrist or lateral cephalogram, etc.), and can be further correlated with dental or chronological age.
- Dental age estimation:
  DAE as defined by the authors of current chapter is "Utilization of single or multiple scientific techniques for determination of age of living or dead individuals by using biological or radiologic samples of teeth is called dental age estimation."

1.2 Introduction to Age Assessment

Age can be considered an indicator of the maturity level for an individual. It can be measured as:

- Chronological age
- Physical age
- Dental age
- Mental age
- Skeletal maturation
- Sexual maturity

Assessment and interpretation of age-related changes in the dead and living are of paramount importance for multiple disciplines [3]. These domains include human biology/evolution, archaeology, pediatrics, palaeo-demography, palaeontology, forensic anthropology, public health, legal medicine [3, 4], and dentistry. The chronological age is ascertained by birth registration in the respective national registries but is subject to a wide divide based on the developing and developed parts of the world. According to recent UNICEF data (2021) on birth registration, North America and Western Europe show 100% registration below the age of 5, followed by Eastern Europe, the Caribbean, Latin America, and Central Asia, showing 94–99% registration, reducing to 40% in the Sub-Saharan African region [5]. Hence, the current scenario, which witnesses higher population migration and crime rate, mandates employing various methods to ascertain age as close to the chronological age as possible for legal renderings. While skeletal age relies more on identifying growth-related changes in the bony skeleton, dental age focuses on the stages of development and calcification of teeth, at multiple levels—histologically, clinically, and radiographically. Dental age estimation (DAE) is a crucial tool not only for growth studies in children and orthodontic treatment planning, but it can also play a pivotal role in forensic identification and anthropological studies. Since these DAE methods are based on the pattern of tooth calcification and eruption, they can allow higher precision in determining chronological age.

Forensic age estimation estimates an individual's true chronologic age by assessing skeletal and dental development and maturation with a sound scientific basis [6]. The accuracy of age estimation varies with different methods in different populations; hence a scientist uses an age range with a corresponding degree of accuracy mentioned for the specific methods involved. Since it better captures the scientific character and inherent uncertainty of the process, forensic professionals are increasingly emphasising that "forensic age estimation" is the most precise and frequently used term within the discipline. The word "estimation" emphasises that establishing age in forensic circumstances does not need to establish a precise chronological age, but rather a likely age range based on biological indications.

1.3 Why Assessment of Age Is Important in Forensics

Forensic age estimation is a crucial aspect of forensic science that determines a person's chronological age in situations where documentary evidence is either disputed, unavailable, or purposefully fabricated. It significantly contributes to both legal and humanitarian contexts by providing an unbiased scientific foundation for decisions related to age and identity verification. Forensic age estimation may be required in several civil and criminal situations, including:

1.3.1 Civil Matters

- Societal norms
- Voting
- Marriage
- Retirement
- Consent
- Labor laws
- Refugees
- Recruitments

1.3.2 Criminal Offenses and Sentences

- Sexual assaults
- Juvenile crimes
- Homicide

Witnessing the current global trend of a rising incidence of disasters (man-made or natural), crime rate, population migration (in reference to the recent Russia-Ukraine conflict), and asylum seekers, it is extremely essential to have a confirmed correct legal identity of an individual. Hence, the estimation of age can be primarily important in three different aspects:

Aspects	Explanation	Possible applications
Comparative assessment	Where the age assessed by dental or skeletal means are matched with the known chronological age of an individual	E.g., possible suspects/victims with known chronological age, age forgery, asylum seekers, etc.
Reconstructive profiling:	Where the deceased or living individual's identity is unknown, and age is one of the measures to ascertain the profile of the individual	E.g., mass disasters, unidentified bodies/body parts, etc.
Age-related research in forensics:	Dental age estimation in correlation with skeletal age or chronological age in different ethnicities and sex. Also, intra-and inter-examiner variations in different methods	E.g., forensic on-field or institution-based research on different age estimation methods, simulation research etc.

1.4 Why Are Teeth Important as Biological Structure for Age Estimation

Defining an appropriate, convenient, and accurate age estimation method is still a worldwide issue [7]. Although various parts of the body can be utilized for the estimation of the age, teeth can serve as an important tool in forensic investigations, especially in paleo-demographic research or in a forensic context (age estimation) [8].

There are various plausible mechanisms which make teeth suitable as biological entities for age estimation:

(a) *Specific patterns of development*: Teeth have set patterns of development from the in-utero stage to adulthood, which can be traced as per formation, calcification, and eruption in different age groups. The sequential formation and eruption of teeth during the first two decades, followed by their regressive changes with advancing age, assist in prediction of age [8, 9]. These have been used in various image-based atlas systems like the Schour and Massler or more recently the London Atlas for determining the age of individuals. They have also been developed into calculative scoring systems like the Demirjian method or the Camariere method, etc., for greater accuracy and objectivity [10].
(b) *Resistant to taphonomic processes*: High mineralization of the tooth structure makes it resistant to extreme conditions such as high temperatures, decomposition, assaults/abuses, disasters (man-made or natural), and pressure, etc. [7]. Additionally, in mass disaster situations where there is a high possibility of soft tissue distortion, the tooth structure remains a stable and reliable means of age determination [8].
(c) *DNA-based age estimation*: Teeth contain DNA, which can help determine the individual's age (using DNA-based age-prediction models), sex, or ethnicity, in addition to identifying them based on their distinctive tooth patterns and characteristics [11].

(d) *More reliable than osseous structures*: Age estimation based on teeth is more reliable than bony age determinations in several ways, as follows:

- Development of bones is completed by the age of 18, whereas tooth development continues up to the 20s (third molar).
- Bone development is influenced by nutritional and environmental factors, whereas tooth development is majorly dependent on genetic factors.
- Bones may not survive the extremes of temperature and pressure as borne by the teeth.

1.5 Introduction to Dental Age Estimation

Dental age estimation techniques have emerged as an imperative and handy component of forensic odontology, along with being an important measure in treatment planning in dentofacial orthodontics or in endocranial and pediatric populations. Various methods of DAE have been used, which can be classified and understood based on different concepts of development, visualization of teeth, methods of examination, or even special situations where dental age shows variations, including craniofacial abnormalities of cleft, Down's syndrome, etc. [12]. These DAE techniques have been classified by various authors based on their understanding of the concept and presented in the last chapter of this book in the form of a mind map.

Growth and maturation are unique to each human and can be used to derive a corresponding age. Presently, DAE techniques are considered the best for assessing the true CA especially during the morphological developmental age range of the dentition [6]. Further, the accuracy and objectivity of the existing methods are enhanced with recent digital solutions such as three-dimensional cone-beam computed tomography (3D-CBCT) or micro CT volumetric assessments of teeth. Furthermore, the applications of artificial intelligence and machine learning on this digital data are also being explored to develop algorithms to further improve the accuracy and automation of age assessment methods.

Still, no single method of DAE is considered the best and applicable for all age groups and ethnicities. Hence, it is imperative to study age with more than one technique and approximate the true age of the individual with the corresponding degree of accuracy.

Therefore, this book reviews and compiles all the principles, methodologies, techniques utilized in forensic dental age estimation to provide the reader a complete overview of the topic. Not only does the book entail each aspect of age estimation in a separate chapter, but it also provides a mind map to enable the readers to comprehend the concepts in a visually illustrative and simple manner.

1.6 Summary and Conclusion

Dental age estimation in forensics has proven its importance in both the comparative and reconstructive profiling of individuals. In criminal, civil, or legal scenarios, DAE is routinely employed to closely match the chronological age of the individual, which is either unknown or is deliberately forged or hidden. The importance of teeth as a measure of estimating the age has been highlighted in the current chapter, keeping in mind the resistance of the hard tissue structure to decomposition under extreme pressure and temperature conditions. Further, teeth have an advantage of depicting distinct developmental stages from childhood till late adulthood. It is estimated by different methods, including radiological, biochemical, or visual, with a varying degree of accuracy. The objectivity and accuracy of various DAE methods have been improved with the advent of newer 3D CBCT/micro CT volumetric assessments. Further, the automation of age assessment based on algorithms generated on digital radiographic data by artificial intelligence and machine learning is also being pursued. Hence, this book aims to highlight all areas related to dental age estimation, from conventional to contemporary methods, and also focuses on recent research areas targeted to reduce the range of accuracy by different DAE methods, and to define the most accurate age estimation for each age group, considering ethnicity and sex.

1.7 Learning Outcomes

- You should be able to understand the importance of age estimation in forensics and the basics of age estimation, and get oriented towards concepts of age assessment.
- You should be able to comprehend the different types of DAE and the correlation of their applications in research and clinical fields.

1.8 Self-Evaluation Questions

- What are the different types of age of an individual?
- Why do we need to estimate the age of an individual?
- What are the different aspects in which age estimation is done, with relevant examples?
- Why are teeth favorable for forensic age estimation?

1.9 Multiple Choice Questions

Q1. Which of the following types of age of an individual?

(a) Dental age
(b) Skeletal age
(c) Mental age
(d) All of the above

Ans: d

Q2. When an unidentified body of an individual is found, whose age is unknown, how do you ascertain the age?

(a) Comparative profiling
(b) Reconstructive profiling
(c) Ethnicity-based research
(d) Antemortem data profiling

Ans: b

Q3. Why are teeth a viable structure for age estimation?

(a) Resistant to high temperature and pressure conditions
(b) Stable in the same stage of development throughout life
(c) Decomposes the DNA contained within the pulp
(d) Influenced mainly by nutritional factors

Ans. a

Q4. Visual comparison of the developmental stage of teeth with standards to estimate the age is done in which method?

(a) Scoring method
(b) Calculation method
(c) Regression formula method
(d) Atlas method

Ans. d

Q5. Age forgery is routinely seen in which case?

(a) Sports quota benefits
(b) Juvenile crime
(c) Retirement benefits
(d) All of the above

Ans. d

References

1. Grover N, Puri N, Arora S, Singh S, Singh N. Age estimation from physiological changes of teeth: a reliable age marker? J Forensic Dent Sci. 2014;6(2):113.
2. Kotecha SD. Dental age estimation in children: a review. Foresic Res Criminol Int J [Internet]. 2016 Nov 11 [cited 2021 Dec 27];3(1). Available from: https://medcraveonline.com/FRCIJ/dental-age-estimation-in-children-a-review.html.
3. Bittles TAAH, Collins KJ, editors. The biology of human ageing. Cambridge: Cambridge University Press; 1986. p. 280. £19.50, ISBN 0 521 30485 7. Ageing Soc. 1986;6(4):524–525.
4. Liversidge HM, Buckberry J, Marquez-Grant N. Age estimation. Ann Hum Biol. 2015;42(4):299–301.
5. Birth Registration [Internet]. Available from: https://data.unicef.org/topic/child-protection/birth-registration.

6. Lewis JM, Senn DR. Forensic dental age estimation: an overview. J Calif Dent Assoc. 2015;43(6):315–9.
7. Marroquin TY, Karkhanis S, Kvaal SI, Vasudavan S, Kruger E, Tennant M. Age estimation in adults by dental imaging assessment systematic review. Forensic Sci Int. 2017;275:203–11.
8. Krishan K, Kanchan T, Garg AK. Dental evidence in forensic identification—an overview, methodology and present status. Open Dent J. 2015;9:250–6.
9. AlQahtani SJ, Hector MP, Liversidge HM. Accuracy of dental age estimation charts: Schour and Massler, Ubelaker and the London Atlas. Am J Phys Anthropol. 2014;154(1):70–8.
10. Kapoor P. Age Estimation from teeth. In: Handbook on forensic odontology: an indian perspective. 1st ed. Century Publications; 2018. p. 18–36.
11. Correia Dias H, Corte-Real F, Cunha E, Manco L. DNA methylation age estimation from human bone and teeth. Aust J Forensic Sci. 2020:1–14.
12. Cherian J, Thomas A, Kapoor S, Kumar R. Dental age estimation using Willems method: a cross-sectional study on children in a North Indian city. J Oral Maxillofac Pathol. 2020;24(2):383.

2 Historical Perspective of Dental Age Assessment

Gabriel M. Fonseca and Cezar Capitaneanu

Abbreviations

ABFO	American Board of Forensic Odontology
DAE	Dental age estimation
IOFOS	International Organization for Forensic Odonto-Stomatology
IOPA	Intra oral periapical radiograph
NAS	United States, National Academy of Sciences
OPG	Orthopantomogram
UK	United Kingdom
UN	United Nations
WW1	World War I
WW2	World War II

2.1 Introduction

Age estimation (also known as "age evaluation", "age determination", "age diagnostics" or "age assessment") [1] of both living and deceased individuals represents a crucial variable in forensic and human rights contexts. In living individuals, it is

G. M. Fonseca (✉)
Centro de Investigación en Odontología Legal y Forense, Faculty of Dentistry, Universidad de La Frontera, Temuco, Chile
e-mail: gabriel.fonseca@ufrontera.cl

C. Capitaneanu
Centro de Investigación en Odontología Legal y Forense, Faculty of Dentistry, Universidad de La Frontera, Temuco, Chile

Cork University Dental School and Hospital, University College Cork, Cork, Ireland

Centre for Forensic and Legal Medicine and Dentistry, School of Dentistry, University of Dundee, Dundee, United Kingdom

© The Author(s), under exclusive license to Springer Nature Switzerland AG 2026

A. Chowdhry, P. Kapoor (eds.), *Dental Age Assessment*,
https://doi.org/10.1007/978-3-032-08788-1_2

frequently associated with adoption or with the imputability of criminal activity, and in recent years, with inappropriate registration of unaccompanied minors in the context of migration and asylum seeking [2]. However, it has been mentioned that age as a focus of judicial investigation will be highly dependent on contextual, phenomenological, and circumstantial variables. The "historicity of age" contains conventions and stipulations with a lot of room for legal discretion dependent on principles and standards in force at the time of study [3]. Regardless of the circumstances of the requirement, achieving certainty for judges and juries regarding chronological age has been a permanent concern, seeking to rely on science to define, beyond a reasonable doubt, the criminal standard of proof [3]. Age estimation plays a fundamental role in the reconstruction of the biological profile. The use of dental tissues for this purpose, dental age estimation (DAE), is one of the most reliable, useful and most cited scientific methods in contemporary literature in forensic odontology [4]. Even considering the theoretical contributions on the topic, DAE has sought from its remote origins to solve situations not only in clinical settings but precisely in conflictive situations of legal nature [4]. The aim of this chapter is to offer a perspective not only to the different DAE methodologies according to their inclusion in a certain time line, but also to place them in their context, reconstructing their historicity, covering the circumstances and processes of their statements [5].

2.2 Visualization of the Dental Emergence

Historically, the age at which someone ceases to be a child and is considered an adolescent or adult has been studied when civic, criminal, or even marital responsibilities that come from adulthood are associated. While for the ancient Greeks, 18 years of age represented the moment in which the child leaves his scholarship, becoming an *ephebian* (a young man training in the arts of war), and then at 20 years of age celebrates the *apaturia* (admitted as a disciplined and responsible citizen), for the ancient Romans the entrance into adulthood was considered when the individual was able to procreate: 14 years old for boys, and 12 years old for girls [6]. Although there is debate among some authors, the wedding stage (even during puberty), or wearing the toga of manhood *(toga virilis)* were the instances that opened up the possibility for young men to do military service, to become orators or priests [6]. In ancient Rome, some dental characteristics offered evidence to establish the age group: Harlow & Laurence state that "[a]n infant was distinguished from older children initially by a lack of teeth", and that the period before the age of 7, the *infantia*, "was defined legally by the coming of the seventh birthday, associated with the physical loss of milk teeth" [7]. Schmeling et al., by citing Müller, mention that it was the complete eruption of the second molar that led to young men being judged fit for military service [8].

Visualization of dental emergence has been the first and most common way to establish the age of an individual [9, 10]. Schmeling & Black (2010) state that hundreds of studies on dental development have focused on eruption, "which incorporates the entire journey of the tooth from its formation in the alveolar crypts to full occlusion", although many of these studies refer to "eruption" when in fact they should refer to "emergence", considering that they are restricted to the moment in which any part of the tooth finally becomes visible in the mouth [1]. According to Demirjian, the frequent and almost universal use of the term "eruption" has been a way "both rapid and convenient" "albeit wrongly, to indicate the clinical appearance of the cusps of a tooth through the gum" [11]. Beyond this terminological digression, it can be stated that dental emergence has been the only criterion for DAE before the advent of X-rays in dentistry [12].

Some authors state that the first formal applications of dental emergence to estimate age date from the early nineteenth century in the United Kingdom (UK), where proving that a child had not reached 7 years of age (age of imputability, and very likely to be sentenced to death by hanging) was extremely difficult due to the irregularity of birth records [13]. According to Miles, one of the few visible signs taken into account by medico-legal experts in 1836 to establish 7 years of age was the emergence of the first permanent molar [13]. Although the Industrial Revolution brought with it a series of technological and scientific advances that completely transformed society and the countries where it took place, these advances did not have the same impact on all social strata. The implementation of technology, although it evidenced an improvement in the production and industrial work methodology, also led to a deterioration in the lives of workers and their families by making labor cheaper, prohibiting the unionization of workers and pushing the families to send their children to work in factories in order to increase income, even with 15-hour work days in dangerous and unhealthy environments [14]. As a way to regulate and improve industrial employment conditions, beginning in 1802, the Parliament of the United Kingdom passed a series of laws known as the Factory Acts. The first acts focused on regulating the working hours and welfare of young children ("apprentices" in the Act) employed in cotton and similar factories [15]. Although the 1802 Act prohibited working hours in excess of 12 hours and night work for children [15], it was the 1819 Act that explicitly prohibited work for children under 9 years of age and limited 12-hour days for children aged between 9 and 16 years [16]. The latter applied only to the cotton industry, but covered all children, whether they were apprentices or not; however, the scarcity of means to comply with it made it inapplicable as its execution was left in the hands of local magistrates [16]. The inefficiencies in the controls of the magistrates, the successive instrumental failures, and the disregarded areas led to intensify efforts to protect children working in the cotton industry leading to the 1833 Factory Act. This Act established that children under the age of 9 years old were not to be employed in factories (except silk factories), while children aged between 9 and 12 years had a limit of 48 hours per week and guarantees of having received at least 2 hours of education per day [17].

Probably one of the most important points of the 1833 Act was that it required the appointment by the Government of four persons as inspectors, who were given the power to enter at will any factory in operation to examine children, make inquiries, call witnesses, or summon any person to testify, forcing themselves to issue reports and meet twice a year to consult on their duties and procedures in order to achieve uniformity of action [17]. Even with the best of intentions, the 1833 Act had few admirers in the textile districts in which it took effect; in 1835, the first report of the inspectors indicated that some clauses were totally impracticable and, furthermore, the work of those inspectors was largely ineffective simply because they were insufficient to supervise the more than 4000 factories on the island [18]. Undoubtedly, this contributed to the lack of appropriate controls; in particular, the mere verification of the child's height to determine age led to worrying situations of abuse and fraud in the industrial districts with evident evasion of parliamentary laws [14]. The recommendations that age should be given based on height were considered by some not only illegal and invasive, but also difficult to implement, making it impossible to properly educate on the age certificates required by the Act [19].

Edwin Saunders, a 23-year-old Londoner, motivated by the mechanical opportunities offered by dentistry (from an early age he showed an aptitude for mechanical gadgets and engineering) and a pupil of a district dentist, proposed to the English Parliament in 1837 "*Teeth a test of age, considered with reference to the Factory Children, addressed to the Members of both Houses of Parliament*", which was considered a reference for permanent use by the inspectors of factories for fraud detection [20]. Taking into account that there were still more than 50 years to go before the use of X-rays became a reality in dentistry, Saunders's work proposes the "discovery" that dental emergence represents "physiological phenomena which may be regarded as the most certain sign by which, in the absence or independently of registration, the age of a child may be determined; possessing, as it does, a most important influence in any legislative enactments of this nature, in securing to the objects for whose protection they are designed, the full benefit of their provisions" [21]. For Saunders, teeth seem to belong "to another and separate economy" as their formation is not influenced by delays in the signs of puberty, nor by congenital or acquired diseases, continuing to grow regularly [21]. Based on a study of 1046 children between 9 and 13 years of age, Saunders proposes dental age eruption tables for Factory Act purposes, which could be used even by relatively untrained people (Fig. 2.1). Although the author considers the emergence of the second molar to be proof of age in this Factory Act, his subsequent observations on 307 children in the

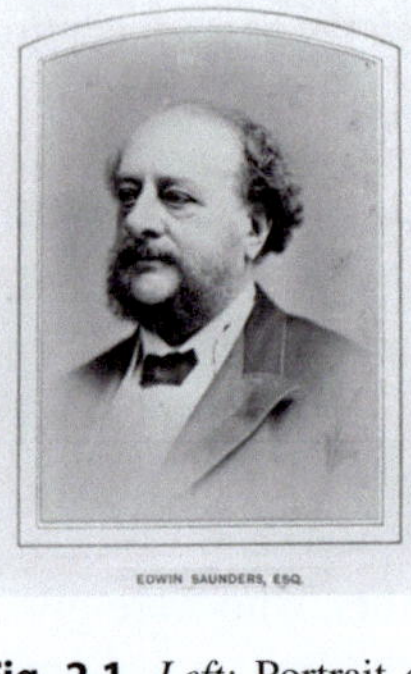

	Years.	
First molar, or large grinder. . .	7	
Central incisor, or front tooth . .	8	
Lateral incisor	9	
First bicuspis, or small grinder . .	10	
Second bicuspis	11	
Cuspidatus, or eye tooth	12	$12\frac{1}{2}$
Second molar, or large grinder . .	$12\frac{1}{2}$	14

Fig. 2.1 *Left:* Portrait of Sir Edwin Saunders (1814–1901) (Photograph by G. Jerrard, 1881, License Creative Commons Attribution CC BY 4.0). Although he practiced as a dentist at the Blenheim Street Infirmary and Free Dispensary from 1834, it was after obtaining his diploma from the Royal College of Surgeons in 1839 that he practiced as dental surgeon and lecturer on dental surgery at St. Thomas' Hospital (a position he held until 1854), that would achieve his greatest recognition. In 1846 he was appointed as dentist to Queen Victoria, the Prince Consort, and the other members of the Royal Family [20]. *Right*: Table of dental eruption for the age 7 to 14 years, according to "*Teeth a test of age...*" [21]

London Orphan Asylum one year later emphasize the differences between the dental characteristics of children aged 9 and aged 13, the first group with an examination that "is exceedingly simple, virtually resolving itself (…) into the observation of the eight teeth situated in the anterior part of the mouth", and the second group with a focus on "canine, and the second molar", although with bicuspids "subject to much variation". The differences in size, shape, configuration, and degree of abrasion in the teeth under study are characteristics that would offer "simple and obvious distinctions, with which anyone may soon render himself familiar by a little practical application, almost the possibility of error will be precluded in the prosecution of this interesting and important subject" [22].

Teeth a Test of Age… led to a great discussion about the reliability of teeth in general and eruption in particular as a means of age estimation [14, 23, 24]. Although the renowned Thomas Bell, an English zoologist and dental surgeon—comparable in popularity and recognition with his friend Charles Darwin —[25], had addressed periods of dental eruption a few years earlier "as a general rule, liable to continual exceptions, not only in the time at which the different teeth appear, but also in the relative order of their precedence" [26] (Fig. 2.2), for some authors the work of Saunders was superior by having "investigated the subject statistically", "with great success" [27]. *Teeth a Test of Age…* would later be published in *The American Journal of Dental Science* in 1847 [28] making it clear that the tables on eruption of permanent teeth were the "*Test of Age*" standard at that time [29].

This trend would continue for several more years. Samuel Cartwright, a British surgeon-dentist recognized as the United Kingdom's first professor of dental surgery and founder of the Odontological Society [30], published in 1857 in the *British Journal of Dental Science* a table based on the study of 3074 school-aged children (Fig. 2.3), in which the author highlights some diseases, inflammatory conditions, anomalous dental positions, root resorption or "abnormal action[s]" as possible

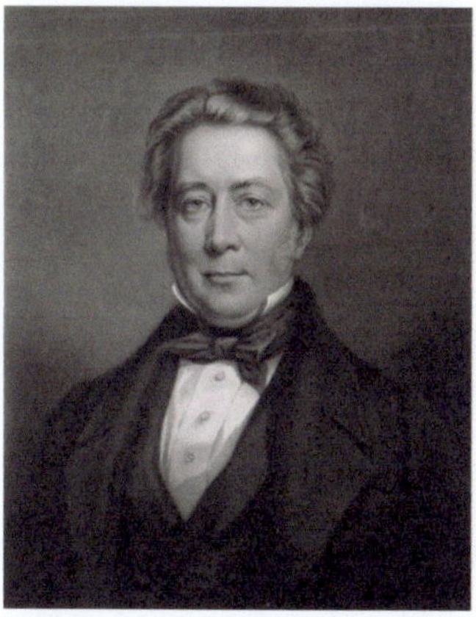

From	5 to 8 months	the four central incisores.
From	7 to 10	the four lateral incisores.
From	12 to 16	the four anterior molares.
From	14 to 20	the four cuspidati.
From	18 to 36	the four posterior molares.

Anterior molares, ...	6½ years.
Central incisores, . . .	7 "
Lateral incisores, ...	8 "
Anterior bicuspides, ...	9 "
Posterior bicuspides, ...	10 "
Cuspidati, ...	11–12 "
Second molares, ...	12–13 "
Third molares, or *dentes sapientiæ*, .	17–19 "

Fig. 2.2 *Left:* Thomas Bell (1792–1880) (Mezzotint by G. Zobel after Taples, 1853–1861, License Creative Commons Attribution CC BY 4.0). *Right:* The progress of dental eruption, according to Bell [26]

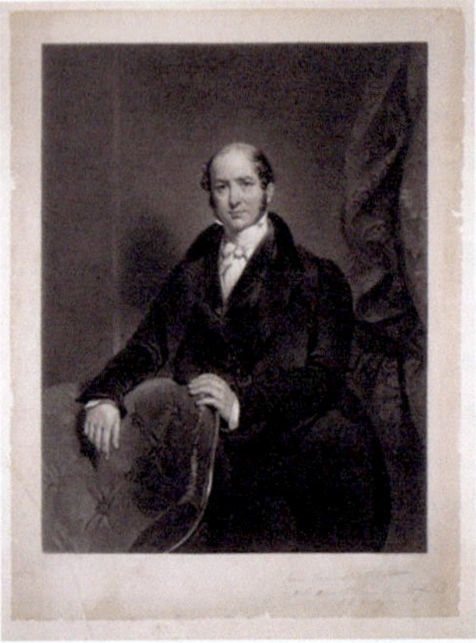

3074 Cases.	Upper Incisors.	Lower "	Upper Cuspids.	Lower "	Upper Anterior Bicuspids.	Lower " "	Upper Posterior Bicuspids.	Lower " "	Upper Anterior Molars.	Lower " "	Upper Posterior Molars.	Lower " "
Between the 5th and 6th birthdays: Out of 170 children	5	17	—	—	—	—	1	—	34	48	—	—
" 6th and 7th Out of 340 children	52	207	—	—	3	1	2	4	182	199	—	—
" 7th and 8th Out of 496 children	180	407	—	—	19	7	3	5	472	479	—	—
" 8th and 9th Out of 530 children	459	524	8	7	85	38	16	12	524	524	—	—
" 9th and 10th Out of 454 children	435	451	20	40	143	60	51	32	453	453	6	11
" 10th and 11th Out of 322 children	318	321	48	98	199	104	110	69	322	322	18	26
" 11th and 12th Out of 303 children	303	303	112	166	231	167	166	123	303	303	51	79
" 12th and 13th Out of 203 children	203	203	136	159	175	149	144	102	203	203	103	1:8
" 13th and 14th Out of 140 children	140	140	115	120	133	116	122	93	140	140	100	113
" 14th and 15th Out of 86 children	86	86	79	83	86	86	79	77	86	86	78	79
" 15th and 16th Out of 30 children	30	30	29	30	30	29	30	28	30	30	30	29

Fig. 2.3 *Left:* Samuel Cartwright (1789–1864) (Mezzotint by S. Bellin after J. Wood, 1800–1899, License Creative Commons Attribution CC BY 4.0). *Right:* Table showing the times of dental appearance, according to Cartwright [31]

factors of anomalous eruptions: "[t]hese periods I find form a moderately fair average. I have particularised them for the sake of affording you some idea of the times of replacement of the various classes of teeth; but exceptions are so frequent that it is not possible to give with accuracy the exact time for their change" [31]. According to Fulton & Price (1954), Cartwright's table served as a scoring model for almost all the research carried out on the topic until well into the twentieth century [29].

In 1880, *The Origin and Formation of the Dental Follicle* [32], was published by one of the most influential researchers at the time, the French Émile Jean Magitot (1833–1897), who—together with Charles Legros (a disciple of the renowned histologist Charles Robin) managed to deepen his research on histology, embryology, and dental development [33]. *The Origin and Formation…* would give rise to the work of experts just a few years later, in one of the most popular identity substitution theories at the time [34, 35]: in June 1894, at the request of Georges Laguerre, lawyer for the descendants of the *Dauphin of France*, the excavation of the alleged remains of Louis-Charles Capet, son of King Louis XVI, was approved, in the Sainte-Marguerite in Paris cemetery. The boy's remains, aged 10 years and 2 months, had been buried in an unmarked grave in 1795, exhumed in 1846, and recognized as belonging to him based on singular traces of decay on bones, on the hair color and on some circumstantial evidence [36] (Fig. 2.4). The second exhumation in 1894 led to the summoning of some recognized experts in anthropological science, who, following strict medical and anthropological protocols, reached some important conclusions.

Magitot was summoned as one of those experts, according to Lipton, thanks to his contribution to *The Origin and Formation…* [34]. The eminent Cuban dentist and professor at the Paris Dental School, Oscar Amoëdo (also summoned in that case), gives a detailed account of the conclusions reached by the experts in his book *L'Art Dentaire en Médecine Légale* [36]:

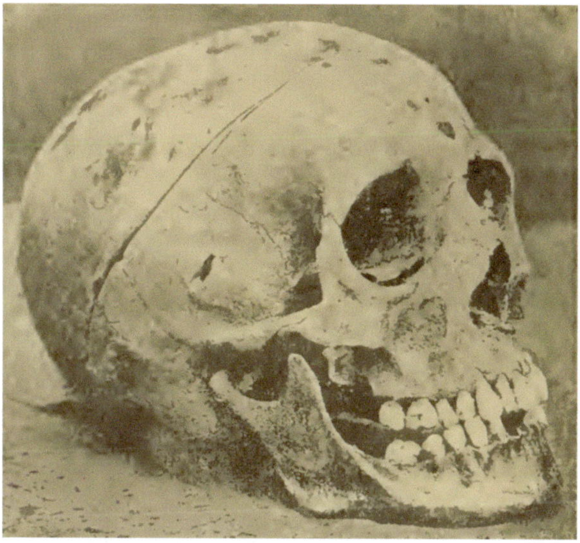

Fig. 2.4 Skull attributed to Louis XVII during the excavations of 1846 (Image obtained *L'Art Dentaire en Médecine Légale* [36], digitized by the Internet Archive in 2010 with funding from Open Knowledge Commons, and belonging to an open digital library)

> *Doctors Magitot and Manouvrier finally gave their conclusions: (1) The skeleton which was submitted to our examination is that of a probably male subject, about 1 meter 63 tall, and certainly between 18 and 20 years old. (2) These findings in no way relate to a child such as the skeleton of the dauphin should be, admitting the historical tradition which places its death and burial at the age of 10 years and 2 months. On June 10, 1894, we went to the Sainte-Marguerite cemetery, in the presence of Mrs. Laguerre and several witnesses. We had no knowledge at the time of the expertise practiced by Magitot. Thus, freed from any prejudice, we were in excellent conditions to carry out our task. Here are our conclusions: (1) Given the wear of the free edge of the incisors; (2) Whereas on the right side of the lower jaw, the space left free by the disappearance of the first large molar (6-year-old tooth) has been filled by the second large molar, which has advanced until it comes into contact with the second small molar, thus promoting the development of the wisdom tooth on this side; (3) Given the presence of two lower wisdom teeth, both of which have perforated the socket (the one on the right side is more developed than the other); (4) Whereas the upper wisdom teeth fell out of the maxilla, after death, which indicates that they were not covered by the alveolar wall, and that, therefore, they were ready to come out; (5) Whereas the enamel of the teeth presents yellow stains; We conclude that the skull examined must have belonged to an individual aged at least 18 years old.*

The findings of the investigation on the exhumed remains attributed to Louis XVII in 1894 at the Sainte-Marguerite cemetery were finally published the same year in the *Archives d'Anthropologie Criminelle de Criminologie et de Psychologie Normale et Pathologique* [37]. The notes detailed the studies carried out on the skeleton, jaws and dentition; in this last case, with the title "*Minimum and Maximum Eruption Dates*", the authors concluded in what could be considered the first forensic historical report on DAE: "[h]owever, according to the documents referred to above, the first trace of the crown of the wisdom teeth (dentin cap) appears in the twelfth year and the eruption outside takes place at the minimum dates of eighteen years and maximum twenty-two or twenty-five years old". The assertions that the skeletal remains belonged to a boy whose age did not fit the identification of Louis XVII, continues to be challenged or confirmed with new studies [35, 38], which still keep the scientific community in suspense.

Regarding the work of Legrot and Magitot, Demirjian stated that histological studies of dental development and eruption chronology, which were very popular in the last years of the nineteenth century, originated standards that enjoyed wide acceptance and use in textbooks and embryology until well into the 1940s [11]. However, for the author, these studies were mostly descriptive and based on histological sections of very small sample sizes, which gave them an unreliable approach that repeatedly persisted for years in other tables, including those by Logan & Kronfeld (1933) [39] or to Schour & Massler (1940) [40, 41]. Regarding the latter, Demirjian speculates that these authors used interchangeable histological and radiographical material in preparing their tables, and that although Schour & Massler warn that "since the x-ray film is a record of density, the stage of tooth development as indicated in histologic sections will be slightly earlier than that indicated by the x-rays" [41], this distinction has often been overlooked [11].

2.3 Evaluation of Dental Development: The Rise of the X-Rays

On November eighth, 1895, on a Friday afternoon, excited by the new findings of the Hungarian Philipp Lenard on photoelectric investigations, the Bavarian physicist Wilhem Conrad Röntgen (1845–1923) produced and detected "a new kind of rays", the X-rays, in a seminal experiment [42]. In 1896, barely a year later, 21 reports had already been published on the application of X-rays in children, and in fact, Heinrich von Ranke, a German paediatrician who had reported on the ossification of the wrist in children [43], proposed the use of hand X-rays of the popular court pianist Raoul Koczalski to corroborate his suspiciously young self-declared age [8]. That same year 1895, while in Germany the dentist Otto Waklhoff took the first dental radiograph with 25 min of X-ray exposure, in the United States. a New York physician, W. J. Morton, used a skull for the same purpose [44]. Quoting again Oscar Amoëdo, the pioneer forensic odontologist already highlighted in his 1898 work, the benefits of X-rays for the medical-legal field: "*[t]oday, radiography has become a valuable aid and will show us the state of the tooth inside the jaw, without the need to make cuts*"; and he added: "*[t]his X-ray also shows us the advantage that X-rays can have in certain disputes in which, for example, a dentist would be accused of having extracted a permanent canine instead of a milk tooth.*". Throughout his book, the author highlighted the use of X-ray to assess the size of pulp chambers, anomalies… and of course, dental eruption and its possible disorders [36].

The entry into the new century brought with it a growth in the popularity of the use of X-rays almost as fast as its technical advances, but also the knowledge of its limitations and risks [44–46]. The complexity and cost of X-ray studies on the one hand, and the relative ease and clinical feasibility of dental emergency evaluation on the other, made the latter still an attractive alternative for DAE researchers [12]. The tabulations evaluating the number of visible teeth in the mouth occupied a lot of research in those years to establish it as a standard that would allow assessing the maturity of children for enrolling in school [47, 48]. Again, let's put this information in context: between 1900 and 1915, more than 15 million immigrants came to the United States—with a vast majority coming from non-English-speaking countries—, and by 1910, three-quarters of the population of New York City were immigrants or children of immigrants [49]. Although the regulations established that only children over 16 years of age carrying an official certificate of age could be employed for factory work, the age was difficult to prove when the parents denied the existence of a birth certificate (unfortunately common in those years, even more in immigrant children or children of immigrants), and dental school records were very inaccurate [50]. Having physiological parameters that characterize the development of the child to be able to remove them from streets and factories [50], and thereby establish their appropriate time of entrance to the graded school [47], again originated proposals to evaluate the teeth as a way to achieve this successfully. In this line, Psyche Cattell, an American psychologist specializing in cognitive development in children and researcher at Harvard University, published in 1928 *Dentition as a Measure of Maturity* [51] (Fig. 2.5). Cattell suggests, "[i]f an index of physiological maturity could be obtained from dentition, it would be free from many of the difficulties noted in connection with anthropometric measurements, the carpal index, and pubescence". The author stated that, although "[t]he determination of physiological age from the Roentgen-ray pictures of the carpal bones of the wrist is the method that up to the present time appears to have been received most favorably", "in a small school or in individual cases the expense of the machine and operator is prohibitive". "The teeth can be seen,

Correlation Coefficients (r) between Mental Age and Dentition

No. of Cases	Age	Sex	r	P.E.
55	6–9	boys	0.12	0.09
47	6–9	girls	0.12	0.09
100	8–6	boys	0.05	0.07
100	8–6	girls	0.05	0.07
100	10–6	boys	0.11	0.07
100	10–6	girls	0.09	0.07
500	5–6 to 10 incl.	boys	0.64	0.02
	age constant		0.11	

Fig. 2.5 Correlations between dental age and mental age, according to Cattell [51]

counted and identified by almost anyone after a little experience and they are either present or absent, therefore, very definite", stated Cattell, underlining the practicality, objectivity, and speed of the method [51].

Although some authors highlight that Cattell's proposal can be considered as the first study assessing dental maturity based on the number of emerged teeth in the mouth [12], Schmeling & Black stated that this work "was a rather crude approach, which received limited scientific support. Very shortly after this date the utilization of radiographs opened up new avenues for visualization of direct dental development in the living and the deceased" [1]. Schmeling & Black cited the publications of Bustin et al. (1929) and Hess et al. (1932), as the first researchers to perform dental X-rays on children, thus consolidating the rise of X-rays on DAE [1]. In particular, precisely Hess et al. (1932) stated: "[t]o our surprise, we have been unable to find any record of a radiographic study of the teeth of infants and children. This circumstance, coupled with the fact that our results have led us to draw certain deductions and conclusions differing to some extent from prevailing opinion, has induced us to publish this report. The reproductions of radiograms taken at various periods of early life from birth to adolescence must be regarded as representing averages at these periods rather than as constituting hard and fast standards". Likewise, the authors stated that "[b]y means of radiograms it is possible to gain information of a quantitative nature in regard to the degree and stage of calcification of the teeth" [52]. X-rays as a diagnostic tool opened up new perspectives for research on dental development, although for Adserias-Garriga, those first studies on DAE had some methodological deficiencies according to current standards [53]. However, observing the different morphological stages of mineralization on the radiographs made it possible to obtain much more reliable, more uniform and gradual correlations, and at the same time less influenced by exogenous factors than the evaluations of dental emergence [10, 54].

Since the development of Coolidge's X-ray tube in 1913, the growth and evolution of dental equipment, films and specific radiographic techniques [44] alternated with the development of the field of diagnostic radiography during the World War I (WWI) [55, 56], but also with stagnation during and World War II (WWII) [42, 43] due to the obvious priorities of its military use. The period between the two world wars favored medical specialization, highlighting a few years later the aforementioned studies by Logan & Kronfeld [39] or those by Schour & Massler [40, 41], widely disseminated, with good precision and updates, beyond the already mentioned limitations [11, 57]. However, it is after WWII that there is an accelerated growth in the need for radiologists with skills developed in the field, the need to regulate radiology (the advent of the bomb and the use of radiation for civilian purposes led to enhanced control and protection measures), and the need for interventional and technological specialties [55, 58]. In 1946, the Finnish Yrjö v. Paatero published a preliminary report of "a new method of X-raying the teeth", the beginning of what for a few years would be his "orthoradial pantomography" (later shortened to "orthopantomography") [59]. Tammisalo stated that Paatero planned "a new method which differs fundamentally from the previous one, making both the X-raying and the diagnosis easier", thereby seeking to optimize the routine work in a Department of Radiology supported exclusively on his own efforts [59]. Paatero pointed out that his preliminary work in Finland led to the development of a prototype for roentgenography (the "Pantomograph") of living subjects in 1950, at the University of Washington (United States). After returning to Finland in 1951, and seeking to solve the problem of combining "the concentric and acentric exposures on a single film, using a single exposure", in 1958 he built a miniature apparatus (the "Orthopantomograph", the author distinguished and explained very well the difference from the previous "Pantomograph") for use on dry skulls, which led to it receiving a grant for building a new prototype [60]. The person responsible for the design and construction of the experimental device was Timo Nieminen, an engineer, with whom Paatero had a close collaboration until Paatero's death in 1963 [61]. In 1959, the first orthopantomograph (OPG) for taking clinical images was completed, a device that from 1961 would be developed on a large scale [59].

Studies on DAE using conventional oral radiographic techniques at that time continued to be developed, with greater or lesser limitations. Gleiser & Hunt, studied in 1955 lateral jaw radiographs of the right side of the face belonging to Bostonian 25 boys and 25 girls, taken at intervals of three months, to evaluate the permanent mandibular first molars and assign them 15 stages of calcification [62]. In 1960, Carmen M. Nolla published the results of her doctoral thesis in a pioneering work on stages of tooth development on 25 girls and 25 boys, 1746 and 1656 serial oral radiographs respectively, all secured for each year of the record at a time approximating the individual's birthday [63]. Moorrees et al. evaluated in 1963 the development of permanent maxillary and mandibular central and lateral incisors by inspecting and staging intraoral radiographs belonging to 48 boys and 51 girls [64]. Coming from Sweden, Liliequist & Lundberg published in 1971 the results of correlating palmar radiographs and full-mouth sets of 148 girls and 139 boys, in the last case assigning developmental stages of the teeth [65]. All these studies, among others, represent the basis of many DAE methods (some of which are still currently being tested), making them unavoidable to mention as part of a historical review, beyond their methodological limitations [66, 67]. However, the market entry of the OPG would substantially expand the possibilities of generating results with much faster methodologies, covering the entire dentition with one exposure. In 1970, Kaarina Haavikko, from the University of Helsinki, used OPGs for dental maturity estimation by assessing 12 crown and root formation stages in all developing teeth, in a sample of Finnish children [68] (seeking to reduce working time, in 1974 the author proposed modifying the method using only a few selected teeth) [69]. In 1972, Leinonen et al. adopt Haavikko's original proposal, although they decrease the number of developmental stages to 7. The authors conclude that OPG is a reliable and rapid method to determine dental age, although "probably cannot be used for children under 5 years of age because it is difficult to keep them motionless during the exposure" [70].

In 1973, "one of the most popular tools for predicting chronological age due to its simplicity, the degree of intraexaminer agreement and the ease of its standardization and reproducibility" [71] is published: *A New System of Dental Age Assessment,* by Demirjian, Goldstein & Tanner [72]. The authors, when estimating dental maturity of French Canadian children—1446 boys and 1482 girls—suggested using OPGs "because they are easier to make than intraoral radiographs in young or nervous children; they give less radiation for a full mouth radiograph (…) and the picture of the mandibular region they produce is little distorted" [72]. The system, based on scoring of the seven left side mandibular teeth and eight stages of calcification for each tooth, was updated in 1976 by including two additional stages and by enlarging the sample [73]. Although it has been reported that the method of Demirjian et al. has technical limitations and is population-specific (causing overestimation when applied to other populations) [10, 74], it is probably the most tested method worldwide [75] and, in fact, it is even described as "an excellent technique for age estimation in children" [74]. Beyond the technical considerations, the influence of this method in proposing OPGs for DAE is also unquestionable, an influence detectable in other currently tested methodologies [76–79], including the evaluation of third molar maturation, one of the most used and tested methodologies today [10, 74, 80, 81]. Armenian born from Istanbul, an immigrant dentist in Canada, and later Professor Emeritus at the University of Montreal [82], Arto Demirjian was honored in 2015 by the Order of Quebec Dentists in consideration of his productivity, his contributions to the evaluation of dental maturation and the creation of his system, which "today has become a world standard" [83]. Unfortunately, Prof. Demirjian passed away on January 22, 2024, in Montreal, Canada.

2.4 The Post-World War II Period and the Need to Identify Adults

> *In deep and everlasting appreciation of the heroic efforts of those who, in keeping their country free, made the supreme sacrifice in World War II, the entire nation has been dedicated to disposing of the mortal remains of those honored dead in a manner consistent with the wishes of their next of kin.* (Harry S. Truman, President of the United States) [84]

Historically the great focus of research on DAE has been identifying parameters applicable to children and young adults. This was determined by the needs and the context of certain social problems, a trend that continues to this day [4]. The global military conflict between 1939 and 1945 left between 50 and 70 million victims, soldiers missing in action, isolated and mass burials, fragments of unidentified bodies and the urgent need to recover these remains to return them to their loved ones [84]. Strategies for this goal were barely coordinated; if the positive identifications could not be supported by clues as tags around the neck, other personal items or any evidence close to the corpse, the intervention of an "identification analyst" ("a combination of detective, gross anatomist, and X-ray and dental technician") looked for identifying evidence involving all physical "deviations from the normal", foreign bodies (e.g. pieces of jewelry embedded in the tissues), and in all cases if possible, the identification analyst recorded fingerprints, and dental charts. Discrepancies and reasonable doubts about the original identification were a constant for these teams. The usefulness of having an officer conduct classes in tooth charting was soon confirmed, and then two dental officers and two dental technicians had to ensure accuracy of data [84].

Particularly in post-war Europe, the need to identify victims placed forensic odontology in a position of great recognition, especially in the Scandinavian countries [85], highlighting the participation of the pioneering forensic odontologists, the Norwegian Ferdinand Ström and the Swedish Gösta Gustafson [86–88]. The eminent Australian Prof. Kenneth A. Brown recalled in 2008: "*My particular interest in forensic odontology, however, was inspired in 1961 when I attended a lecture arranged jointly by the Dental Board of South Australia and the Law society, presented by visiting Professor Gösta Gustafson, Professor of Oral Pathology at the Dental School, University of Lund, Malmo, Sweden, on the subject "Dental Aspects of Forensic Medicine". I was fascinated by his graphic accounts of the cases he had undertaken, particularly those during the second world war when, as Sweden had maintained its neutrality, his expertise in identification had been utilised by both warring sides*" [89]. Karl Gustaf "Gösta" Gustafson, graduated in Odontology in 1932 at the Ludwig-Maximilians-University in Munich, and in 1934 in Stockholm. He published in 1947 *Microscopic Examination of Teeth as a Means of Identification in Forensic Medicine* [90], an article in which he exposed one of the many collaborations made with the aforementioned Prof. Ström. In this study, Gustafson proposed: "An important question in this connection is the age of the victims. By study of peculiarities such as periodontosis, secondary dentin and cement coating on the root, it is possible to make an approximate estimate of the age. In the course of the present investigation, I tried to estimate age with the aid of the teeth, and I found that it often is possible to determine age—at least approximately—n this way. It is rather difficult to lay down any principles for such a determination. Extensive experience with tooth preparations is required in order to make such determinations with sufficient reliability" [90].

Although the idea of linking regressive tooth changes with the age of the individual already had sufficient historical precedent [91, 92], Gustafson's proposal would be made that same year, 1947 [90], and then formally crystallized in 1950 as a method of six features (attrition, periodontosis, secondary dentin, cementum apposition, root resorption, and transparency of the root orifice) [93] (Fig. 2.6), which has been considered "a more systematic and statistical approach to dental age estimation", by publishing "a scoring system with the use of a regressive model" [1]. Schmeling & Black [1] stated that, although Gustafson's method received subsequent criticism due to its small sample size (41 teeth with known ages, 11–69 years) or some statistical deficiencies, its parameters have been the basis for subsequent lines of research that have resulted in considerable improvements to DAE for adults' methodologies [94–97]. In 1992, Lamendin et al. published a simplified alternative to the Gustafson method (the model only uses root translucency height and periodontal height) [98], which has been considered more accurate, less invasive, and more effective in various contexts compared to the original method, which is currently validated in different population groups [99, 100]. In 1995, Kvaal et al. presented a technique based on only one of Gustafson's parameters, the secondary dentine formation, which is examined in intra oral periapical radiograph (IOPA), avoiding tooth extraction and destruction, and allowing age estimation in living adult individuals [101]. This trend continues to this day, with different technical and technological modifications that have offered very satisfactory results when considering the apposition of secondary dentine and the possibility of measuring the pulp-tooth ratio in an imaging environment and therefore, non-destructive [102, 103].

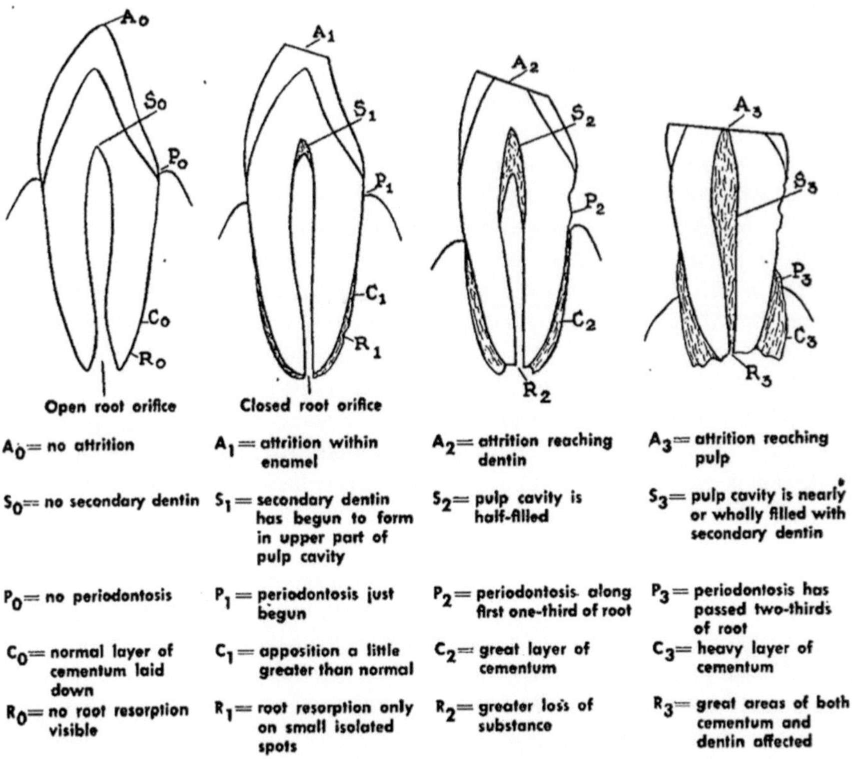

Fig. 2.6 Standard dental features for DAE in adults, according to Gustafson [93]

The legacy of Prof. Gösta Gustafson is undeniable. While publishing his method in 1950, he directed the Department of Oral Histopathology at the Faculty of Dentistry at Lund University, Sweden until 1972. In 1966 he published his best-seller "*Forensic Odontology*" [87], and thanks to that work, the combined terms forensic and odontology were used for the first time in the Oxford Dictionary. Gösta Gustafson was a co-founder and first honorary president of the *International Society for Forensic Odontology* (later named as *International Organization for Forensic Odonto-Stomatology*—IOFOS). Throughout his career, Gustafson collaborated with coroners, forensic pathologists, and police officers from many countries. Between 1944 and 1950, he served as an advisor to the police in Gothenburg, Sweden [104]. In July 1962, at the Second International Conference on Oral Biology held in Bonn (West Germany), Gustafson concluded his introduction to the session on "*Forensic Dentistry*" with words that sought to highlight the odontologist's responsibility in carrying out scientific and accurate forensic identification: "*The United States War Department requested after World War 2 that 274,000 bodies of its soldiers be identified and taken home. This number of bodies required certain methods so that among all these soldiers each could be characterized and found-methods that have not yet been developed*" [105].

2.5 A Critical New View to Scientific Standards

In 1967, Griffith asserted that for personal identification "[p]ossibly the most important factor is assessing the age of a person" [106]. Since the end of the 1960s and during the 1970s, the influence of Gustafson as well as that of other notable researchers around the world (the Danish Keizer-Nielsen also stands out with his important contributions to the recognition of the specialty and the standardization of dental identification) [107, 108]—not only established theoretical bases but also the possibility of genuinely linking forensic odontologists with fieldwork. Those years marked a period of genuine development of the discipline, encompassing its different work areas and highlighting the importance of the dental expert's opinion [109]. The foundation and growth of scientific societies sought not only to generate enthusiastic dentists, but also to promote education, research, and the appropriate certification of experts [110]. The triumphal entry of forensic odontology onto the scene, with a wide media coverage of some of its successful interventions [110, 111] should inevitably bring precautionary suggestions, and above all, more research to give appropriate foundations to this "new discipline" [112, 113]. Specifically on DAE, Biggerstaff already mentioned in 1977 that all available material should be carefully evaluated even if rapid results were required by the police or other agencies, prioritizing the criteria, experience and training of the odontologist "to provide the precise age data" [114]. In 1978, Demirjian advised not to fall into "experimental pitfalls" when seeking to develop more precise and scientific methods [11]. Although there was an increase in publication of case reports on identification and age estimation [115–117], other authors complained about the scant original research in contrast to the excess of these case reports, even mentioning that "[o]f all the problems in forensic dentistry the one of age at death has received more attention than other" [118]. Along the same line, Katz & Cottone, reviewing the publication trends in forensic odontology from 1980 to 1987, highlighted that, although DAE received considerable attention, mass disaster identification and bite mark analysis (the latter "[o]ne of the fastest growing areas of forensic odontology") became the great attraction of the discipline [119].

The start of the 1990s turned history around. The 1989 genetic exoneration of Gary Dotson and David Vazquez, convicted based on forensic evidence, *The Innocence Project* in 1992, *Daubert v. Merrell Dow Pharmaceuticals Inc.* in 1993 [120], the alarming number of wrongful convictions for forensic evidence in the following years, the growing questions about the accuracy of traditional forensic sciences, and finally the pivotal report *Strengthening Forensic Science in the United States: a Path Forward*, by the United States National Academy of Science (NAS) in 2009 [121], all had an overwhelming impact on forensic sciences in general [122] and forensic odontology in particular [110, 123]. Bush & Delattre stated in 2013 that "[m]any forensic odontologists are dental practitioners and not researchers", and that the necessary stimulus to attract these experts towards scientific research should come from institutional funding [124]. The authors, under the title "Needed Research", highlighted the results of a survey carried out by the American Board of Forensic Odontology (ABFO) in 2007 in which the most prominent research topics were injury/bite mark analysis and dental identification, in first and second place respectively. DAE was described as one of the least needed topics for future research, just above "dental jurisprudence" and "facial approximation" [124]. Interestingly, different reviews of the literature on forensic odontology in the last 20 years have reported that the areas and topics most chosen by researchers do not correspond to those identified as priorities in 2007: DAE has been (and still is) the most studied topic with a significant annual increase, it represents between 35% and 41% of worldwide publications and, in fact, the most cited articles in forensic odontology are original research papers related to DAE [4, 125, 126]. Papadoupolos et al. [126], taking these data into account, interpreted that the interest in DAE is the result of the great demand for precise methods, and of the greater "popularity" of DAE in relation to other topics which are more debatable or called for discussion due to their questioned admissibility, opinion shared by Espinoza-Silva et al. [4].

It has been claimed that *Daubert v. Merrell Dow Pharmaceuticals Inc.* and the resulting "era of validation and scientific rigor" have forced the reformulation of methodological strategies for DAE [127]. With regards to the *known error rate* (undoubtedly one of the most discussed *Daubert* factors), Lewis & Kasper emphasized that the scientifically acceptable error threshold should be 95%, which is expressed in DAE as the age interval containing 95%, of the population [74]. However, Page et al. [128] stated that the *Daubert* factors do not really constitute a definitive checklist, and that after the *Kumho* sentence [129], the judge may consider admission of evidence, even with lower confidence level. Likewise, the authors concluded that in DAE (as in any forensic technique), declaring the error rate is highly desirable and that the accuracy rates should be as high as possible [128]. This search for improving accuracy and reliability on DAE methods has led in recent years to the growth and development of highly attractive methodological proposals, all tested in different populations worldwide, whether in neonates, children, adolescents and adults. These include methodological proposals for quantitative measurement through computer-assisted image analysis to eliminate the subjectivity of observations [77, 130, 131], with proposals based on the correction of methodological deficiencies of previous charts/atlases [74, 77], with the resurgence of histological-based [132] or biochemical-based [133] techniques, with the development and validation of technological tools applied to DAE [134, 135] (including the very current artificial intelligence-based approaches with process automation) [136], or simply with the improvement and standardization of DAE protocols and reports [137, 138], DAE continues to be one of the most important contributions and "hot research topic" in forensic odontology [53].

The critical view of scientific standards established by the *Daubert* challenge has brought the DAE back onto the scene. In 2000, Ritz-Timme et al. reported the increase in the need for accurate methods for age estimation, for two fundamental reasons: the increasing number of corpses and unidentified human remains, and the increase in cases of living individuals without proper birth records, the latter in particular related to the phenomenon of illegal immigration in Europe [139]. A similar assessment is made by Schmeling et al. noting that before the 1990s, European forensics were rarely required to report age estimates on living individuals with accurate birth records, but that the "flood of immigrants from extracommunitarian countries" has led to especially complex situations, even more so in the case of unaccompanied minors [10]. Although the migratory phenomenon is not new, it has changed significantly in volume and nature, leading some authors to highlight the particular challenges in Europe, due to the heterogeneity of the migrants but also of the countries which receive them [140]. Specifically on DAE, this European problem could explain the leadership of Europe, of some of its institutions and of its researchers in this topic in recent years: Italy, Belgium, the United Kingdom and Croatia are among the most productive on this topic worldwide [4]. These same authors have highlighted that DAE in the living has become extremely relevant not only in relation to migration, but also to other critical areas such as age of criminal responsibility, human trafficking, child pornography (enhanced with the introduction of the Internet) or even confirmation of appropriate age for sport competitions [1, 67, 141–143].

Despite the significant historical background in answering questions related to chronological age, Lewis & Kasper stated that DAE was possibly the least used discipline within forensic odontology, and that this underutilization lies in the "failure to fully understand how the science can be fully applied", both by forensic odontologists and the legal community. The authors stated that the possibility of resolving these questions quickly and cheaply, in both deceased and living individuals, is being wasted by the forensic community [74]. We agree with the point of view of Adserias & Tejada: DAE is probably the best contribution of forensic odontology to the identification and reconstruction of the biological profile, both in forensic and archaeological cases. The authors add that some considerations must be taken into account: that each case will determine the age estimation method selected; that whenever possible DAE should be combined with skeletal and biochemical methods to obtain more accurate results; and that the international database cross-referencing can be extremely useful, considering that the effect of population depletion on accuracy and precision of the method can impact the estimates [2]. Age is a matter of great importance in the human rights context, and there is still need for agreement, dispute resolution and a 'holistic" multidisciplinary approach in the developing research [144].

2.6 Learning Outcomes

- You should be able to recognize the various historical events that favored the development of specific techniques and the resources available at those times for DAE.
- You should also understand the role played by key researchers in those historical events, as well as the legacy they have left in many techniques currently in use.

2.7 Self-Evaluation Questions

- What was the historical context that favored Edwin Saunders' proposal to visualize dental emergence for the DAE?
  Ans: The Industrial Revolution and the child labor.

- What important discovery made the study of dental development for DAE possible?
  Ans: The X-Rays.
- What historical context has established the need for identification and DAE in adults?
  Ans: The post-World War II period.
- Why was a new critical standard for forensic science defined since 1989?
  Ans: Because that year the entry into the forensic scene of genetics set those new standards.

2.8 Multiple Choice Questions

Q1. Visualization of dental emergence:
(a) Is synonymous with dental eruption, according to Demirjian
(b) Was proposed for DAE in London in 1837, but was not officially recognized
(c) Allowed for the regulation and protection of child laborers
(d) Is highly reliable because it is not affected by external variables

Ans: c

Q2. What was the impact of X-rays on DAE?
(a) They allowed for a more reliable assessment of dental morphological variables
(b) They enabled the development of simpler systems for chronological prediction
(c) They ensured the proposal of worldwide validated standards
(d) All of the above

Ans: d

Q3. What was the historical event when Gustafson proposed his technique for estimating the age of unidentified deceased adults?
(a) The post Swedish-Norwegian War (1814)
(b) The post-World War I (1914–1918)
(c) The post-World War II (1935–1945)
(d) The post-Congo Crisis (1960–1965), with Sweden as a member of the UN

Ans: c

Q4. What was the event that reshaped the way in which forensic science should be evaluated in the United States, and with it, the thorough validation of the methodological strategies for DAE?
(a) The genetic exoneration of Gary Dotson and David Vazquez, convicted based on forensic evidence (1989)
(b) The Innocence Project (1992)
(c) Daubert v. Merrell Dow Pharmaceuticals Inc. (1993)
(d) The report of the United States National Academy of Sciences (2009)

Ans: d

2.9 Mind Map (Fig. 2.7)

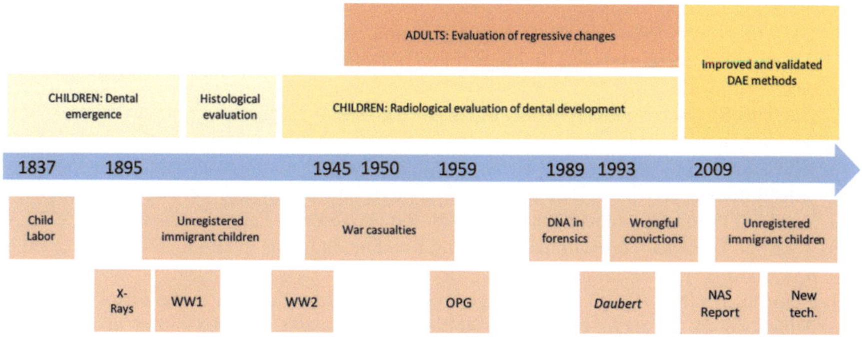

Fig. 2.7 Milestones and historical phenomena (*below*) that provided context and promoted the development of the different DAE methods (*above*)

References

1. Schmeling A, Black S. An introduction to the history of age estimation in the living. In: Black S, Payne-James J, Aggrawal A, editors. Age estimation in the living. Chichester: Wiley-Blackwell; 2010. p. 1–18.
2. Adserias-Garriga J, Tejada J. Dental aging methods and population variation. In: Parra RC, Zapico SC, Ubelaker DH, editors. Forensic science and humanitarian action: interacting with the dead and the living. Hoboken: John Wiley & Sons; 2020.
3. Pande I (2020) Sex, law, and the politics of age. Child marriage in India, 1891–1937. University Press, Cambridge.
4. Espinoza-Silva PV, López-Lázaro S, Fonseca GM. Forensic odontology and dental age estimation research: a scoping review a decade after the NAS report on strengthening forensic science. Forensic Sci Med Pathol. 2023;19:224–35.
5. Girola L. Historicidad y temporalidad de los conceptos sociológicos [Historicity and temporality of sociological concepts]. Sociológica (Mex). 2011;26:13–46. Spanish.
6. Jassogne G. Adolescence during antiquity: the Greek and Roman periods. Psychiatr Danub. 2020;32:164–6.
7. Harlow M, Laurence R. Growing up and growing old in ancient Rome. A life course approach. London: Routledge Taylor and Francis Group; 2002.
8. Schmeling A, Reisinger W, Geserick G, Olze A. Forensic age estimation of live adolescents and young adults. In: Tsokos M, editor. Forensic pathology reviews, Vol 5. Totowa: Humana Press; 2008.
9. Livy J. On the periods of eruption of the permanent teeth as a test of age. Br Med J. 1885;2:241–4.
10. Schmeling A, Garamendi PM, Prieto JL, Landa MI. Forensic age estimation in unaccompanied minors and young living adults. In: Duarte NV, editor. Forensic medicine-from old problems to new challenges. Rijeka: InTech; 2011.
11. Demirjian A. Dentition. In: Falkner F, Tanner JM, editors. Human growth. Boston: Springer; 1978.
12. Demirjian A. Dental development: a measure of physical maturity. In: Johnston FE, Roche AF, Susanne C, editors. Human physical growth and maduration. Methodologies and factors NATO Advanced Study Institutes Series, vol. 30. Boston: Springer; 1980. p. 83–100.
13. Miles AEW. Dentition in the estimation of age. J Dent Res. 1963;42:255–63.
14. No authors listed. The teeth a test of age. Br Foreign Med Rev. 1838;5:205–7.

15. Raithby J. The statutes of the United Kingdom of Great Britain and Ireland, vol. I. London: Containing the Acts 41 Geo. III (1801) and 42 Geo. III (1802). Eyre and Strahan, printers to the King; 1822.
16. UK Parliament (2024) Early factory legislation. https://www.parliament.uk/about/living-heritage/transformingsociety/livinglearning/19thcentury/overview/earlyfactorylegislation. Accessed 30 Jan 2024.
17. Hutchins BL, Harrison A. A history of factory legislation. London: 2nd ed. Rev. King & Son, Orchard House; 1911.
18. UK Parliament (2024) The 1833 Factory Act. https://www.parliament.uk/about/living-heritage/transformingsociety/livinglearning/19thcentury/overview/factoryact/. Accessed 30 Jan 2024.
19. Ward JT. The factory movement 1830–1855. 1st ed. Toronto: Palgrave Macmillan; 1962.
20. Young N. Dictionary of National Biography. London: 2nd Supp. 3. Smith, Elder & Co.; 1912. p. 269–70.
21. Saunders E (1837) Teeth a test of age, considered with reference to the factory children. Addressed to the members of both houses of parliament, Royal College of Physicians Edinburg. Thomas C Savill, London.
22. Saunders E. The teeth a test of age. In: Wakley T, editor. Lancet 1837–1838, vol. 2nd. London: George Churchill; 1838. p. 492–6.
23. Harris CA. The Dental Art a practical treatise on dental surgery. Baltimore: Armstrong & Berry; 1839.
24. Mata P. Cirugía y medicina legal [surgery and legal medicine], vol. 1. 2nd ed. Spanish; 1846. p. 314–5.
25. Doubleday FN. The contributions of King's college, London, to the science of dentistry. Proc R Soc Med. 1949;42:783–90.
26. Bell T (1830) The anatomy, physiology, and diseases of the teeth. Carey & Lea, Philadelphia.
27. Tomes J (1848) A course of lectures on dental physiology and surgery, delivered at the Middlesex hospital School of Medicine. John W. Parker, West Strand, London.
28. Saunders E. The teeth a test of age, considered with reference to the factory children. Am J Dent Sci. 1847;7:330–75.
29. Fulton JT, Price B. Longitudinal data on eruption and attack of the permanent teeth. J Dent Res. 1954;33:65–79.
30. Gelbier S. 125 years of developments in dentistry, 1880–2005. Part 5: dental education, training and qualifications. Br Dent J. 2005;199:685–9.
31. Cartwright S. A course of lectures on dental surgery delivered at King's college. Lecture IV, Brit J Dent Sc. 1857;1:346.
32. Legros C, Magitot E. The origin and formation of the dental follicle. The first memoir on the development of the teeth. In: Trad. Dean MS, editor. . Chicago: Jansen, McClurg & Company; 1880.
33. Sanz Serrulla J. Émile Magitot (1833–1897). Maxillaris; 2006. Feb. Spanish.
34. Lipton BE, Murmann DC, Pavlik EJ. History of forensic odontology. In: Senn DR, Weems RA, editors. Manual of forensic odontology. 5th ed. Boca Raton: CRC Press; 2013.
35. Puech PF. Portrait of the 'Temple child', a missing-link in the case of Louis XVII. Int J Legal Med. 1995;107:209–12.
36. Amodëo O. L'Art Dentaire en Médecine Légale [the dental art in legal medicine]. Paris: Masson et Cie Editeurs; 1898. French
37. Magitot E, Manouvrier L. In: Storck A, Masson G, editors. Notes et observations medico-légales: Age probable d'un squelette exhumé le 6 juillet 1894 et attribué à Louis XVII [Notes and medico-legal observations: Probable age of a skeleton exhumed on July 6, 1894 and attributed to Louis XVII], vol. 9. Archives D'anthropologie Criminelle de Criminologie et de Psychologie Normale et Pathologique; 1894. p. 597–604. French.
38. Merheb M, Matar R, Hodeify R, Siddiqui SS, Vazhappilly CG, Marton J, Azharuddin S, Al Zouabi H. Mitochondrial DNA, a powerful tool to decipher ancient human civilization from domestication to music, and to uncover historical murder cases. Cells. 2019;8:433.
39. Logan WHG, Kronfeld R. Development of the human jaws and surrounding structures from birth to the age of fifteen years. J Am Dent Assoc. 1933;20:379–428.

40. Schour I, Massler M. Studies in tooth development: the growth pattern of human teeth. Part I. J Am Dent Assoc. 1940;27:1778–93.
41. Schour I, Massler M. Studies in tooth development: the growth pattern of human teeth. Part II. J Am Dent Assoc. 1940;27:1918–31.
42. Thomas AMK, Banerjee AK. The history of radiology. Oxford: University Press; 2013.
43. Willich E, Ebel KD. The history of paediatric radiology in Germany. In: Kaufmann HJ, Ringertz H, Sweet E, editors. The first 30 years of the ESPR. The history of pediatric radiology in Europe. Berlin: Springer-Verlag; 1993.
44. Iannucci JM, Howerton LJ. Dental radiography: principles and techniques. 5th ed. St. Louis: Elsevier; 2017.
45. Price W. The science of dental radiography. The Dental Cosmos. 1901;43:483–503.
46. Clark CA. Radiographs of the teeth and associated parts. Proc R Soc Med. 1909;2:39–46.
47. Beik AK. Physiological age and school entrance. The Pedagogical Seminary. 1913;20:277–321.
48. Bean RB. The eruption of the teeth as a physiological standard for testing development. The Pedagogical Seminary. 1914;21:596–614.
49. Library of Congress (2024). Immigrants in the Progressive Era. https://www.loc.gov/classroom-materials/united-states-history-primary-source-timeline/progressive-era-to-new-era-1900-1929/immigrants-in-progressive-era/. Accessed 30 Jan 2024.
50. Trinkley CG. Child labor in America: an historical analysis. Buff Envtl LJ. 1993;13:59–93.
51. Cattell P. Dentition as a measure of maturity. Harvard monographs in education, No. 9. Cambridge: Harvard University Press; 1928.
52. Hess AF, Lewis JM, Roman B. A radiographic study of calcification of the teeth from birth to adolescence. Dent Cosmos. 1932;74:1053–61.
53. Adserias-Garriga J. Evolution of methods and state-of-the-art in dental age estimation. In: Adserias-Garriga J, editor. Age estimation, a multidisciplinary approach. San Diego: Academic Press; 2019.
54. Frucht S, Schnegelsberg C, Schulte-Mönting J, Rose E, Jonas I. Dental age in Southwest Germany. A radiographic study. J Orofac Orthop. 2000;61:318–29.
55. Hessenbruch A. A brief history of x-rays. Endeavour. 2002;26:137–41.
56. Eckert WG, Garland N. The history of the forensic applications in radiology. Am J Forensic Med Pathol. 1984;5:53–6.
57. Liversidge HM, Herdeg B, Rösing FW. Dental age estimation of non-adults. A review of methods and principles. In: Alt KW, Rösing FW, Teschler-Nicola M, editors. Dental anthropology, fundamentals, limits and prospects. Vienna: Springer-Verlag; 1998.
58. Ferris CM. The development of specialisation in diagnostic radiography: concepts, contexts and implications. A thesis submitted in partial fulfilment of the requirements of Sheffield Hallam University for the degree of Doctor of Philosophy. ProQuest LLC; 2017. https://shura.shu.ac.uk/3193/2/10700846.pdf. Accessed 30 Jan 2024
59. Tammisalo EH. Professor yrjö v. Paatero—the pioneer of panoramic oral tomography. Dentomaxillofac Radiol. 1975;4:53–6.
60. Paatero Y. Pantomography and orthopantomography. Oral Surg Oral Med Oral Pathol. 1961;14:947–53.
61. Hallikainen D. History of panoramic radiography. Acta Radiol. 1996;37:441–5.
62. Gleiser I, Hunt EE Jr. The permanent mandibular first molar: its calcification, eruption and decay. Am J Phys Anthropol. 1955;13:253–83.
63. Nolla CM. The development of the permanent teeth. J Dent Child. 1960;27:254–66.
64. Moorrees CF, Fanning EA, Hunt EE Jr. Age variation of formation stages for ten permanent teeth. J Dent Res. 1963;42:1490–502.
65. Liliequist B, Lundberg M. Skeletal and tooth development. A methodologic investigation. Acta Radiol Diagn (Stockh). 1971;11:97–112.
66. AlQahtani S. Dental age estimation in fetal and children. In: Adserias-Garriga J, editor. Age estimation, a multidisciplinary approach. San Diego: Academic Press; 2019.
67. Cummaudo M, De Angelis D, Magli F, Minà G, Merelli V, Cattaneo C. Age estimation in the living: a scoping review of population data for skeletal and dental methods. Forensic Sci Int. 2021;320:110689.
68. Haavikko K. The formation and the alveolar and clinical eruption of the permanent teeth. An orthopantomographic study. Suom Hammaslaak Toim. 1970;66:103–70.

69. Haavikko K. Tooth formation age estimated on a few selected teeth. A simple method for clinical use. Proc Finn Dent Soc. 1974;70:15–9.
70. Leinonen A, Wasz-Höckert B, Vuorinen P. Usefulness of the dental age obtained by orthopantomography as an indicator of the physical age. Proc Finn Dent Soc. 1972;68:235–42.
71. Paz Cortés MM, Rojo R, Alía García E, Mourelle Martínez MR. Accuracy assessment of dental age estimation with the Willems, Demirjian and Nolla methods in Spanish children: comparative cross-sectional study. BMC Pediatr. 2020;20:361.
72. Demirjian A, Goldstein H, Tanner JM. A new system of dental age assessment. Hum Biol. 1973;45:211–27.
73. Demirjian A, Goldstein H. New systems for dental maturity based on seven and four teeth. Ann Hum Biol. 1976;3:411–21.
74. Lewis JM, Kasper KA. Assessment of dental age. In: David TJ, Lewis JM, editors. Forensic odontology: principles and practice. San Diego: Academic Press; 2018.
75. Butti AC, Clivio A, Ferraroni M, Spada E, Testa A, Salvato A. Häävikko's method to assess dental age in Italian children. Eur J Orthod. 2009;31:150–5.
76. Willems G, Van Olmen A, Spiessens B, Carels C. Dental age estimation in Belgian children: Demirjian's technique revisited. J Forensic Sci. 2001;46:893–5.
77. AlQahtani SJ, Hector MP, Liversidge HM. Brief communication: the London atlas of human tooth development and eruption. Am J Phys Anthropol. 2010;142:481–90.
78. Cameriere R, Ferrante L, Cingolani M. Age estimation in children by measurement of open apices in teeth. Int J Legal Med. 2006;120:49–52.
79. Wang J, Dou J, Han J, Li G, Tao J. A population-based study to assess two convolutional neural networks for dental age estimation. BMC Oral Health. 2023;23:109.
80. Lewis JM, Senn DR. Dental age estimation. In: Senn DR, Weems RA, editors. Manual of forensic odontology. 5th ed. Boca Raton: CRC Press; 2013.
81. Haglund M, Mörnstad H. A systematic review and meta-analysis of the fully formed wisdom tooth as a radiological marker of adulthood. Int J Legal Med. 2019;133:231–9.
82. Elkouri R. Un café avec… le Dr Arto Demirjian. 2022, La Presse, 18 Sept 2022 https://www-lapresseca/contexte/2022-09-18/un-cafe-avec-le-dr-arto-demirjian/la-deuxieme-chancephp. Accessed 30 Jan 2024.
83. Cision (2015) L'Ordre des dentistes du Québec remet le prix Hommage 2015 au Dr Arto Demirjian. 25 May 2015. https://www.newswire.ca/fr/news-releases/lordre-des-dentistes-du-quebec-remet-le-prix-hommage-2015-au-dr-arto-demirjian-517744701.html. Accessed 30 Jan 2024.
84. Steere E, Boardman TM. Final disposition of World War II dead. QMC Historical Studies Series II, N° 4. Washington DC: Office of the Quatermaster General; 1957.
85. Lake AW (2015) History of forensic odontology in Australia. The Australian Society of Forensic Odontology 9 Aug 2015 http://wwwausfoorgau/welcome-to-ausfo-inc/history-of-forensic-odontology-in-australia/. Accessed 30 Jan 2024.
86. Gustafson G. Forensic odontology. Aust Dent J. 1962;7:293–303.
87. Gustafson G. Forensic odontology. London: Staples Press; 1966.
88. Taylor J. A brief history of forensic odontology and disaster victim identification practices in Australia. J Forensic Odontostomatol. 2009;27:64–74.
89. Brown KA (2024) Studies in forensic odontology. https://digital.library.adelaide.edu.au/dspace/bitstream/2440/59199/2/Brown2008_DDSc.pdf. Accessed 30 Jan 2024.
90. Gustafson G. Microscopic examination of teeth as a means of identification in forensic medicine. J Am Dent Assoc. 1947;35:720–4.
91. Bödecker CF. A consideration of some of the changes in the teeth from youth to old age. Dental Cosmos. 1925;67:543–9.
92. Lehner J, Plenk H. Die Zähne [the teeth]. In: Bargmann W, Heiss R, Lehner J, Patzelt V, Plenk H, editors. Verdauungsapparat. Handbuch der Mikroskopischen Anatomie des Menschen. Berlin: Springer; 1936. German.
93. Gustafson G. Age determination on teeth. J Am Dent Assoc. 1950;41:45–54.
94. Dalitz GD. Age determination of adult human remains by teeth examination. J Forensic Sci Soc. 1962;3:11–21.

95. Johanson G. Age determinations from human teeth: a critical evaluation with special consideration of changes after fourteen years of age. Odontol Revy Suppl. 1971;22:1–126.
96. Solheim T. Dental root translucency as an indicator of age. Scand J Dent Res. 1989;97:189–97.
97. Solheim T. Amount of secondary dentin as an indicator of age. Scand J Dent Res. 1992;100:193–9.
98. Lamendin H, Baccino E, Humbert JF, Tavernier JC, Nossintchouk RM, Zerilli A. A simple technique for age estimation in adult corpses: the two criteria dental method. J Forensic Sci. 1992;37:1373–9.
99. Parra RC, Ubelaker DH, Adserias-Garriga J, Escalante-Flórez KJ, Condori LA, Buikstra JE. Root dentin translucency and forensic international dental database: methodology for estimation age-at-death in adults using single-rooted teeth. Forensic Sci Int. 2020;317:110572.
100. Garizoain G, Parra RC, Escalante-Flórez KJ, Aranda CM, Luna LH, Condori LA, Valderrama-Leal CI, Retana-Milán F. Age-at-death estimation in adults using three forensic methodologies: a Lamendin's technique approach for Latin American context and the extension of a forensic international dental database. J Forensic Sci. 2021;66:2456–68.
101. Kvaal SI, Kolltveit KM, Thomsen Ib O, Solheim T. Age estimation of adults from dental radiographs. Forensic Sci Int. 1995;74:175–85.
102. Bosmans N, Ann P, Aly M, Willems G. The application of Kvaal's dental age calculation technique on panoramic dental radiographs. Forensic Sci Int. 2005;153:208–12.
103. Cameriere R, Ferrante L, Belcastro MG, Bonfiglioli B, Rastelli E, Cingolani M. Age estimation by pulp/tooth ratio in canines by peri-apical X-rays. J Forensic Sci. 2007;52:166–70.
104. Arbeitskreises für Forensische Odonto-Stomatologie (AKFOS). Newsletter. 2002;9:45–6.
105. Gustafson G. Introduction to the session. J Dent Res. 1963;42:252–4.
106. Griffiths TK, Knott NJ. Identification by teeth. Police J. 1967;40:209–13.
107. Kieser JA, Taylor JA, Khouri Z, Churton M. Foundation knowledge in forensic odontology. In: Taylor JA, Kieser JA, editors. Forensic odontology, principles and practice. West Sussex: John Wiley & Sons; 2006.
108. Rötzscher K. History of forensic and legal dentistry. In: Rötzscher K, editor. Forensic and legal dentistry. Speyer: Springer; 2014.
109. Hodson JJ. Forensic odontology and its role in the problems of the police and forensic pathologist. Med Sci Law. 1970;10:247–51.
110. Fonseca GM, Briem-Stamm AD, Cantín M, Lucena J, Bentkovski A. Odontología Forense I: Las Huellas de Mordedura [forensic dentistry I: bite Marks]. Int J Odontostomat. 2013;7:149–57. Spanish
111. Eckert WG, Furst G. Forensic odontology in 1980. The year in review. Am J Forensic Med Pathol. 1981;2:253–5.
112. Moenssens AA. Admissibility of scientific evidence—an alternative to the Frye rule. Wm & Mary L Rev. 1984;25:545–75.
113. Giannelli PC. The admissibility of novel scientific evidence: Frye v. United States, a half-century later. Columbia Law Rev. 1980;80:1197–250.
114. Biggerstaff RH. Forensic dentistry and the human dentition in individual age estimations. Dent Clin N Am. 1977;21:167–74.
115. Holt JK. Forensic odontology—assistance in a problem of identity. J Forensic Sci Soc. 1981;21:343–6.
116. Levine S. Forensic odontology—identification by dental means. Aust Dent J. 1977;22:481–7.
117. Owens JF. Forensic odontology with care report. Ir J Med Sci. 1970;3:137–47.
118. Whittaker DK. Research in forensic odontology. Ann R Coll Surg Engl. 1982;64:175–9.
119. Katz JO, Cottone JA. The present direction of research in forensic odontology. J Forensic Sci. 1988;33:1319–27.
120. Daubert v. Merrell Dow Pharmaceuticals (509 US 579 (1993)).
121. Committee on Identifying the Needs of the Forensic Sciences Community, National Research Council. Strengthening forensic science in the United States: a path forward. Washington DC: National Academies Press; 2009.
122. Fradella HF, O'Neill L, Fogarty A. The impact of Daubert on forensic science. Pepp L Rev. 2004;31:323–61.

123. Salazar-Aguilar P, Zaror-Sánchez C, Fonseca GM. Forensic odontology: wrong convictions, "bad apples" and "the innocence files". J Forensic Leg Med. 2023;96:102528.
124. Bush MA, Delattre VF. Science and forensic odontology. In: Senn DR, Weems RA, editors. ASFO manual of forensic odontology. 5th ed. Boca Raton: CRC Press; 2013.
125. Sengupta N, Sarode SC, Sarode GS, Gadbail AR, Gondivkar S, Patil S, Patil S. Analysis of 100 most cited articles on forensic odontology. Saudi Dent J. 2020;32:321–9.
126. Papadopoulos CK, Bouzala A, Stavrianos C, Stavrianou P. Trends in forensic odontology publications: 2000–2015. Int J Forensic Odontol. 2018;3:12–6.
127. Cameriere R, Cunha E, Wasterlain SN, De Luca S, Sassaroli E, Pagliara F, Nuzzolese E, Cingolani M, Ferrante L. Age estimation by pulp/tooth ratio in lateral and central incisors by peri-apical X-ray. J Forensic Leg Med. 2013;20:530–6.
128. Page M, Taylor J, Blenkin M. Commentary on: De Luca S, Bautista J, Alemán I, Cameriere R. Age-at-death estimation by pulp/tooth area ratio in canines: study of a 20th-century Mexican sample of prisoners to test Cameriere's method. J Forensic Sci 2011;56(5):1302–1309. J Forensic Sci. 2012;57:556. author reply 557–559
129. Kumho Tire Co Ltd v Carmichael 526 US 137, 1999.
130. Liversidge HM, Lyons F, Hector MP. The accuracy of three methods of age estimation using radiographic measurements of developing teeth. Forensic Sci Int. 2003;131:22–9.
131. Cameriere R, Ferrante L, Cingolani M. Variations in pulp/tooth area ratio as an indicator of age: a preliminary study. J Forensic Sci. 2004;49:317–9.
132. Pinto PHV, Fares LC, Silva RHAD. Dental age estimation by cementum incremental lines counting: a systematic review and meta-analysis. Forensic Sci Int. 2022;341:111492.
133. Matteussi GT, Jacometti V, Franco A, da Silva RHA. Age estimation in humans through the analysis of aspartic acid racemization from teeth: a scoping review of methods, outcomes, and open research questions. Forensic Sci Int. 2022;331:111154.
134. Barbosa MG, Franco A, de Oliveira RDB, Mamani MP, Junqueira JLC, Soares MQS. Pulp volume quantification methods in cone-beam computed tomography for age estimation: a critical review and meta-analysis. J Forensic Sci. 2023;68:743–56.
135. De Tobel J, Hillewig E, Bogaert S, Deblaere K, Verstraete K. Magnetic resonance imaging of third molars: developing a protocol suitable for forensic age estimation. Ann Hum Biol. 2017;44:130–9.
136. Vila-Blanco N, Varas-Quintana P, Tomás I, Carreira MJ. A systematic overview of dental methods for age assessment in living individuals: from traditional to artificial intelligence-based approaches. Int J Legal Med. 2023;137:1117–46.
137. ABFO (2021) Standards and Guidelines for Dental Age Assessment. http://abfo.org/wp-content/uploads/2021/02/ADA-Technical-Report-No.-1077_July_2020.-02-2021.pdf. Accessed 30 Jan 2024.
138. IOFOS (2022) Recommendations for Quality Assurance: Dental age estimation. https://iofos.eu/wp-content/uploads/2022/12/Age_estimation_final.pdf. Accessed 30 Jan 2024.
139. Ritz-Timme S, Cattaneo C, Collins MJ, Waite ER, Schütz HW, Kaatsch HJ, Borrman HI. Age estimation: the state of the art in relation to the specific demands of forensic practise. Int J Legal Med. 2000;113:129–36.
140. Villalonga-Olives E, Kawachi I, von Steinbüchel N. Pregnancy and birth outcomes among immigrant women in the US and Europe: a systematic review. J Immigr Minor Health. 2017;19:1469–87.
141. Cameriere R, De Angelis D, Ferrante L, Scarpino F, Cingolani M. Age estimation in children by measurement of open apices in teeth: a European formula. Int J Legal Med. 2007;121:449–53.
142. Thevissen PW, Kvaal SI, Willems G. Ethics in age estimation of unaccompanied minors. J Forensic Odontostomatol. 2012;30(Suppl 1):84–102.
143. Galić I, Lauc T, Brkić H, Vodanović M, Galić E, Biazevic MG, Brakus I, Badrov J, Cameriere R. Cameriere's third molar maturity index in assessing age of majority. Forensic Sci Int. 2015;252:191.e1–5.
144. Aynsley-Green A, Cole TJ, Crawley H, Lessof N, Boag LR, Wallace RM. Medical, statistical, ethical and human rights considerations in the assessment of age in children and young people subject to immigration control. Br Med Bull. 2012;102:17–42.

The Significance of Dental Age Assessment

3

Douglas H. Ubelaker

Concepts and Definitions

- Dental formation: The development of the crowns and roots of the teeth.
- Dental eruption: The emergence of the tooth through the alveolus to reach the occlusal plane
- Taphonomic factors: Conditions that impact postmortem change of bones and teeth

3.1 Why Should Dental Age Assessment Be Preferred Over Other Methods?

Dental age assessment is an important aspect of forensic analysis of human remains for two primary reasons:

1. Teeth are very durable and resist postmortem, taphonomic, destructive factors.
2. Assessment of dental formation in juveniles provides more accurate age estimates than other methods.

In many soils and other forensic environments, skeletal remains can be markedly reduced and/or altered by taphonomic factors. Such factors include time, temperature, soil acidity, soil composition, exposure to scavengers, sun exposure, applications of caustic materials, and fluvial contexts. In cases of extreme fragmentation and decomposition, teeth (and frequently the petrous portion of the temporal bone)

D. H. Ubelaker (✉)
Department of Anthropology, National Museum of Natural History, Smithsonian Institution, Washington, DC, USA
e-mail: ubelaked@si.edu

© The Author(s), under exclusive license to Springer Nature Switzerland AG 2026

A. Chowdhry, P. Kapoor (eds.), *Dental Age Assessment*,
https://doi.org/10.1007/978-3-032-08788-1_3

may be the only tissues available for forensic analysis. In such cases, dental age assessment may be the only method possible.

In juveniles, prior to the complete formation of the third molars, assessment of the stage of dental formation is the most accurate method of age estimation. Although dental eruption, long bone growth and maturation, epiphyseal closure, and other skeletal indicators offer some age-related information, they incorporate more variation than dental formation and are thus less accurate age indicators. The method of age estimation utilizing dental formation requires an accurate classification of the stage of formation of the tooth crown and roots, accurate recognition of which specific tooth is being examined, and differentiation between deciduous from permanent teeth.

3.2 Comparative Analysis

Although dental formation exhibits less variation than other methods for juvenile remains, differences do exist in varying magnitudes in the timing of dental formation across different populations. For this reason, it is important to utilize the method of dental analysis most relevant for the individual case. For example, in the past, many forensic scientists have utilized the Schour and Massler dental chart published by the *American Dental Association* (1941) [1]. This chart was originally compiled from a small North American sample and visually presents information on dental formation and eruption. Ubelaker (1974) demonstrated that age estimates generated from dental formation differ markedly from those derived from dental eruption, especially when applied to human remains from populations that differ from those the methods were developed from [2]. In 1978, Ubelaker produced a new dental chart similar in format to that of Schour and Massler but based on the published literature available at that time [3]. Comparison of the two charts reveals differences in the timing of dental formation and eruption, reflecting variation in the populations represented.

The need for dental age estimation is global in scope and practice. Practitioners in all countries face challenges related to human identification and age assessment in various scenarios. Since the timing of age changes in dental tissues varies globally, local standards are vitally needed to support accurate assessments. This need is being met through research, which reveals complex variables that induce variations in dental age changes. Research also provides data on age changes within local and regional samples that facilitate region-specific age estimation.

3.3 Why Use More Than One Method?

Selection of methods in age assessment depends largely on the samples and tissues available. When multiple tissues are present, more than one method should be employed to provide a comprehensive overview of the age-related changes. Special consideration must also be given to the accuracy of the individual methods employed and the samples upon which they are based.

For example, Baccino et al. (1999) tested seven methods of age estimation on a French sample of individuals with documented ages at death [4]. These methods included:

1. The Lamendin dental method assessing periodontal tissue and root translucency, [5]
2. The Kerley bone microscopy method, [6]
3. The Suchey-Brooks pubic symphysis method
4. The Iscan sternal rib end technique, [7] and three combined methods that integrated the results of individual techniques

The study demonstrated that all the combined methods outperformed the individual methods. In addition, results documented the importance of examiner experience with each technique.

3.4 Summary and Conclusion

Dental age estimation methods provide comparatively accurate results, especially when applied to juveniles. In juvenile applications, assessment of dental formation is preferred over dental eruption. Selection of methods should consider the tissues available and the population represented. Utilizing more than one method provides comprehensive information on age changes and facilitates accurate age assessment.

3.5 Learning Outcomes

- You should understand the importance of dental age estimation in forensic analysis.

You should understand the importance of population variation in dental age estimation and the value of using more than one method.

3.6 Self-Evaluation Questions

- Why should dental age assessment be preferred over other methods?
- How does population variation affect dental age estimation?
- Is it better to use one method or more than one method to estimate age?

3.7 Multiple Choice Questions

Q1. In cases involving extreme decomposition and fragmentation, which structures are most likely to survive and be available for age estimation?

(a) Long bones
(b) Teeth
(c) Metacarpals
(d) The pelvis

Ans: b

Q2. In estimating the age at death of juveniles, which information provides the most accurate estimate?

(a) Long bone lengths
(b) Dental eruption
(c) Epiphyseal union
(d) Dental formation

Ans: d

Q3. Which of the following approaches facilitates the most accurate age estimation?

(a) Consideration of multiple methods utilizing all tissues available.
(b) Relying only on the method of measuring long bone lengths.
(c) Using your favorite method since they are all of equal accuracy.
(d) Using a method developed from a population sample very different from the population reflected in the case being considered.

Ans. a

3.8 Mind Map

Dental age estimation	
Why preferred method?	Comparative analysis
Teeth survive taphonomic processes	Methods vary in accuracy
More accurate method for juveniles	Methods are population specific
Less variation than in other tissues/ methods	Use of multiple methods provides a comprehensive assessment

References

1. Schour I, Massler M. The development of the human dentition. J Am Dent Assn. 1941;28:1153–60.
2. Ubelaker DH. Reconstruction of demographic profiles from ossuary skeletal samples: a case study from the Tidewater Potomac. Smithsonian Contr. to Anthro. 18, 1974. Smithsonian Institution. Washington, DC.

3. Ubelaker DH. Human skeletal remains: excavation, analysis, interpretation. In: Aldine manuals on archeology. Chicago: Aldine Publishing Company; 1978.
4. Baccino E, Ubelaker DH, Hayek LC, Zerilli A. Evaluation of seven methods of estimating age at death from mature human skeletal remains. J For Sci. 1999;44(5):931–6.
5. Lamendin H, Baccino E, Humbert JF, Tavernier JC, Nossintchouk RM, Zerilli A. A simple technique for age estimation in adult corpses: the two criteria dental method. J For Sci. 1992;37:1373–9.
6. Kerley ER. The microscopic determination of age in human bone. Am J Phys Anthro. 1965;23(2):149–63.
7. Iscan MY, Loth SR. Determination of age from the sternal rib in white females: a test of the phase method. J For Sci. 1986;31:990–9.

Methods of Dental Age Assessment

4

Cezar Capitaneanu and Gabriel M. Fonseca

Abbreviations

CA	Chronological age
CBCT	Cone beam computed tomography
CT	Computed tomography
DAA	Dental age assessment
DAE	Dental age estimation
PA	Periapical radiograph
OPG	Orthopantomogram
2D	Two-dimensional
3D	Three-dimensional

C. Capitaneanu (✉)
Centro de Investigación en Odontología Legal y Forense, Faculty of Dentistry, Universidad de La Frontera, Temuco, Chile

Cork University Dental School and Hospital, University College Cork, Cork, Ireland

Centre for Forensic and Legal Medicine and Dentistry, School of Dentistry, University of Dundee, Dundee, United Kingdom
e-mail: capitaneanucezar@yahoo.co.uk

G. M. Fonseca
Centro de Investigación en Odontología Legal y Forense, Faculty of Dentistry, Universidad de La Frontera, Temuco, Chile
e-mail: gabriel.fonseca@ufrontera.cl

© The Author(s), under exclusive license to Springer Nature Switzerland AG 2026

A. Chowdhry, P. Kapoor (eds.), *Dental Age Assessment*,
https://doi.org/10.1007/978-3-032-08788-1_4

4.1 Introduction

"How old are you?" or "What is your age?" are usual questions addressed in our life.

So, "What is the age of an individual?" In the living, it is a measure of how long a person has been alive since they were born, expressed in years. In the deceased, it is a measurement of time from birth to the day of death [1, 2].

Dental age assessment (DAA) is not only needed in the forensic context of identifying victims in mass disasters but also in legal contexts where documents are unavailable or inadequate in relation to criminal responsibility, migration and asylum seeking, adoption, etc. [1]. The process of age assessment needs to be based on current guidelines and must follow national, legal, and ethical requirements.

The aim of this chapter is to provide an outline of DAA methods which can be used to estimate the age of an individual. However, not all existing DAA methods are covered in this section.

4.2 Dental Age Assessment Methods

Dental age assessment has as objective the prediction of the chronological age (CA) of an individual, using the available evidence. The process involves the use of age-related variables/parameters which change throughout life (see Fig. 4.1) [1].

There are several classifications of DAA methods, described below.

Related to the investigated subject, these methods can be used in living and/or deceased individuals.

According to the age interval/group, the DAA methods can be applied in four groups [3]:

1. Prenatal (fetal/intra-uterine human development).
2. Children (from birth to the time of the last primary tooth being normally exfoliated; this includes the early period of mixed primary and permanent dentitions, e.g., the presence of the developing, developed, and resorbing of primary dentition as well as the initial development of the permanent dentition).
3. Adolescents (begins after all primary teeth are normally lost, and the permanent teeth are developing or developed, and ends when all permanent teeth present are fully developed).
4. Adults (begins when all permanent teeth are completely developed and continues throughout life).

Dental age assessment methods can be categorized as non-radiological and radiological methods [4].

Non-radiological methods can be classified in three categories:

1. Visual methods—include clinical observation of stages of eruption of teeth and evidence of changes due to function such as attrition, presence or absence of mamelons, and presence/absence of tooth/teeth [5].

2. Histological methods—based on microscopic regressive changes of tooth and adjacent structures such as attrition, secondary dentin apposition, cementum apposition, root resorption, root transparency, periodontal attachment, as well as enamel, dentine, and cementum increments, etc. (e.g., Gustafson 1950 [6], Bang and Ramm 1970 [7], Johanson 1971 [8], Maples 1978 [9], Lamendin et al. 1992 [10], Prince and Ubelaker 2002 [11]).
3. Biochemical methods—based on life changes within the biochemical structure of tooth (e.g., determination of aspartic acid racemization in dentine [12, 13], radiocarbon analysis [14]).

Radiological methods are used to record developmental stages of dentition (e.g., Moorrees et al. 1963 [15], Demirjian et al. 1976 [16], Mincer et al. 1993 [17], Cameriere et al. 2006 [18]) and morphological measurements of the tooth/teeth (e.g., Kvaal et al. 1995 [19], Cameriere et al. 2004 [20], Cameriere et al. 2007 [21]).

Two-dimensional (2D) or three-dimensional (3D) imaging can be employed depending on the radiological/medical imaging technique. Periapical radiographs (PA) and panoramic radiographs/orthopantomograms (OPGs) are currently used as two-dimensional imaging, and cone beam computed tomography (CBCT), computed tomography (CT), and magnetic resonance imaging (MRI) are used as three-dimensional imaging, respectively [1, 22, 23].

According to the type of assessment, the DAA methods can be divided in two categories:

1. Comparative methods (Atlas methods)—based on the comparison of the status of the developing tooth/teeth from the medical image with an atlas (e.g., Schour and Massler 1941 [24], Ubelaker 1989 [25], AlQahtani et al. 2010 & 2014 [26, 27]).
2. Calculative methods (scoring system, formula)—based on scoring the stages of tooth/teeth development (e.g., Demirjian et al. 1976 [16], Willems et al. 2001 [28])or on using different formulae/equations (e.g., Gustafson 1950 [6], Bang and Ramm 1970 [7], Johanson 1971 [8], Maples 1978 [9], Lamendin et al. 1992 [10], Kvaal et al. 1995 [19], Cameriere et al. 2004 [20], Cameriere et al. 2007 [21]).

Considering the availability of teeth and the reason for performing age assessment, there is a choice of different DAA methods using a single tooth or a combination of teeth, or a specific tooth/teeth position or jaw(s) (e.g., Lamendin et al. 1992 [10], Kvaal et al. 1995 [19], Cameriere et al. 2004 [20], Demirjian et al. 1976 [16], Willems et al. 2001 [28], Schour and Massler 1941 [24], Ubelaker 1989 [25], AlQahtani et al. 2010 & 2014 [26, 27]).

4.2.1 Dental Age Assessment Methods in the Prenatal Period

The atlas method is used in the prenatal age interval/group. This method is based on a graphic and diagrammatic representation of the morphology of developing tooth structures (e.g., Schour and Massler 1941 [24], Ubelaker 1989 [25], AlQahtani et al. 2010 & 2014 [26, 27]) and can be used in both living and deceased individuals.

4.2.2 Dental Age Assessment Methods in Children

In children, DAA methods are based on examination of the developmental stage(s) of dentition, primary or permanent, using medical images (e.g., Schour and Massler 1941 [24], Ubelaker 1989 [25], AlQahtani et al. 2010 & 2014 [26, 27], Moorrees et al. 1963 [15], Demirjian et al. 1976 [16], Willems et al. 2001 [28], Cameriere et al. 2006 [18]). These methods can also be applied in estimating the age in living and deceased individuals, respectively.

Biochemical methods can be used in deceased individuals only.

4.2.3 Dental Age Assessment Methods in Adolescents

Adolescent DAA methods are based on medical images examination of the developmental stage(s) of dentition toward the second half of the dental maturation process (e.g., Moorrees et al. 1963 [15], Demirjian et al. 1976 [16], Mincer et al. 1993 [17], Cameriere et al. 2006 [18]) and can be utilized in living or deceased individuals.

Biochemical methods can be used in deceased individuals only.

4.2.4 Dental Age Assessment Methods in Adults

In adults, DAA methods are based on medical images evaluation of tooth/teeth morphology or microscopic evaluation of regressive changes of the tooth and adjacent structures. Some methods can be used in living or deceased individuals (e.g., Kvaal et al. 1995 [19], Cameriere et al. 2004 [20]) while other methods involving extraction or extraction and sectioning of the tooth can be used in deceased individuals only (e.g., Gustafson 1950 [6], Bang and Ramm 1970 [7], Johanson 1971 [8], Maples 1978 [9], Lamendin et al. 1992 [10], Cameriere et al. 2007 [21]).

Biochemical methods can be used in deceased individuals only.

4.3 Learning Outcomes

- You should be able to understand the utility of dental age assessment methods and their applicability in a forensic context.
- You should be able to understand the classification of dental age assessment methods and how to utilize the appropriate method(s) in different circumstances.

4.4 Self-Evaluation Questions

- How can be Dental age assessment methods classified according to the age interval/groups?
  Answer: Prenatal, Children, Adolescents, Adults
- Can all Dental age assessment methods be applied in the deceased individual?
  Answer: Yes
- Can Dental age assessment methods published in the original peer-reviewed papers be modified when the forensic odontologist is performing age estimation?
  Answer: No
- What is the medical image most used in dental age assessment?
  Answer: Two-dimensional

4.5 Multiple Choice Questions

Q1. Dental age assessment methods should be used considering?

(a) National requirements
(b) Legal requirements
(c) Ethical requirements
(d) All of the above
Answer: d

Q2. Non-radiological Dental age assessment methods are?

(a) Visual
(b) Biochemical
(c) Histological
(d) All of the above
Answer: d

Q3. Radiological Dental age assessment methods are based on?

(a) Two-dimensional (2D) or three-dimensional (3D) imaging
(b) Two-dimensional (2D) imaging only
(c) Three-dimensional (3D) imaging only
(d) None of the above
Answer: a

Q4. Dental age assessment methods can be used in?

(a) Living
(b) Deceased
(c) Living or deceased
(d) None of the above
Answer: c

4.6 Mind Map

DENTAL AGE ASSESSMENT METHODS				
	PRENATAL (FETAL)	CHILDREN	ADOLESCENTS	ADULTS
DEVELOPMENTAL	ATLASES Schour and Massler 1941 Ubelaker 1989 AlQahtani et al. 2010 & 2014	ATLASES & Moorrees et al. 1963 Demirjian et al. 1976 Willems et al. 2001 Cameriere et al. 2006 Living or Deceased	ATLASES & Moorrees et al. 1963 Demirjian et al. 1976 Mincer et al. 1993 Willems et al. 2001 Cameriere et al. 2006 Mincer et al. 1993 Living or Deceased	
MORPHOLOGICAL				Kvaal et al. 1995 Cameriere et al. 2004 or 2007 Living or Deceased
POSTFORMATION CHANGES				Bang and Ramm 1970 Johanson 1971 Maples 1978 Lamendin et al. 1992 Prince and Ubelaker 2002 Deceased
BIOCHEMICAL		Aspartic Acid Racemization Radiocarbon Analysis (14C) Deceased		

Fig. 4.1 Mind map illustrating the classification of Dental age assessment methods

References

1. Brkic H, Lessig R, Alves da Silva RH, Pinchi V, Thevissen P. Textbook of forensic odonto-stomatology by IOFOS, Naklada Slap, Jastrebarsko. 2021.
2. Parekh S. Dental age assessment – developing standards for UK subjects. 2011. https://core.ac.uk/download/pdf/1882903.pdf. Accessed 09 Feb 2024.
3. ABFO. ABFO standards and guidelines for dental age assessment. 2021. http://abfo.org/wp-content/uploads/2021/02/ADA-Technical-Report-No.-1077_July_2020.-02-2021.pdf. Accessed 09 Feb 2024.
4. Tyagi A, Srivastava N, Rana V, Kaushik N. Radiological and nonradiological methods of dental and skeletal age assessment: a narrative review. J Oral Maxillofac Radiol. 2022;10:1–7.
5. Sue B, Aggrawal A, Payne-James J. Age estimation in the living: the practitioner's guide. 1st ed. Oxford: Wiley; 2010.
6. Gustafson G. Age determination on teeth. J Am Dent Ass. 1950;41(54):45–54.
7. Bang G, Ramm E. Determination of age in humans from root dentin transparency. Acta Odontol Scand. 1970;28:3–5.
8. Johanson G. Age determination from human teeth. Odontol Revy Suppl. 1971;22:1–26.
9. Maples WR. An improved technique using dental histology for estimation of adult age. J Forensic Sci. 1978;23(4):764–70.
10. Lamendin H, Baccino E, Humbert JF, Tavernier JC, Nossintchouk RM, Zerilli A. A simple technique for age estimation in adult corpses: the two criteria dental method. J Forensic Sci. 1992;37(5):1373–9.
11. Prince DA, Ubelaker DH. Application of Lamendin's adult dental aging technique to a diverse skeletal sample. J Forensic Sci. 2002;47(1):107–16.
12. Alkass K, Buchholz BA, Ohtani S, Yamamoto T, Druid H, Spalding KL. Age estimation in forensic sciences: application of combined aspartic acid racemization and radiocarbon analysis. Mol Cell Proteomics. 2010;9(5):1022–30.

13. Alkass K, Buchholz BA, Druid H, Spalding KL. Analysis of 14C and 13C in teeth provides precise birth dating and clues to geographical origin. Forensic Sci Int. 2011;209(1-3):34–41.
14. Ohtani S, Yamamoto T. Age estimation by amino acid racemization in human teeth. J Forensic Sci. 2010;55(6):1630–63.
15. Moorrees CF, Fanning EA, Hunt EE. Age variation of formation stages for ten permanent teeth. J Dent Res. 1963;42:1490–502.
16. Demirjian A, Goldstein H. New system for dental maturity based on seven and four teeth. Annals of Hum Biol. 1976;3(5):411–21.
17. Mincer HH, Harris EF, Berryman HE. The A.B.F.O. study of third molar development and its use as an estimator of chronological age. J Forensic Sci. 1993;38(2):379–90.
18. Cameriere R, Ferrante L, Cingolani M. Age estimation in children by measurement of open apices in teeth. Int J Legal Med. 2006;120(1):49–52.
19. Kvaal SI, Kolltveit KM, Thomsen IO, Solheim T. Age estimation of adults from dental radiographs. Forensic Sci Int. 1995;74(3):175–85.
20. Cameriere R, Ferrante L, Cingolani M. Variations in pulp/tooth area ratio as an indicator of age: a preliminary study. J Forensic Sci. 2004;49:317–9.
21. Cameriere R, Ferrante L, Belcastro MG, Bonfiglioli B, Rastelli E, Cingolani M. Age estimation by pulp/ tooth ratio in canines by periapical X-rays. J Forensic Sci. 2007;52:166–70.
22. Pinchi V, Pradella F, Buti J, Baldinotti C, Focardi M, Norelli GA. A new age estimation procedure based on the 3D CBCT study of the pulp cavity and hard tissues of the teeth for forensic purposes: a pilot study. J Forensic Leg Med. 2015;36:150–7.
23. De Tobel J, Phlypo I, Fieuws S, Politis C, Verstraete KL, Thevissen PW. Forensic age estimation based on development of third molars: a staging technique for magnetic resonance imaging. J Forensic Odontostomatol. 2017;35:117–40.
24. Schour I, Massler M. Development of human dentition. J Am Dent Assoc. 1941;20:379–427.
25. Ubelaker DH. Human skeletal remains: excavation, analysis, interpretation. 2nd ed. Washington: Taraxacum; 1989.
26. AlQahtani SJ, Hector MP, Liversidge HM. Brief communication: the London atlas of human tooth development and eruption. Am J Phys Anthropol. 2010;142:481–90.
27. AlQahtani SJ, Hector MP, Liverside HM. Accuracy of dental age estimation charts: Schour and Massler, Ubelaker, and the London Atlas. Am J Phys Anthropol. 2014;154:70–8.
28. Willems G, Olmen AV, Spiessens B, Carels C. Dental age estimation in Belgium children: Demirjian's technique revisited. J. Forensic Sci. 2001;46:893–6.

Dental Age Estimation Methods for Prenatal and Postnatal Periods

5

P. Sema Aka

Abbreviations

CH	Crown height
CrT	Crown thickness
CT	Computed tomography
DAE	Dental age estimation
DNA	Deoxyribonucleic acid
EU	Extra uterine
HC	Head circumference
IU	Intra uterine
LL	Labio-lingual
MD	Mesio-distal
N	Neonatal
NL	Neonatal line
NR	Neonatal ring
Pre-N	Pre-natal
Post-N	Post-natal
RH	Root height
SEM	Scanning electron microscope

Prof. Dr. Sema P. AKA's surname was "*Kedici*" between years 1976–2004.

P. S. Aka (✉)
Department of Prosthodontics & Unit of Forensic Odontology, Faculty of Dentistry, Ankara University (retired), Ankara, Türkiye

Forensic Odontology Commission of Turkish Forensic Scientists Society, Ankara, Türkiye

Indo Pacific Academy of Forensic Odontology, Patiala, India

Independent Researcher at Present, Ankara, Türkiye

© The Author(s), under exclusive license to Springer Nature Switzerland AG 2026

A. Chowdhry, P. Kapoor (eds.), *Dental Age Assessment*,
https://doi.org/10.1007/978-3-032-08788-1_5

TH	Tooth height
VirDent-ID	Virtual dental identification

Concepts and Definitions

- *Dental Age Formula:*
  The dental age formula is the equation used to calculate dental age.
- *Fetus and Dentition Period of the Fetus*:
  The term *fetus* refers to a living embryo during the intrauterine (IU) prenatal developmental period, between the embryonic stage and birth. *Foetus* is an alternative spelling, and *fetuses* is the plural form. The fetus becomes a neonate, or new born, at birth. Dentition Period of the Fetus is the first prenatal phase of primary dental development, which begins approximately at the 13th week after conception and continues until birth. During this time, calcification and crown formation of the primary teeth take place [1].
- *Neonatal Line*:
  The neonatal line (NL) is a band-shaped landmark that occurs as a result of the interruption of dental tissue development between the Pre-Natal (Pre-N) and Post-Natal (Post-N) periods due to the stress associated with birth. It indicates whether the fetus is alive at the time of birth [2].
- *Oral Autopsy*:
  Oral Autopsy is defined by Aka PS and Canturk N (2014) as "*A forensic odontological entirety of transactions to identify unknown individuals or human remains, which comprises; the extra oral examination, followed by an access to the oral cavity, intra oral examination, photographing, collection of; data, oral evidence as DNA (Deoxyribonucleic Acid), tooth germs, teeth, saliva, and surrounding tissues, then recording of all data obtained.*" [3]
- *Odontometric age estimation methods*:
  Age estimation based on measurements of teeth [1].
- *Osteometric age estimation methods*:
  Age estimation based on measurements of bone [4].
- *Virtual Dental Identification*:
  It is an indirect digital dental image measurement method, proposed by authors PS Aka and Canturk N as "VirDent-ID." [5].

5.1 Introduction to Dental Age Estimation for Prenatal and Postnatal Periods

Dental age estimation (DAE) is typically studied in deceased people, although it is occasionally performed in living people as well. Estimating age at death, including the fetal period, is one of the most important basic research topics for a forensic scientist during identification research conducted on unidentified deceased individuals and human remains [1]. DAE of the fetus and newborn at the time of death is momentous in terms of criminal or inheritance law. In general, following intrauterine (IU) 210 days of pregnancy, the fetus is expected to be capable of living separately from the mother after the moment of birth [6]. In case the fetus or newborn is not alive, the mode of its delivery—such as normal birth, caesarean section, or stillbirth—and the age of the unidentified deceased individual can be assessed by forensic dental examinations performed on the tooth specimens that are obtained at the oral autopsy [2]. The dental samples, which are collected from the oral cavity after the extraoral and intraoral examinations, are the most significant sources of evidence. It has been stated that the estimation of age from dental structures is more precise than from the bones [7]. For this reason, a "Forensic Dentistry Unit" should be located within all morgue departments.

5.2 Oral Autopsy Procedures

Oral autopsy procedures are generally simpler and less complicated for fetal or infant cases, depending on their muscle weakness. There are some actions that need to be taken in this regard. There is a special oral autopsy protocol called "Aka-Canturk Oral Autopsy Method" for fetus or newborn cases, which is a gentle tooth germ extraction method that does not require any skin dissection or jaw removal for identification purposes [3]. The application steps of the mentioned oral autopsy protocol and the required equipment are as follows:

- The first condition of this protocol to obtain the samples to be examined is to receive written legal and ethical official permissions.
- Consecutive double swabs, moistened with sterile distilled water, must be taken to maximize DNA extraction, air-dried at room temperature, and sent for analysis as soon as possible. Swabs can be stored at room temperature for the first 4–6 h, if stored for more than 6 h; they must be stored in the refrigerator without freezing [8].
- X-ray images must be recorded.
- Tooth germ extraction should be performed after curved incisions of the maxillary and mandibular alveolar crests and the separation of the periosteum using surgical hand instruments such as elevators and retractors. The straight and curved elevators must be applied from the mesial aspects of the periodontal sockets, without contact with the tooth germ. Then, the tooth germ must be photographed with an ABFO number 2 scale, measured with callipers and gauges.
- The extracted tooth specimens must be conserved in labelled containers or test tubes filled with 10% formalin or 1% phenol solution [9, 10].
- The test tubes must be marked with case numbers and identifying codes.
- If an erupted tooth is present, it should be measured in situ [3].
- In case the determination of the viability of the deceased fetus at the time of birth is required, the selected tooth specimens should be sent for scanning electron microscope (SEM) examinations for neonatal line (NL) detection [2].
- A detailed oral autopsy report must be prepared after the completion of the dental forms and charts. Copies of all the original documents related to the case must be saved by the forensic odontologist. Despite all, it has been denoted that oral autopsy protocols can be modified depending on the requirement of the case [11].

5.3 Determination of the Mode of Birth

Tooth development occurs by the activity of two groups of cells; mainly, enamel tissue forms from the ameloblasts of ectodermal origin, dentine and pulp tissues forms from the dentinoblasts of mesodermal origin [12]. These tissues are configured throughout dental development at a constant rate of a circadian rhythm, which is interrupted by the metabolic changes of birth, where a distinctive line called the neonatal line (NL) is formed between the Pre-N and Post-N dental tissues [13]. NL is a band-type landmark that occurs when the formation of dental tissues is blocked in between the ameloblastic secretion and its recurrence, due to birth trauma, as the fetus passes from intrauterine (IU) to extrauterine (EU) life [14]. The NL indicates the time of birth and can be detected in each primary tooth and first permanent molar by examining the SEM images in vertical or horizontal sections, where the NL in vertical sections appears as a ring in horizontal sections and called neonatal ring (NR).

The SEM studies must be performed according to the following procedures: Each dental sample, which was kept in a labelled test tube containing preserving solution, must be embedded in acrylic methyl methacrylate blocks ($CH_2 = C (CH_3) COOCH_3$). Vertical and horizontal sections of these dental samples must be prepared and polished, etched with 37% orthophosphoric acid for 3 minutes, washed, dried, and coated with a gold-palladium alloy. By measuring and comparing the NL and NR thicknesses on the SEM images of these sections, the mode of birth can be determined as normal, caesarean, or stillbirth. The presence of hypo-mineralized NL can be detected only in normal birth and caesarean section cases between 200× and 2000× magnifications as dark lines, where the NL of normal delivery cases was found significantly thicker (mean 9.2 μm in vertical and 6.2 μm horizontal sections) than the NL of caesarean section cases (mean 2.7 μm in vertical and 2.1 μm horizontal sections), due to the completion of the childbirth process in a shorter period. On the contrary, stillbirth cases show no signs of NL [2].

5.4 Dental Age Estimation (DAE) Methods

Teeth are the hardest tissues of the body, which are certainly resistant to postmortem changes therefore, age estimation from dental analysis is a very reliable method. Furthermore, it is stated that tooth mineralization stages provide more precise information about chronological age than bones, as the mineralization stages of teeth are found not to be much affected by variations in nutrition and endocrine status when compared to bone mineralization [15]. In addition, dental development of the primary dentition undergoes a series of changes in a chronological order. The following differentiation steps occur during the intrauterine (IU), Pre-N dental development: Initiation (bud stage), proliferation (cap stage), histo-differentiation, and morfo-differentiation (bell stage), apposition and calcification, enamel and dentine formation before eruption [12]. The IU, Pre-N period comprises the calcification and crown formation of teeth, which initiate with the mineralization of incisors at the 13th week of pregnancy and continues through the extrauterine (EU), post-natal period, which covers the eruption of these teeth (after their root heights reach 2/3 of their final formation), nascency of the supporting periodontal ligaments and alveolar bone tissues, and finally, the development of primary dentition concludes with the completion of roots of the primary second molars circa at age 3 after birth (birth to 36 months). All these developmental phases provide precise age indicators for each stage. Serial photographs of fetal pre-natal, and infant post-natal teeth in six aspects: Labial, Lingual, Mesial, Distal, Incisal, and Root direction surfaces, with all details observable from the text and atlas of "*Primary Tooth Development in Infancy*" [16].

In the field of dentistry, DAE systems such as the "atlas method", "scoring method", "odontometric method" and "odontometric—osteometric method" have been applied for a long time to determine the developmental stages of teeth. The first two systems are both based on evaluations of radiographic images such as peri-apical, lateral, cephalometric x-rays, or panoramic radiographs (orthopantomograms); however, the other metric systems calculate individual measurements to assess the age. One of the earliest studies on the atlas method was Kronfield's (1935) numerical dental development chart, where the first mineralization stages of the primary dentition initiate from intrauterine (IU) 4–5 months [17]. The atlas method was facilitated with the scoring method applied on panoramic radiographs, for the age range 3–17 years, where the dental maturity score was obtained by the sum of the scores of 8 development stages of the 7 lower left quadrant tooth, from the first appearance of dental calcified points to the closure of the root apexes, which do not need any accurate measurements [18]. The accuracy and universal applicability of odontogenic chronological DAE methodologies have been tested, repeated, and rated by researchers on different ethnic groups. One study evaluated the accuracy of the original Demirjian method on a Belgian Caucasian population sample (age range of 2.3–18 years) and detected significant overestimation of dental age due to varying rates of dental growth in different populations, and established a more specific revised method for DAE of the Belgian population [19]. It has been reported that, based on the original Demirjian 8-teeth method, a comprehensive DAE chart entitled "*DAEcc8*" was proposed for its simplicity in understanding and application [20]. It has also been shown that new dental age tables are needed for different ethnic groups due to different results obtained [21]. Another effective approach for determining chronological age was found to be comparable to previous age estimation techniques, based on the linear relationship between age and the open apices of seven left mandibular teeth, measured on digitized X-ray images taken from children (age range 5–15 years), which showed significant correlations on a computer-aided drafting program, and linear regression formulas for both sexes were generated [22]. In addition, a detailed atlas, integrating both tooth formation and alveolar eruption stages (for age range IU 28 weeks—23 years), was created [23]. All techniques covered by this topic will be discussed in full details in the following chapters. Hereafter, the above-mentioned metric DAE methods will be presented, which consists of direct and indirect approaches specific for the pre-natal and post-natal periods of primary teeth.

5.4.1 Metric DAE Methods

5.4.1.1 Direct Odontometric DAE Method

Odontometric age estimation methods are preferred to be performed on the central incisors, which develop and erupt first among the primary dentition, starting around the IU fourth month and completes its development by the EU, at age 2, with full root formation. Central incisors have proven to be the most decisive teeth for age estimation, with a minimum margin of error (±2.42 weeks) [1]. Direct measurements can be taken from the extracted tooth germs or from the erupted teeth Fig. 5.1.

Case measurements on unerupted teeth: The age of a deceased person whose central primary teeth have not yet erupted can be estimated from examination, analysis, and measurements of the diagnostic tooth germ removed during oral autopsy procedures for diagnostic purposes. The mesio-distal (MD), labio-lingual (LL), crown height (CH), root height (RH), and tooth height (TH) dimensions can be measured from the extracted tooth germs. Due to morphological changes, the crown thickness (CrT) dimensions of the extracted tooth germ can be measured until root formation starts; after this time, the RH can be measured instead of CrT. Two types of callipers (sensitive to 0.1 mm) can be used for this purpose; digital Vernier calliper (*Mitutoyo, Japan*), used for LL, MD, CH, RH and TH dimensions, and dental thickness calliper (*Fara Dental, Germany*) used for CrT dimension Figs. 5.2 and 5.3.

The age of the individual can be calculated by placing the dental measurements taken from various dimensions of tooth structures into tooth age regression formulas (which are derived from the regression analysis of the statistically processed data). The cross-sectional time for age calculations from the central tooth is found to be 44.45 ± 0–2 weeks, which can be considered as 40 weeks from conception under normal conditions, plus 4–5 weeks after birth. This is the cut-off point for age estimation between CrT and RH. The RH measurements of teeth were found statistically significant for DAE ($p < 0.01$). For this reason, four age formulas entitled ATA[1] were derived to give the relationship between age from conception to 44 weeks and after 44 weeks [1]. Dental age of a deceased pre-natal (Pre-N) and post-natal

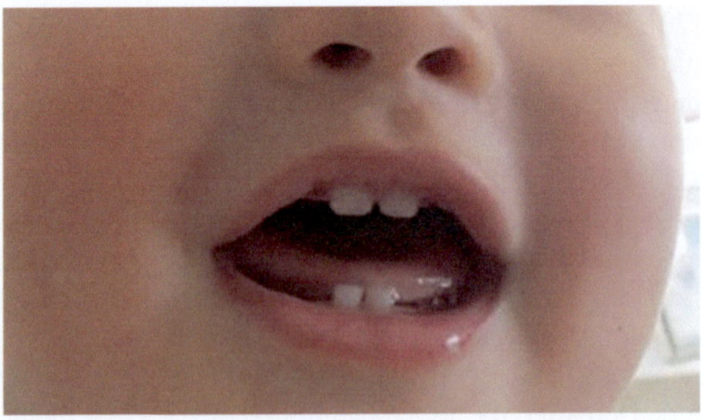

Fig. 5.1 A 17-month-old infant with erupted primary central teeth

[1]ATA is the special name given to the dental age formulas in honour of the great Turkish leader Mustafa Kemal Ataturk (1881–1938) [1].

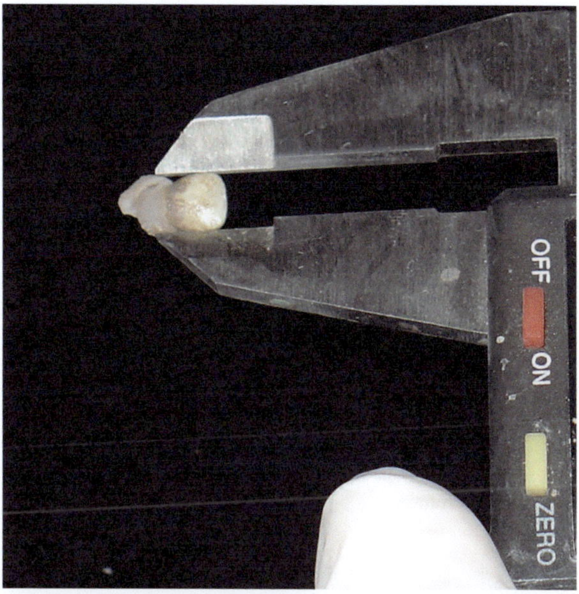

Fig. 5.2 Mesio-distal measurement of a tooth using a Vernier calliper

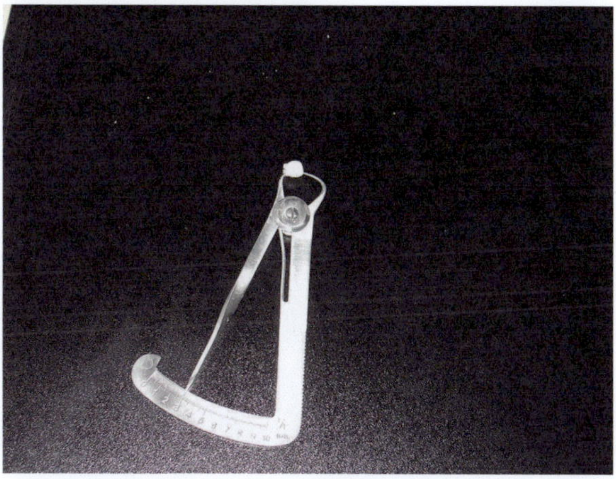

Fig. 5.3 Crown thickness measurement of a tooth using a dental thickness calliper

(Post-N) can be calculated from the formulas given in Table 5.1 with an accuracy of ±0–2 weeks [1]. It is important to preserve the tooth germ evidence in the archive of the case in the event of burial or cremation of the body.

5.4.1.2 Direct Odontometric and Osteometric DAE Method

It is found that, based on correlation analysis, the head circumference (HC) of a fetus or infant of both sexes and the LL, MD and CH dimensions of their upper central tooth—as seen in Fig. 5.1—were strongly correlated. HC is a circular measurement in centimetres taken by a metric band, which must contact to the glabella and external occipital protuberance points Fig. 5.4. In case the primary central teeth

Table 5.1 Age estimation regression parameters for maxillary and mandibular central incisors for the first 44-week period starting with conception and after 44 weeks

Age formulas	Time interval	Equation
	From conception to 44 weeks	
ATA 1	Age for the maxillary central incisor	Age = 17.785–2.026sex[a] + 4.978LL + 0.744CrT
ATA 2	Age for the mandibular central incisor	Age = 20.703–3.293sex[a] + 5.407LL + 1.671CrT
	After 44 weeks	
ATA 3	Age for the maxillary Central incisor	Age = 43.419 + 6.997RH
ATA 4	Age for the mandibular central incisor	Age = 8.434CH + 5.671RH

[a]In the formula, the sex code was given as 2 for girls and 1 for boys

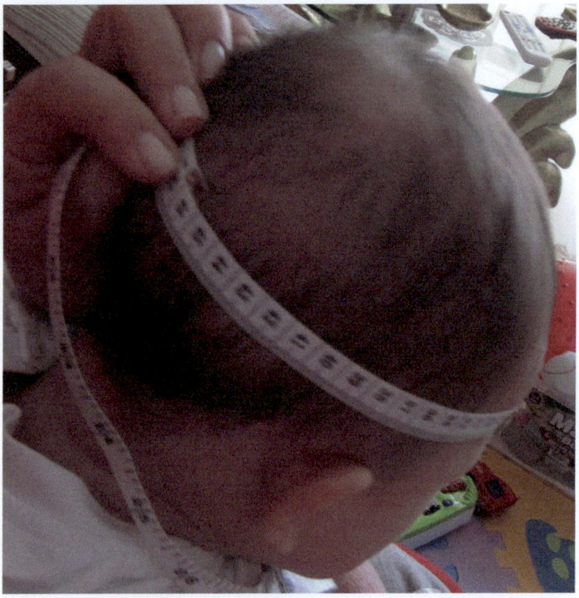

Fig. 5.4 Measurement of the head circumference

are erupted, measurements can be recorded in-situ. The linear combination of these measurements may provide the best estimation for age, giving the minimum age estimation error (±1.56 weeks) for both sexes. The following age regression formulas are derived from HC and LL, MD, and CH tooth dimensions for age estimation of fetuses or infants [24] Table 5.2.

Table 5.2 Selected regression formulas with head circumference and labio-lingual, mesio-distal, crown height and tooth height measurements for dental age estimation

Tooth variables	Regression formulas for age estimation including head circumference and tooth measurements
LL	Log (age) = 2.149 + 0.051*HC-0.154*LL + 0.003*HC*LL
MD	Log (age) = 2.178 + 0.049*HC-0.104*MD + 0.002*HC*MD
CH	Log (age) = 2.25 + 0.039*HC-0.066*CH + 0.003*HC*CH
TH	Log (age) = 2.235 + 0.031*HC + 0.071*TH

After finding natural Log (Age) by substituting the related measurements, the Anti-logarithm value of the above equation must be found as given below:

If Log (Age) equals to 3.3345, then the age will be estimated with its Anti-logarithm value = $e^{3.3345}$ = 28.06 weeks or (7 Months).

5.4.2 Indirect Metric DAE Methods

It is also possible to find out the age of a pre-natal (Pre-N) or post-natal (Post-N) forensic case from the indirect dental measurements, either measured from plaster dental models or from computed tomography (CT) digital maxillofacial images. In a study, it was reported that 76% of 164 missing persons were aged correctly with CT analyses and examinations [25]. The analysis of digital images in the field of autopsy is known as the "Virtopcy" method, which is derived from the phrase "Virtual Autopsy" and is indicated as a conservative means for identifying dental evidence from captured images instead of invasive oral autopsies that involve forensic interventions [26].

Dental analysis from digital images is also a reliable method entitled as Virtual Dental Identification (VirDent-ID) [5, 27]. The indirect tooth measurements—LL, MD, TH and CrT—can be obtained from each tooth on the sagittal, coronal and axial three planes of the CT digital images, with precise electronic callipers sensitive to 0.01 mm Fig. 5.5. It has been proven that the longest vertical dimension TH, is the most precise tooth dimension for age estimation, and the best formula for age estimation is derived from the TH with LL dimension measurements (R^2 = 98.1), where reliable age estimation results were found with a margin of error equal to ±1.07 weeks [27] Table 5.3.

Indirect age estimation studies have given a more accurate result for upper central primary teeth than for lower central primary teeth. Therefore, upper central primary teeth should be preferred for statistical extraction of data. However, it was found that the sex factor did not contribute to this statistical model ($p > 0.05$) [27].

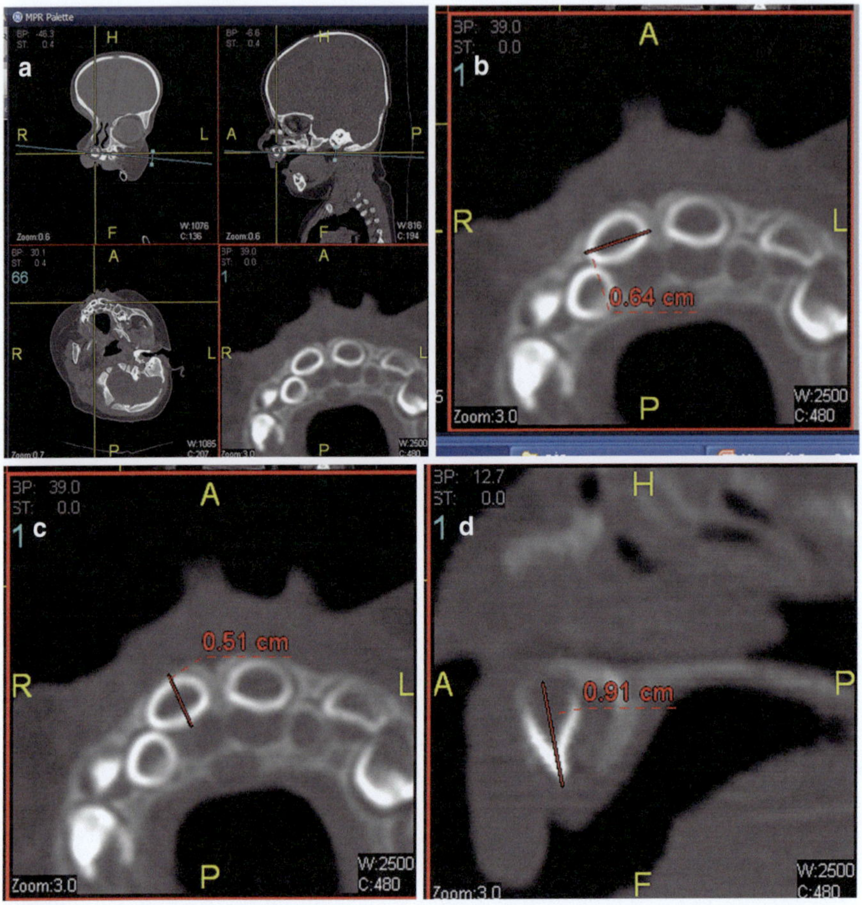

Fig. 5.5 Computed tomography (CT) image of a post natal 4-month-old case. (**a**) Axial plane of the CT image. (**b**) Axial MD measurement of the upper central tooth. (**c**) Axial LL measurement of the upper central tooth. (**d**) Sagittal TH measurement of the upper central tooth

Table 5.3 Regression formulas entitled "*Virtual Dental Identification Formulas*" for age estimation from each dental measurement on the sagittal, coronal and axial computed tomography directions

Tooth variables for log (age)	Regression formulas for age estimation		
	Computed tomography directions		
	Sagittal	Coronal	Axial
LL	−1.009 + 0.902xLL	–	−2.352 + 1.286xLL
MD	–	−7.095 + 1.712xMD	−6.236 + 1.579xMD
TH	−0.205 + 0.335xTH	−0.007 + 0.315xTH	–
CrT	−1.491 + 1.622xCrT	−1.801 + 1.803xCrT	–
LL & TH	0.601 + 0.27xLL + 0.287xTH	–	–

5.5 Summary and Conclusion

Forensic scientists deal with estimating the age of unidentified individuals from dental evidence for identification purposes, including the fetal period, which is an important research topic especially for criminal or inheritance law cases. When the fetus or newborn is deceased, the mode of delivery of the unidentified deceased—such as normal birth, caesarean section or stillbirth—and the age of the case can be determined by examining the neonatal line from the scanning electron microscope images, which is performed on the oral autopsy tooth samples. The oral autopsy procedures for fetus or newborn cases entitled "*Aka-Canturk Oral Autopsy Method*" are described in this chapter.

Estimation of age from dental analysis is a very reliable method as teeth undergo a series of changes in chronological order throughout life, besides being the hardest and most durable tissues of the body. Direct and indirect metric dental age estimation methods, including osteometric and odontometric measuring procedures, are defined. The direct method covers measurements of the tooth germ extracted from oral autopsy operations or measurements of erupted teeth in situ with callipers, and the indirect method includes tooth measurements from plaster dental models or from computed tomography digital images with precise electronic callipers, followed by calculation of the age of the case by placing these measurements in the age formulas.

5.6 Learning Outcomes

- You must be able to perform an oral autopsy.
- You can determine the mode of delivery of the unidentified deceased individual—such as normal birth, caesarean section, or stillbirth—from the scanning electron microscope images of the oral autopsy tooth samples.
- You can estimate age from the direct measurements of the dental structures of prenatal and postnatal deceased individual or from the indirect measurements taken either from digital tooth images or from plaster dental models.
- You should be able to calculate dental age by using the direct or indirect measurement data and age formulas.

5.7 Self-Evaluation Questions

- What are the steps for performing an oral autopsy on a deceased pre- or postnatal case?
- What information does a neonatal line give about a deceased neonate or postnatal individual?
- How can dental age be estimated from the direct measurements of the dental structures.
- How can dental age be estimated from the indirect measurements of the dental structures.

5.8 Multiple Choice Questions

Q1. Which is the most decisive primary tooth for age estimation?

(a) Central incisors.
(b) Canine tooth.
(c) First molar.
(d) Second molar.
(e) First Premolar.

Ans: a

Q2. Which calliper must be used for the direct age estimation method?

(a) Sliding.
(b) Vernier.
(c) Spreading.
(d) None of the choices in a, b, or c.
(e) All of the choices in a, b, or c.

Ans: b

Q3. To what stage of tooth development can crown thickness be measured for calculating tooth age?

(a) Until Initiation (bud stage).
(b) Until proliferation (cap stage).
(c) Until morfo-differentiation and histo-differentiation (bell stage).
(d) Until the root formation starts.
(e) Until the formation of the periodontal ligament.

Ans: d

Q4. Which of the following is the cut-off point for age estimation between crown thickness and root height of a central tooth?

(a) 36.45 ± 0–2 weeks
(b) 22.45 ± 0–2 weeks
(c) 44.45 ± 0–2 weeks
(d) 88.45 ± 0–2 weeks
(e) 11.45 ± 0–2 weeks.

Ans: c

Q5. Which osteometric body dimension is strongly correlated with primary tooth size for age estimation of a fetus or infant?

(a) There is a strong correlation between tooth dimensions and bi-orbital breadth (external orbital breadth).
(b) There is a strong correlation between tooth dimensions and interorbital breadth (internal orbital breadth).
(c) There is no correlation between tooth dimensions and osteometric body dimensions.

(d) There is a strong correlation between tooth dimensions and the head circumference (HC).
(e) There is a strong correlation between tooth dimensions and biparietal breadth.

Ans: d

Q6. Which of the following storage medium solutions is used for placing and keeping the dental samples in tube containers?

(a) 10% formalin solution
(b) 37% orthophosphoric acid
(c) 20% hydrogen peroxide
(d) 1% sulfuric acid
(e) 10% lactic acid.

Ans: a

Q7. Which of the following etching solutions is used for etching the sectioned dental samples of scanning electron microscope (SEM) studies?

(a) 20% sodium chloride
(b) 10% formalin solution
(c) 37% orthophosphoric acid
(d) 1% sulfuric acid
(e) 10% citric acid.

Ans: c

Q8. If the neonatal line is not detected on the scanning electron microscopy image of the tooth section, what does this prove?

(a) Absence of neonatal line shows normal delivery cases.
(b) Absence of neonatal line shows caesarean section cases.
(c) Absence of neonatal line shows normal birth cases.
(d) Absence of neonatal line shows stillbirth.
(e) The absence of the neonatal line indicates that the baby was alive when born.

Ans: d

Q9. Which of the following is an indirect digital dental image measurement method?

(a) Dental measurements with Vernier calliper on dental samples.
(b) Dental measurements from computed tomography images.
(c) In situ dental measurements.
(d) None of the above items is an indirect digital dental image measurement.
(e) All of the above items are indirect digital dental image measurements.

Ans: b

Q10. From which indirect digital dental image measurement can the best formula for age estimation be generated?

(a) From tooth height with labio-lingual dimension.
(b) From mesio-distal with labio-lingual dimension.
(c) From crown height with mesio-distal dimension.
(d) From crown thickness with labio-lingual dimension.
(e) From root height with mesio-distal dimension.

Ans: a

5.9 Mind Map (Fig. 5.6)

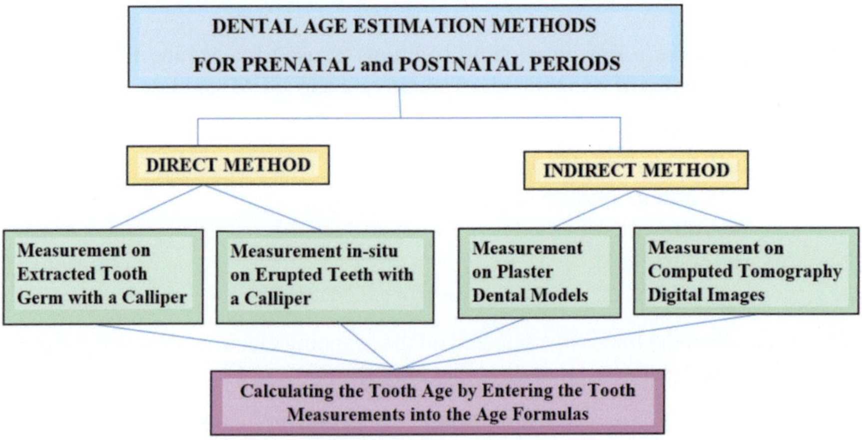

Fig. 5.6 Mind map describing the applicable metric systems for dental age estimation of prenatal and postnatal periods of primary dentition

References

1. Aka PS, Canturk N, Dagalp R, Yagan M. Age determination from central incisors of fetuses and infants. Forensic Sci Int. 2009;184(1–3):15–20. https://doi.org/10.1016/j.forsciint.2008.11.005.
2. Canturk N, Atsu SS, Aka PS, Dagalp R. Neonatal line on fetus and infant teeth: an indicator of live birth and mode of delivery. Early Hum Dev. 2014;90(8):393–7. https://doi.org/10.1016/j.earlhumdev.2014.05.002.
3. Aka PS, Canturk N. Aka Canturk Oral autopsy method for the dental identification of fetus and infant cases. Forensic Med Anat Res. 2014;2:48–50. https://doi.org/10.4236/fmar.2014.23009.
4. Iscan MY, Steyn M. The human skeleton in forensic medicine. 3rd ed. Springfield: Charles C. Thomas; 2013. p. 66. ISBN 978-0-398-08878-1.
5. Aka PS, Yagan M, Canturk N, Dagalp R. Direct and indirect forensic age estimation methods for deciduous teeth. J Forensic Res. 2015;6(2):273–5. https://doi.org/10.4172/2157-7145.1000273.
6. Soysal Z, Eke MS, Cagdır AS. Post-mortem examination of babies [Bebegin postmortem incelenmesi]. In: Forensic autopsy [Adli Otopsi], vol. 3. Istanbul: Press and Movie Center of University of Istanbul; 1999. p. 1054.
7. Eckert WG. Introduction to forensic sciences, 2nd ed., CRC Press, Boca Raton. 1997:306.
8. American Board of Forensic Odontology. Diplomates reference manual, 2014: p.111. [Internet]. Available from: http://www.abfo.org/wp-content/uploads/2012/08/ABFO-Reference-Manual-1-22-2013-revision.pdf.
9. Lee JJ, Marbell AN, Cook A, Pimenta LAF, Leonard R, Ritter AV. Using extracted teeth for research: the effect of storage medium and sterilization on dentin bond strengths. J Am Dent Assoc. 2007;138(12):1599–603. https://doi.org/10.14219/jada.archive.2007.0110.
10. Van Beek, GC. Dental morphology: an illustrated guide. 2nd Edition, Elsevier, Philadelphia. 2008:7.
11. Stimson PG. Oral Autopsy Protocol. Dent Clin North Am. 2013;21:177–9.
12. Pinkham JR, Casamassimo PS, Mc Tigue DJ, Fields HW, Nowak AJ. Pediatric dentistry. Infancy through adolescence. 4th ed. St. Louis: Elsevier Inc; 2005. p. 172–97.
13. Berkovitz BKB, Holland GR, Moxham BJ. Oral anatomy, histology and embryology. 4th ed. Edinburg: Mosby Elsevier; 2009. p. 105–28.
14. Sabel N, Johansson C, Kühnisch J, Robertson A, Steiniger F, Norén JG, et al. Neonatal lines in the enamel of primary teeth—a morphological and scanning electron microscopic investigation. Arch Oral Biol. 2008;53(10):954–63.
15. Willems G. A review of the most commonly used dental age estimation techniques. J Forensic Odontostomatol. 2001;19:9–17.
16. Aka PS, Yagan M, Canturk N, Dagalp R. Primary tooth development in infancy: a text and atlas. 1st ed. Boca Raton: CRC Press, Taylor & Francis Group; 2015. ISBN 9781482238518.
17. Kronfeld R. Development and calcification of the human deciduous and permanent dentition. Bur. 1935;15:18–25.
18. Demirjian A, Goldstein H, Tanner JM. A new system of dental age assessment. Hum Biol. 1973;45(2):211–27.
19. Willems G, Van Olmen A, Spiessens B, Carels C. Dental age estimation in Belgian children: Demirjian's technique revisited. J Forensic Sci. 2001;46(4):893–5.
20. Kapoor P, Jain V. Comprehensive chart for dental age estimation (DAEcc8) based on Demirjian 8-teeth method: simplified for operator ease. J Forensic Leg Med. 2018;59:45–9.
21. Phillips VM, van Wyk Kotze TJ. Testing standard methods of dental age estimation by Moorrees, Fanning and Hunt and Demirjian, Goldstein and Tanner on three South African children samples. J Forensic Odontostomatol. 2009;27(2):20–8.
22. Cameriere R, Ferrante L, Cingolani M. Age estimation in children by measurement of open apices in teeth. Int J Legal Med. 2006;120:49–53. https://doi.org/10.1007/s00414-005-0047-9.
23. AlQahtani SJ, Hector MP, Liversidge HM. Brief communication: the London atlas of human tooth development and eruption. Am J Phys Anthropol. 2010;142(3):481–90.

24. Dagalp R, Aka PS, Canturk N, Kedici I. Age estimation from fetus and infant tooth and head measurements. Int J Legal Med. 2014;128(3):501–8. https://doi.org/10.1007/s00414-013-0935-3.
25. O'Donnell C, Iino M, Mansharan K, Leditscke J, Woodford N. Contribution of postmortem multidetector CT scanning to identification of the deceased in a mass disaster: experience gained from the 2009 Victorian bushfires. Forensic Sci Int. 2011;205(1–3):15–28.
26. Tejaswi KB, Periya EA. Virtopsy (virtual autopsy): a new phase in forensic investigation. J Forensic Dent Sci. 2013;5(2):146–8.
27. Canturk N, Aka SP, Dagalp R, Uzun C, Canturk G, Fitoz S. Age estimation from primary teeth through virtual dental identification. Aust J Forensic Sci. 2015;47(3):293–305.

Dental Age Assessment Methods in Children and Adolescents

6

Cristiana Palmela Pereira

Abbreviations

ABFO	American Board of Forensic Odontology
ADA	American Dental Association
AGFAD	Study Group on Forensic Age Diagnostics
ALARA	As low as reasonably achievable
CBCT	Cone Bean Computed Tomography
CC	Portuguese Civil Code
CNN	Convolutional Neural Networks
CPU	Central Processing Unit
CRC	Convention on the rights of the Child
CT	Computed Tomography
DL	Decree Law

C. Palmela Pereira (✉)
President of the International Organization for Forensic Odonto-Stomatology, IOFOS, Zagreb, Croatia

Tenured Professor from the School of Dental Medicine, University of Lisbon, Lisbon, Portugal

Integrated Researcher from the Centre of Statistical and its Application CEAUL, University of Lisbon, Lisbon, Portugal

Chair of the Executive Committee of Forensic Experts from the Portuguese Dental Association (OMD), Porto, Portugal

Forensic Odontologist of the Portuguese DVI team, Portuguese National Institute of Legal Medicine and Forensic Sciences,
Lisbon, Portugal

National Representative of Portugal to the INTERPOL DVI Sub-Working Group on Forensic Odontology, Lisbon, Portugal

Forensic Expert on Forensic Odontology for the Courts, Lisbon, Portugal
e-mail: cpereira@edu.ulisboa.pt

© The Author(s), under exclusive license to Springer Nature Switzerland AG 2026
A. Chowdhry, P. Kapoor (eds.), *Dental Age Assessment*,
https://doi.org/10.1007/978-3-032-08788-1_6

EASO	European Asylum Support Office
EU	European Union
GPU	Graphics Processing Units
I_{2M}	Second molar maturity index
I_{3M}	Third molar maturity index
IOFOS	International Organization for Forensic Odonto-Stomatology
ISO	International Organization for Standardization
LPCJP	Law for the Protection of Children and Young People in Danger
OSAC-NIST	Organization of scientific area committees for forensic science by National Institute of Standards and Technology
UN	United Nations

Concepts and Definitions

Dental age

Is the age inferred from tooth development stages or structural dental changes, used to approximate chronological age.

Age markers

Physiological features that pass through distinguishable stages, each associated with a specific chronological age range.

Dental age range (interval) assessment

Processes using dental information and relating it to chronological age.

Dental age assessment technique

Method used for dental age assessment.

Dental data

Analysis of an individual's dental condition in their current or previously documented state.

Chronological age:

Actual time elapsed since birth.

Biological age:

Reflects the level of physiological maturity or development of an individual, inferred from biological markers (e.g. dental, skeletal) relative to normative reference data.

Estimated age:

Is the inferred value (or interval) of chronological age derived from biological markers and scientific models when the actual date of birth is unknown.

Dental age assessment:

The processes used to produce an estimation of an individual's biological age using dental markers and subsequently correlate biological age to chronological age.

Infant/child dental age interval:

The interval in human dental development that begins at birth, includes the presence of the developing, developed and resorbing primary dentition as well as the initial development of the permanent dentition. This interval includes the early period of mixed primary and permanent dentitions and ends when the last primary tooth is exfoliated normally.

Adolescent's dental age interval:

The interval in human dental development that begins after all primary teeth are normally shed, and the permanent teeth are developing or developed. The adolescent interval ends when all permanent teeth present are fully developed.

6.1 General Considerations on the Importance of Age at the Forensic Level on This Group (Children and Adolescents)

The beginning of this chapter deals with the relevance of age in the forensic field. The legal interest of this parameter, age, results from the importance of criminal law in knowing the age of the individual. In the light of most European legal system, the minor individual does not have his personality completely formed and, since the judicial-criminal guilt consists of a judgment of ethical-social censorship that falls on the personality of the agent, it is concluded that the minor under the age of 16 years has no capacity for guilt (the Portuguese criminal age threshold; in the world judicial systems there are significant variations in this criminal age; but the concept is identical for each legal age threshold). Thus, any offense committed by young people below this age limit of criminal imputability can only lead to the establishment of protective or educational measures. This question arises with special relevance in the field of juvenile delinquency, whose perpetrators of criminal offenses are, as a rule, young adolescents, or pre-adolescents, aged between 12 and 16 years[1], with particular attention to 14 years of age (according to the Portuguese Criminal Law).

Other important aspect of age is the majority of age at civil law. The age of Portuguese civil majority begins at the age of 18, becoming the person fit for the activities of civil life that do not require a special limit. This limit was not the one adopted in the Portuguese Civil Code (CC) of 1966.[2] Despite continuously changing, age is an innate characteristic of one's identity. As part of the personal status of a person, it determines the relationship between the state and the person. As such, changes in age may trigger specific rights and obligations, for example being considered an adult when someone turns 18. However, the age of 18 is not always the

[1] The article No. 19 of Código Penal (Portuguese Criminal Code) provides that "those under 16 years of age are not liable". Imputability can be defined as the capacity of the agent, at the time of perpetration of the fact, to assess the illegality of the fact or to determine in accordance with that assessment.

[2] It should be noted that, in the validity of the Código Civil (Portuguese Civil Code) from 1966 this age of majority is foreseen in the article No. 130 where it reads, "He who reaches twenty-one years of age acquires full capacity to exercise rights, being entitled to rule his person and dispose of his goods". This has been amended by the Portuguese Law DL N°. 496/77, of 25 November. Currently, we read "Who have 18 years of age acquires full capacity to exercise rights, being able to govern his person and to dispose of his owns goods".

determining factor for acquiring new rights and obligations or full capacity in some aspects such as military service, the emancipation age, the minimum age of criminal responsibility, the age of consent for marriage, or the age for employment or sexual relations. As we could explain until now, depending on national legislations, these thresholds may be reached at an earlier chronological age.

The other important field of age estimation is in asylums seekers that are undocumented, unaccompanied, and minors. This is the most present and controversial situation at European and international levels. The granting of asylum or subsidiary protection is provided by the Portuguese Law N°. 27/2008, from 30 June, amended by Law N°. 26/2014, which establishes the conditions and procedures for granting asylum or subsidiary protection and the status of asylum seeker, refugee, and subsidiary protection, transposing the Directives of the European Parliament and of the Council N°. 2011/95/EU, from 13 of December, 2013/32/EU, from 26 of June, and 2013/33/EU, from 26 of June. However, the treatment of this type of cases is different when the age of the individual is less than 18 years (paragraphs l) and m) of the article No. 2).

In these cases, persons younger than 18 years old, there is an additional judicial consideration for the protection of asylees, undocumented persons, and minors—the Law for the Protection of Children and Young People in Danger (LPCJP, Law N°. 147/99, from 01 of September), as amended by Law N°. 23/2017. Under this law, protective measures are applied until the age of 16.

The article 3 from the LPCJP, *Legitimacy* of the intervention, justifies, in its paragraph 2, "*The child or young person is considered to be in danger when, in particular, he is in one of the following situations: a) He is abandoned or lives surrendered to himself; (b) Does not receive the care or affection appropriate to his age and personal situation; (e) It is obliged to activities or work that are excessive or inappropriate to its age, dignity and personal situation or that are detrimental to its formation or development...*".

Based on those laws, the judge order opening an investigation, which justifies the examination of age, for lack of documents and the need for promotion and protection; proceeding immediately to its protection, which shall continue until the end of the instructive process.[3]

The importance of age at the level of the process of medico-legal identification of a body with unknown identity is the last field. In this process, the age parameter is important for the reconstructive phase of the cadaver, and in order to exclude possible disappearances based on the age parameter. This facilitates the identification

[3]Article 106th of the Legal Code for Children and Young People (LPCJP)[Decree-Law N°. 164/2019, from 25 of October, establishes the regime for the implementation of residential care, a measure to promote the rights and protection of children and young people in danger, provided for in point f) of paragraph 1 of article 35th and articles 49 to 51 of the Law on the Protection of Children and Young People in Danger, approved by Law N°. 147/99, from 1 of September.

process, particularly when the number of missing persons and bodies is very large. The identification of the cadavers is a goal of the medico-legal autopsy.[4]

6.1.1 Circumstances of Dental Age Assessment for Age Estimation in Children and Adolescents (Particularly in Cases of Unaccompanied, Unidentified and Minor's Asylum Seekers)

Age is an essential element of a child's identity. The European Union (EU) acquis—as well as—the Convention on the Rights of the Child (CRC)—defines childhood by reference to age (article 1):[5]

A child/minor is any person below 18 years of age.

Two main consequences derive from this definition. The first one is that the convention applies to every person under 18 years of age. Secondly, as established in the EU acquis, any international protection applicant under 18 years of age is entitled to child-sensitive procedural safeguards and special reception conditions. This is important in the situations of cases of asylum seekers of unaccompanied, unidentified, or minors.

Before, we continue this chapter, we have already discussed different concepts for child. The methods for age dental assessment include prenatal, infant/child, adolescent, and adult. This chapter includes children and adolescents.

For dental age assessment, the concept *Infant/Child Dental Age Interval* is the one defined by American Board of Forensic Odontology (ABFO) [1]. The interval in human dental development that begins at birth, includes the presence of the developing, developed, and resorbing primary dentition, as well as the initial development of the permanent dentition. This interval includes the early period of mixed primary and permanent dentition and ends when the last primary tooth is exfoliated normally. However, as we know, during the adolescent age and adult dental age intervals, primary teeth may be atypically retained for various reasons. The concept *Adolescent Dental Age Interval* refers to human dental development that begins after all primary teeth are normally shed, and the permanent teeth are developing or developed. The adolescent interval ends when all permanent teeth are fully developed [2].

The European Union (EU) concept of Child encompasses the two concepts of intervals of dental age assessment: child/adolescent.

---

[4] Regarding the medico-legal identification we can read in Palmela Pereira C, Costa Santos J. "How to identify single cases according to the Quality Assurance from IOFOS. The positive identification of an unidentified body by dental parameters: A case of homicide". *Journal of Forensic and Legal Medicine* 2013; volume 20(issue 3): pages 169–173, as recommendations of the International Organization for Forensic Odontostomatology (IOFOS).

[5] From the Directive 2013/33/EU of the European Parliament and of the Council of 26 June 2013 laying down standards for the reception of applicants for international protection (recast). It has also been cited as the 'reception conditions directive' recast).

Age assessment in living individuals is the process by which the authorities seek to estimate the chronological age range of a person in order to establish whether an individual is a child or an adult. The correct identification of an individual as a child or adult is crucial to ensure that children's rights are protected and guaranteed, as well as to prevent adults from being placed among children to take advantage of additional rights or safeguards such as access to education, appointment of a guardian, etc. [3].

6.2 Definitions and Concepts of Age Related to This Group (Children and Adolescents)

6.2.1 Difference Between Chronological Age and Biological Age

Chronological age refers to the age that is calculated through the time elapsed since the date of birth. It is one of the key elements that regulates the civil identification of each person, it is the concept used at the legal level, it is irreversible, and and does not suffer influences.

Civil identification appears in the Portuguese Civil Code[6] in the section Personality and legal capacity. The article 66th defines the beginning of the personality and the article 68th the term of personality.[7] This is an example as other European Countries.

This civil identification is regulated by Law N°. 33/99, from18 May (amended by Decree-Law N°. 194/2003, from 23 of august). In article first named, object and general principles, we can read "Civil identification has obligation the collection, processing and keeping of the individualizing personal data of each citizen in order to establish each own civil identity".

The Law N°. 7/2007, from 5 February (amended by Law N°. 91/2015, from 12 of August) creates the Portuguese citizen card (as almost European countries). The visible elements that must be included are designated in the article 7[8], including the date of birth.

Thus, the normative assumptions for the definition of chronological age are found. It is this, the concept, which is the identifying element of any individual and which includes the time elapsed since the day he/she was born, that is, that he/she acquires legal personality, and which runs until the day of his/her death, when his/her legal personality ceases.

[6] Decree-Law No. 47344, from 25-11-1966.

[7] Article 66 of the Portuguese Civil Code: "Personality is acquired at the moment of complete birth and with life," and art. 68°, "Personality ceases with death".

[8] Art. 7.° Law N° 7/2007, quoted, "The citizen card contains the following visible identification elements of its holder: a) Surnames; (b) proper name(s); (c) affiliation; (d) nationality; (e) *Date of birth*; (f) sex; (g) height; (h) Facial image; (i) signature; (j) civil identification number; (l) VAT identification number; (m) health services number; (n) Number of social security identification".

However, since human longevity is closely linked to the aging process and vulnerability to disease and death, the existence of a high percentage of elderly people in a population is an index of progress and development of the society in which it operates. As it is not possible to measure aging directly, there is a need to identify parameters that allow as reliable an evaluation as possible, designated as biological markers of the aging of the human organism.

Thus, the concept of biological age arises, associated with the knowledge of the changes that various organic and functional parameters undergo as time passes. However, this concept has limitations, including the selection of markers, since being organic substances suffer, like the developing organism, the influence of genetic and environmental factors.

6.2.2 Estimated Age

Thus, in the medico-legal context, as in other contexts, such as archaeological and clinical, the concept of estimated age appears. It is the evaluation of continuous processes of development of the individual from birth to maturity, assuming that this type of development occurs in all individuals regardless of the time elapsed. There is, therefore, an intimate relationship between the indicators of chronological age and biological age, but these are neither linear nor constant.

In the application of biological age to a normative question, it is important to choose the indicators for the estimation of age. Another crucial factor in the application of biological age has to do with the moment of life at which this estimate is made: in the developmental phase or in the aging phase. Finally, another key factor is its application, in this case in the forensic field, since it differs depending on whether it is a living individual or a corpse.

It is important to safeguard that in the estimation of medico-legal age, the concept that is intended to be estimated through biological age is chronological age—a normatively defined concept. It is not intended in this application, when requested, for example, in the context of the instructive phase of a process, to estimate age, to use the psychological assessment of age, since this does not translate the normative concept of chronological age. This may, at a later stage of the process, when in certain situations, namely in the living, and in undocumented individuals and minors, be used for contextualization of the child and/or adult. But, never to estimate the chronological age in the first phase of instruction, when it is necessary to respond in a quick and scientific way to the question without violating the assumption: the legal situation is the absence of individual identification; the forensic experts answer on civil identification related to age estimation, which does not exist.

6.3 Age Estimation Methods Related to This Group (Children and Adolescents)

6.3.1 Considerations on the Estimation of Age in the Living Individual, and in the Corpse

Age estimation appeals to different methods, depending on whether we are estimating the age of a corpse or a living individual.

In the living individual, within the scope of age estimation in cases of asylum seekers, undocumented, unaccompanied, and minors, performing the dental medical forensic examination, the underlying principles are the best interests of the child, the benefit of the doubt (presumption of minority), autonomy (informed consent), and the application of non-invasive methods, non-maleficence, beneficence and justice.[9] They are the principles underlying any medical Act [4].

The principle of the best interests of the child is deeply rooted in the European human rights and asylum legislation and the international legal framework. The benefit of the doubt is a key principle and safeguard in the field of age assessment since none of the current methods of age assessment are able to determine a specific age with certainty. The individual shall be considered and treated as a child throughout the forensic process for age assessment:

- If any of the methods applied during the age assessment obtain a result indicating childhood, the assessment shall stop there, and the lowest age of the range is to be taken as valid;
- If after the process has ended the results are still inconclusive, age assessment shall consider the lowest age of the range as valid.

The right to information starts prior to the examination of the individual for international protection, the child must receive all the relevant information in a language that the individual is able to understand. The informed consent refers to a free, voluntary, and informed decision.

The use of radiation to perform complementary radiological imaging diagnostic tests for age estimation is based on the principle of *ALARA* (as low as *reasonably achievable*), that is, using radiation as low as reasonably feasible. This is important for justice and to protect the children. We cannot protect an individual who is supposed to be a child as a true child if the means used for the estimation of age are not

[9] We recall that, regarding the relationship between the principle of autonomy and the principle of beneficence (and not non-maleficence) in medical bioethics present in the medico-legal examination, we can read Cristiana Palmela Pereira, Catarina Pereira Escobar, Jorge Costa Santos. "*Age Estimation of Unaccompanied Minors*: A Portuguese Overview". *Annals of Forensic Research and Analysis* in 2015; 2 (1):1012–1015. Those principles apply as long as the age estimation examination in forensic clinic is performed by a doctor/dentist, who is responsible for bioethical behavior. They do not apply to forensic professionals other than doctors/dentists. This is a reason that justifies only age estimation in living persons by doctors and dentists.

the most appropriate and accurate. The use of radiation is framed in the true interests of the child[10] [3].

There is a variability of methods, which are not used in the same way by all professionals, leading to considerable heterogeneity in the estimation of age in undocumented living individuals in Europe. In recent years, in certain Portuguese research institutions related to age estimation, they have been working on more equitable methods of application in order to promote objective 16 of the 17 Sustainable Development Goals proposed by the UN, Peace, Justice and Strong Institutions. In recent years, certain Portuguese research institutions involved in age estimation have been working on more equitable methods of application in order to promote Goal 16 ("Peace, Justice and Strong Institutions") of the United Nations Sustainable Development Goals (SDGs).[11]

As a reflection of the above, both international and European legal frameworks identify the following standards and safeguards necessary for age assessment:

Besides the lack of harmonization in the application of methods, there are methods which, because they are not accurate, should not be used.

In corpses, the age estimate respects the principles of the medico-legal examination itself, namely the ethics underlying an examination carried out on a corpse. It is fundamental in establishing the *postmortem* profile of corpses of unknown identity. In estimating the age parameter in a corpse of unknown identity there is the possibility of using invasive and destructive methodologies. These may be an alternative or complementary to the direct and indirect, but non-invasive and non-destructive methodologies used in living individuals. However, all methodologies that are chosen in the medico-legal examination of a corpse must be in accordance with the recommendations contained in the 2005/26 resolution on human rights and forensic sciences.[12]

[10] In 1959, more than 10 years after the Universal Declaration of Human Rights of 1948, the UN issued the Universal Declaration of the Rights of the Child, which enshrined at the international level the rights of the child. In 1989, the most important "Convention on the Rights of the Child" was approved, proclaimed by the General Assembly at the United Nations on 20 November, of obligatory compliance, where the child is considered a subject of law.

[11] United Nations. Sustainable Development Goal 16: Peace, Justice and Strong Institutions. In: The 17 Sustainable Development Goals (SDGs) of the 2030 Agenda for Sustainable Development. United Nations; 2015.

[12] Human Rights Resolution 2005/26: Human Rights and Forensic Science Document E/CN.4/RES/2005/26—"Noting that the practice of forensic science includes examinations and identification procedures of both dead and living persons, and underlines the importance of dignified handling of humans remains, including their proper management and disposal, as well as of for the needs of families."; "Also recommends that the Office of the High Commissioner encourage, as appropriate, the dissemination and use of the principles, best practices and referred manuals to in the present resolution and the promotion of forensic capacity-building, including training where necessary, particularly in countries without sufficient expertise in forensic science and related fields."

6.3.2 Methods Variability and Accuracy

The biological indicators, bone and tooth, are those that allow, among other macroscopic biological parameters, the best accuracy of the estimate of biological age framed within any medico-legal circumstance [5]. However, when comparing the two indicators at the level of precision, the teeth have a lower influence of genetic and environmental factors on their dental maturity, so they are more accurate.

At this point in the chapter, we introduce to the discussion other biological parameters used in the estimation of age in living individuals, which raise significant controversy between countries, especially in the examinations of age estimation of asylum seekers, as well as in the estimation of age by sexual maturity and physical development (somatic evaluation). Additionally, the estimation of age by psychological interview and age assessment interview is also discussed.

In fact, when we talk about the estimation of age, by age assessment interview and/or by psychological interview, we are talking about non-medical methods included in a methodology of estimating age by a holistic approach. This holistic approach is advocated by some countries as a preventive methodology for the child, minimizing the impact of true age estimation exclusively by medical methods [3].

As the author of this chapter, I give myself permission to be able to present several points of disagreement with this methodology, based on science and the norm. This view is also shared by many countries, notably the Nordic countries. When it comes to the holistic approach, we are being more intrusive and without obtaining the results sought, which are the purpose of the requested forensic examination. That is, the estimate of the person's age. In these cases of undocumented individuals claiming to be minors, the estimate of age must be as accurate as possible, as close as possible to the chronological age, because the chronological age of an individual is defined clearly in the civil code.

What we intend is to use a biological method that allows the biological age to be the most representative of the chronological age of this individual, through estimation. The assessment of psychological age and, what they call an age assessment interview, do not translate into reality the chronological age of the individual, but the psychological age, which falls within a parameter other than the normative. This evaluation will and should be employed. But at a later stage, for the social framework of the individual, whether he is a minor or not. It should not be used, in a normative sense of law enforcement, and for speedy realization.

Well, let's see.

This is a situation of duality. One should not use a radiographic method, because we are exposing the individual to radiation and, it is considered by some to be intrusive. But, if this method uses the principle of ALARA, and that in an age group it presents the most accurate results, and with this results, it is possible to produce a more reliable result for law enforcement; what is the reason not to use? But we can use a psychological assessment of age to estimate the age at a stage of the examination of an undocumented individual's asylum application, which does not respond to the normative question, that is, the chronological age (because we don't know this).

Is the principle of the best interests of the child, which is deeply rooted in European human rights legislation, not protected with a precise and standard-bound result? Is not the true child protected and the rights of the child respected, according to the result obtained? Even, because in reality the benefit of the doubt throughout the age assessment process is present. Beneficence and justice are bound. Non-maleficence is left without a figure, and becomes abstract, when we are protecting the true rights of children. Is it not maleficence, by presenting a bad result, to place an adult individual as a child? And, or a child as an adult?

Let's raise the discussion, with the introduction of the evaluation of sexual maturity and physical development, such as medical examinations. Is it an intrusive or invasive act?

Although they use these two concepts equally, it is important to clarify their differences in the classification of age estimation methods in a technical-scientific way. An invasive method is considered any method that requires a cutting instrument. It is a method that cuts the limit between internal and external boundaries. It is, for example, extracting a tooth. It is an invasive method. It is allowed in estimating the age of a body. An intrusive method is understood as evaluating the perception of this method by the individual. How this affects the way of being of each one.

After this previous discussion on the possible biological indicators, we will keep the present chapter linked to the two macroscopic biological indicators that are considered to be more accurate: bones and teeth.

Thus, age estimation methods can be divided into bone methods and dental methods for this group of age discussed in this chapter.

For bones and teeth, the methods can be applied to sub-adults and adults, depending on the age group for which they are intended. The methods may be dependent on sex and population affinity. They may be influenced by genetic and environmental factors.

Dental methods can be divided into direct methods and indirect methods. The direct ones include, for example, the estimation of age by observing the clinical characteristics of the oral cavity. The indirect ones use imaging tests, particularly radiographic ones, to observe certain characteristics to estimate age. Other classification of dental methods is the classification into invasive and non-invasive methods. Noninvasive methods include the previous examples. The invasive method is for example the extraction of the tooth to estimate the age of an unknown corpse. In the classification of invasive methods, we can divide them into destructive and non-destructive methods. Extraction of the tooth from the alveolus is an invasive and non-destructive method. If the tooth is cut, it is already an invasive and destructive method.

All dental methods used in most forensic situations are called morphological methods because they evaluate or quantify dental morphological characteristics to estimate dental age. They can be macroscopic methods and microscopic methods. According to how we observe and/or quantify the morphology: with the naked eye or with a microscope with staining. There are also chemical methods.

The choice of dental methods for age estimation will depend on the age group. In the sub-adult age group, we have several age groups: newborn, child, adolescence and late adolescence. This applies to living individuals or corpses. For each dental method there are several methodologies.

Evaluating the biological evidence for forensic application, in this particular case, evaluating the tooth for the medico-legal age estimation through a certain methodology, we evaluate [5]:

- Reliability: The forensic method must demonstrate coherent results in order to draw the desired conclusions.
- Repeatability: The ability to obtain the same results and conclusions from the same method and under the same conditions. It refers to the reliability of measurements or conclusions by a particular examiner under the same conditions.
- Reproducibility: This is the other form of reliability of measurements or conclusions by different examiners under the same conditions.
- Objectivity: This is evaluated by the sensitivity, specificity, independence, and size of the study population.
- Precision: This is the degree of agreement between the measured values obtained by repeated measurements on the same or similar objects, under specific conditions; it is the variability of the results in a series of measurements.
- Accuracy: This is the degree of agreement between a measured value and the generally accepted value based on a standard reference. It is the quality or state of being correct or precise.

Thus, when we evaluate the methodologies that exist for the estimation of age, we evaluate the objectivity of the method (rational and impersonal), reliability (consistent and precise, that is, inter-examiner reliability or reproducibility) and repeatability (intra-examiner reliability) [6].

According to Schmeling et al. 2008, for an age assessment method used as reference material to be accurate, it must fulfill certain requirements: adequate sample size, verified ages of test persons, uniform age distribution, separation by gender, details on date of examination, clear definition of characteristics studied, exact description of methodology, details on reference population relative to genetic-geographic origin, socioeconomic status, state of health and details of group size, mean or median value and a measure of variation for each characteristic studied [4].

Faced with a variability of methods and with different accuracies, several countries are trying to harmonize some methods for age estimation. One of the international governmental bodies that evaluate the standardization of the various areas of knowledge for application in the forensic sciences is the OSAC administered by the NIST in the United States of America. One of the scientific areas for forensic sciences is forensic odontology. This working group has the normalization of age estimation by dental assessment. Since July 2020 the document *ADA TR 1077* for *Human Age Assessment by Dental Analysis*[13, 14] is a technical report [2].[15]

[13] OSAC-NIST, the Organization of Scientific Area Committees for Forensic Science by the National Institute of Standards and Technology. Searchable at: https://www.nist.gov/topics/organization-scientific-area-committees-forensic-science

[14] Dentistry is one of the 25 subcommittees of OSAC. Searchable at: https://www.nist.gov/topics/organization-scientific-area-committees-forensic-science/odontology-subcommittee

[15] In the WG14.3 working group for this document, the University of Lisbon, namely the Faculty of Dental Medicine, participated as an observer by Professor Cristiana Palmela Pereira.

Another example to evaluate the scientific evidence of the methods for estimating age through biological parameters was the one carried out by the Norwegian government on the two biological parameters, teeth, and bones. For the teeth, the government asked to perform a systematic review of Demirjian's method. They established the question that had to be answered and systematically and objectively sought all the information, through systematic review. It was then evaluated by a group of experts in order to summarize the evidence obtained from this systematic review [7].[16]

They concluded that the studies that evaluated and used the Demirjian methodology did not present reliable results when they distributed the chronological age by the Demirjian stages from A to H in the third molar. Based on the variability of methods and small samples, it is recommend for age estimation by dental assessment for each individual, an age range and the accuracy rate of the method should be calculated; this means that it should be indicated how often the chronological age falls within the estimated age range.[17]

The other method on which the Norwegian government requested a systematic review was the bone atlas of Greulich and Pyle and its correlation with chronological age. After the systematic review in 2017 they concluded that there continues to be a good correlation between the biological bone age estimated by the Greulich and Pyle atlas in current populations. However, the individual variation of development within each population and the heterogeneity between studies is very significant [7].[18, 19]

In 2020, a new document was proposed on the Designation System for Tooth Developmental Stages (ISO/NP 5365). The scope of this document is to provide a single unified coding system and vocabulary to allow for the unambiguous assessment of dental age development stages and interoperability between methods. Also, it will allow for the easy comparison of the data tables of numerous methods of age assessment by dental means currently used. This means that the multiple scoring systems currently combined with multiple methods using this scoring system will be substituted by one scoring system.

---

[16] Demirjian A, Goldstein H, Tanner JM. A New System of Dental Age Assessment. Wayne State University Press [Internet]. 1973; 45:211–27. Available from: https://www.jstor.org/stable/4145986

[17] Report carried out in 2017 and published by the institute the Norwegian Public Health Policy. Searchable at https://www.fhi.no/en/publ/2017/demirjians-utviklingsstadier-pa-visdomstenner-for-estimering-av-kronologisk/

[18] William Walter Greulich, S. Idell Pyle. *Radiographic Atlas of Skeletal Development of the Hand and Wrist*. first Edition, Palo Alto, California: Stanford University Press 1959.

[19] Report carried out in 2017 and published by the institute the Norwegian Public Health Policy. Searchable at https://www.fhi.no/en/publ/2017/samsvar-mellom-kronologisk-alder-og-skjelettalder-basert-pa-greulich-og-pyl/

6.3.3 Bone Methods and Dental Methods (Combined Methods)

This part of the chapter aims at the very brief description of the various methods of age estimation using bone and tooth as a biological marker for age assessment in children and adolescents. It is not intended to provide an exhaustive explanation of the methods themselves which should be approached from a more specialized and more advanced perspective, in particular in more technical chapters for the field. However, when a forensic expert, mainly forensic odontologist, performs dental age assessment in this period of time, they use complementary bone age assessment. The goal of this chapter is to privilege the focus on dental methods (dental development, dental eruption, morphological and chemical methods) and their interrelation with the various stages of age; and whether it is a living individual and/or a corpse.

As for bone methods, it is important to mention, among other aspects, the relevance of the development of the hand and wrist, which are already used as a competence for dentists in the evaluation of growth for clinical purposes, namely at the orthodontic level through imaging examinations. Finally, in a necessarily brief way some aspects of the various methods will be addressed: direct, indirect, invasive, and destructive.

6.3.3.1 Bone Methods Used in Combination with Dental Methods

Ossification Center

Left Hand and Wrist Ossification Parameters by Radiographs

The assessment of bone age can be performed by the primary ossification centers and by the fusion of the epiphyses—the union of the secondary ossification centers to the primary centers. The estimation of bone age by fusion of epiphyses is a methodology that applies morphological and macroscopic characteristics and is applied, for example, to the hand and left wrist. This methodology is applied to non-adult individuals and is a method with great application in living individuals. There are several methods that use this methodology. They are indirect methods because they require radiographic imaging. One of these methods is a method still used at present and is a standard reference at an international level: the Greulich and Pyle method of 1959 [8]. The authors drew an atlas with photographs of radiographs of skeletal development of the hand and left wrist for males (up to 19 years) and females (up to 18 years). This atlas was built in 1959 based on a population of children from Ohio between 1930 and 1940. They selected 100 radiographs of different individuals with the same chronological age. They ordered the radiographs according to the state of skeletal development from the least developed to the most developed. They chose an X-ray that, in their opinion, was the most representative of the central tendency of each chronological age.

The radiography chosen by each age group was not always the closest to the midpoint of the 100 radiographs. The age assigned to each photograph in the atlas is called skeletal age or bone age and is broken down by sex: male up to 19 years and female up to 18 years [8].

There are reference studies that report that a high level of medical and economic development accelerates ossification rates, whereas a low modernization level delays ossification. They conclude that if radiological age diagnostic uses the Greulich-Pyle standards for persons originating from a country with a comparatively low modernization status, the age of that person will be underestimated. According to Schmeling (2008) when performing age estimations, the forensic expert conclusion should therefore draw attention to the issue of different modernization levels [4].

The other method that uses the same morphological macroscopic methodology of the development and fusion of the epiphyses in the left hand and wrist is the Tanner and Whitehouse method. The estimate of bone age is made in the same way as the previous method; however, the 20 bones of the zone are individually classified into eight or nine stages, then assigned one degree per bone, the various degrees are added,[20] and the corresponding bone age is obtained by sex [9].

Clavicular Ossification Classification by Radiographs

According to the recommendations of the Study Group on Forensic Age Diagnostics (AGFAD) the bone development age assessment is important to be performed with dental development age assessment [4, 10]. If the skeletal development of the hand is completed, an additional examination of the clavicles should be carried out. The methods should be used together to increase the diagnostic accuracy and to improve the identification of age-relevant for the justice. Schmeling et al. in 2004 developed a five-stage classification system for characterization of clavicular ossification (Fig. 6.1) [11]:

- Stage 1: Non-ossified ossification center.
- Stage 2: Ossified ossification center with non-ossified epiphyseal cartilage.
- Stage 3: Partially ossified epiphyseal cartilage.
- Stage 4: Fully ossified epiphyseal cartilage with discernible epiphyseal line.
- Stage 5: Non-discernible epiphyseal line.

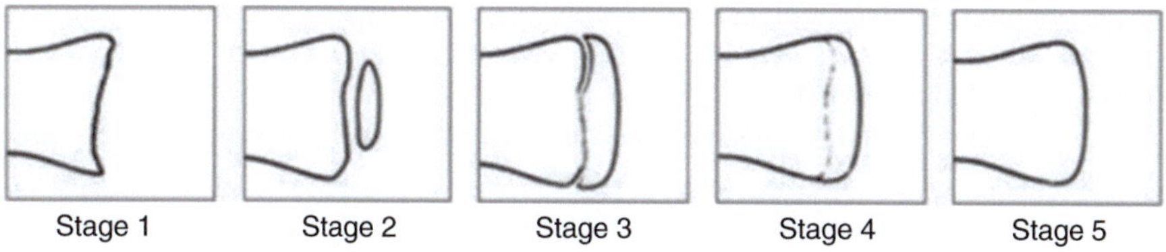

Fig. 6.1 Main stages of clavicle ossification. Stage 1: non-ossified epiphysis; stage 2: isolated ossified epiphysis; stage 3: partial bony fusion between epiphysis and metaphysis; stage 4: complete bony fusion between epiphysis and metaphysis with definable epiphyseal scar; Stage 5: complete bony fusion between epiphysis and metaphysis without visible epiphyseal scar

[20] Tanner JM, Whitehouse RH, Healy MJR. *A New System for Estimating Skeletal Maturity from the Hand and Wrist, with Standards Derived from a Study of 2600 Healthy British Children.* Paris: International Centre de l'Enfance, 1962.

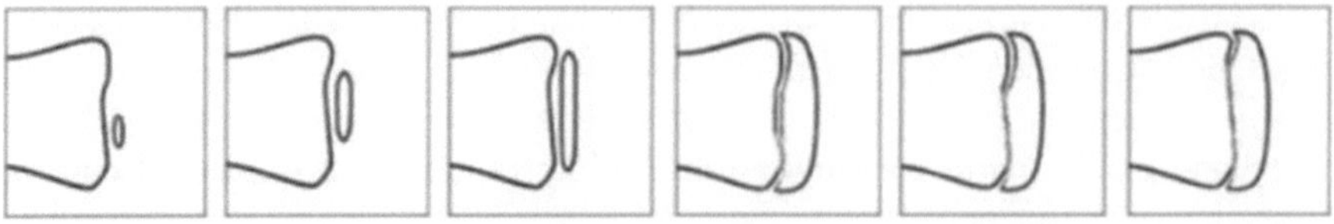

Fig. 6.2 Substages of clavicle ossification. Stage 2a: the length of ossified epiphysis is maximally one-third the metaphysis width; stage 2b: the epiphysis length is between one-third and two-thirds [maximum] the metaphysis width; stage 2c: the epiphysis length is more than two-thirds the metaphysis width; stage 3a: a maximum of one-third of the epiphyseal plate is ossified; stage 3b: between one-third and two-thirds [maximum] of the epiphyseal plate is ossified; stage 3c: more than two-thirds of the epiphyseal plate is ossified

According to Schmeling (2010) the stages 2 and 3 can each be divided into three substages (a, b and c). The sub-classification stages were defined as follows (Fig. 6.2) [12]:

Stage 2a: The lengthwise epiphyseal measurement is one third or less compared to the widthwise measurement of the metaphyseal ending.

Stage 2b: The lengthwise epiphyseal measurement is over one third until two thirds compared to the widthwise measurement of the metaphyseal ending.

Stage 2c: The lengthwise epiphyseal measurement is over two thirds compared to the widthwise measurement of the metaphyseal ending.

Stage 3a: The epiphyseal-metaphyseal fusion completes one third or less of the former gap between epiphysis and metaphysis.

Stage 3b: The epiphyseal-metaphyseal fusion completes over one third until two thirds of the former gap between epiphysis and metaphysis.

Stage 3c: The epiphyseal-metaphyseal fusion completes over two thirds of the former gap between epiphysis and metaphysis.

According to the authors, stage 3c indicates a minimum age of 19 years, while stage 4 indicates a minimum age of 21 years.

Of the currently available imaging methods for determining the ossification stage of the medial clavicular epiphysis, thin-slice CT is the method of choice.

6.3.3.2 Dental Methods

The assessment of dental age must be considered in two different periods: until 23 years of age and after 23 years of age, this means, in a period of sub-adult age (including childhood and adolescent) and on the adulthood [13].

The second division we must consider is the type of forensic cases: in living individuals and/or in corpses. In corpus as an integral part of the medico-legal examination of identification, as part of the reconstructive phase, namely to draw the *post-mortem* profile of the cadaver. We can't omit that the dental methodologies that are chosen and the dental methods depend on this division.

Atlas of Dental Development, Scoring Systems, and Other Dental Age Assessment Methods

The most commonly used dental methodology in a sub-adult (child and adolescent) population in living individuals, with application in forensic examinations of cadavers, is a macroscopic and indirect radiographic morphological methodology (or, with other imaging examination) based on dental development. There are several methods including several atlas of dental development applying to imaging techniques.

Dental development, formation and mineralization of the dental tissues, begins at the most occlusal and incisal part of each tooth and continues until each root tip is fully formed. At the same time with tooth formation is the movement of the forming tooth through the alveolar bone toward the surface of bone and the overlying gingival tissues into the oral cavity. This movement, normally continuing to the level of occlusion with teeth in the opposing jaw. Dental development begins before birth and can continue for until 23 years old [14].

There are several scoring systems based on the tooth development stages. They are various degrees in the development of human teeth that represent specific points of mineralization discernible through a variety of diagnostic imaging exams.

Different dental age assessment techniques use different tooth development scoring systems. Currently, there is no consensus on what staging system is better. Dental development staging systems are method dependent, and it is recommended that they be used based on the appropriate reference study.

The selection of dental age assessment methods must take into account the independent variables such as sex, population affinity and environmental and genetic factors (although these have less influence on dental age assessment than on the bone age assessment) [4].

Environmental factors are verified in the forensic expert examination of the living individuals for age estimation at the time of the anamnesis (collection of the biographical information of the individual), such as nutrition, general health status and oral health, medications any other environmental or cultural factors that may have affected skeletal, oral, or dental development or contributes to post-development skeletal, oral, or dental changes [4].

Atlas-based dental age assessment methods utilize graphic and diagrammatic representations of the morphology of developing tooth structures. Some include the associated emergence patterns. Those ones that use emergence through alveolar bone should be used where indicated over those techniques that are dependent on tooth emergence through soft tissues. Most, but not all, atlas techniques are non-sex specific and have a limited number of population-specific data sets resulting in a higher degree of variability, particularly in mid-childhood through adolescence. Atlas methodologies are often based on mixed population and ethnic data.

For the purpose of forensic dental age assessments, the infant/child dental age interval has been defined as begins at birth, includes the presence of the developing, developed and resorbing primary dentition as well as the initial development of the permanent dentition. This interval includes the early period of mixed primary and permanent dentitions and ends when the last primary tooth is exfoliated normally.

However, there are persons that retained atypically the primary teeth for various reasons. The dental age assessment for this period of time uses techniques based on radiographic evaluation (normally, but can be other imaging examinations such as CBCT, Dental Scan or CT) to stage the degree of dental morphologic development of the primary or permanent dentition.

The second definition important for this chapter is adolescent dental age interval. This interval has been defined as the interval in human dental development that begins after all primary teeth are normally shed, and the permanent teeth are developing or developed. The adolescent interval ends when all permanent teeth present are fully developed. The adolescent dental age assessment techniques utilize radiographic evaluation (or other imageology images) to stage the degree of dental development toward the latter half of dental morphologic maturation. Although the third molar exhibits the highest degree of morphologic developmental variability, it remains extremely useful in the assessment of age [15].

The Schour and Massler atlas[21] describe 21 chronological stages corresponding to dental development, from 5 months in-utero to 21 years of age (Fig. 6.3). It has an additional stage, which would be the 22nd and corresponds to the age of 35 years. However, there is no change in relation to stage of 21 years. This atlas was designed in 1941, and in 1944 a reprint was made with the permission of the ADA.[22] This method is one of the oldest and was designed to be a guide for dentists in clinical practice. It is used in the field of dental anthropology in an archaeological way, in the version of Ubelaker's 1989,[22] published by Buikstra and Ubelaker in 1994 (Fig. 6.4) [15].[23]

The Schour and Massler atlas was designed based on a very small sample of 25 individuals with known chronological ages. It is applied to both sexes. The drawings are outlines of dental development and eruption relative to the gingival line and the corresponding age. Despite having 21 stages of development there is omission of several categories where dental development is very variable, between 12 and 15 years of age [15].

The stages are consecutive until the age of 12 and then there is only the category at 15 years of age. On the other hand, it does not have stages only for the third molar, which is the only tooth available to assess certain legal ages.

A more recent atlas is the London Atlas from AlQahtani from 2010 [16]. This atlas was developed as a comprehensive, evidence-based atlas covers from the chronological age of 28 weeks[24] in utero to 23 years of age. The atlas uses the Moorrees stage scoring from Moorrees, Fanning, and Hunt method from 1963 (Fig. 6.5) [17] The atlas was designed for age prediction, is tooth specific and illustrates tooth development and eruption for 31 age categories. It was built with a

---

[21] Schour I, Massler M. Development of human dentition. *J Am Dent Assoc* 1941; 20:379–427.

[22] American Dental Association.

[23] Buikstra, J. E., & Ubelaker, D. H. (1994). Standards for data collection from human skeletal remains. Fayateville, AR: Arkansas Archaeological Survey Research. Series No. 44.

[24] AlQahtani, S.J., Hector, M.P., Liversidge, H.M., 2010. Brief communication: the London Atlas of Human Tooth Development and eruption. Am. J. Phys. Anthropol. 142, 481–490.

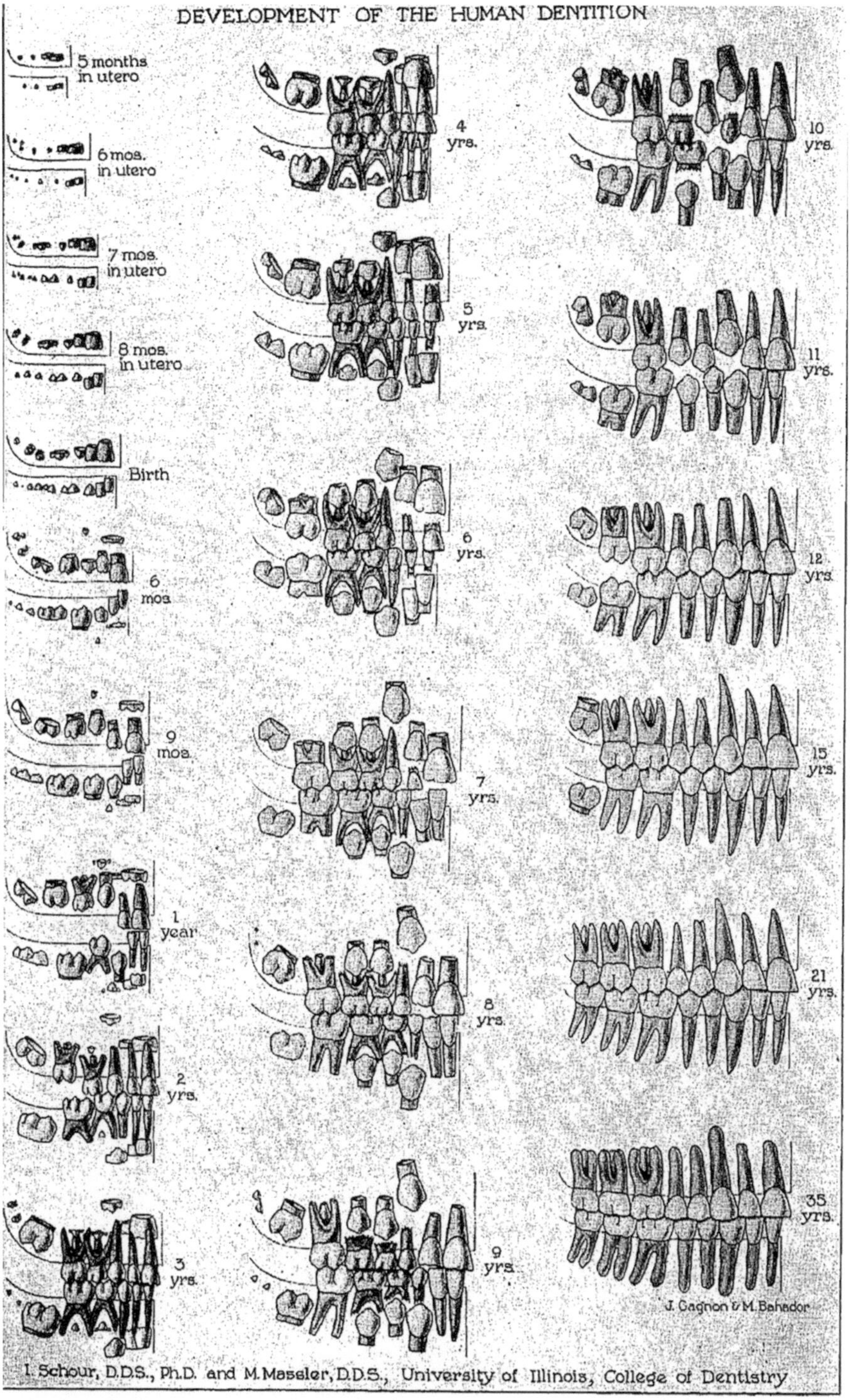

Fig. 6.3 Schour and Massler Atlas: The development of the human dentition. Bureau of Public Relations, 1944

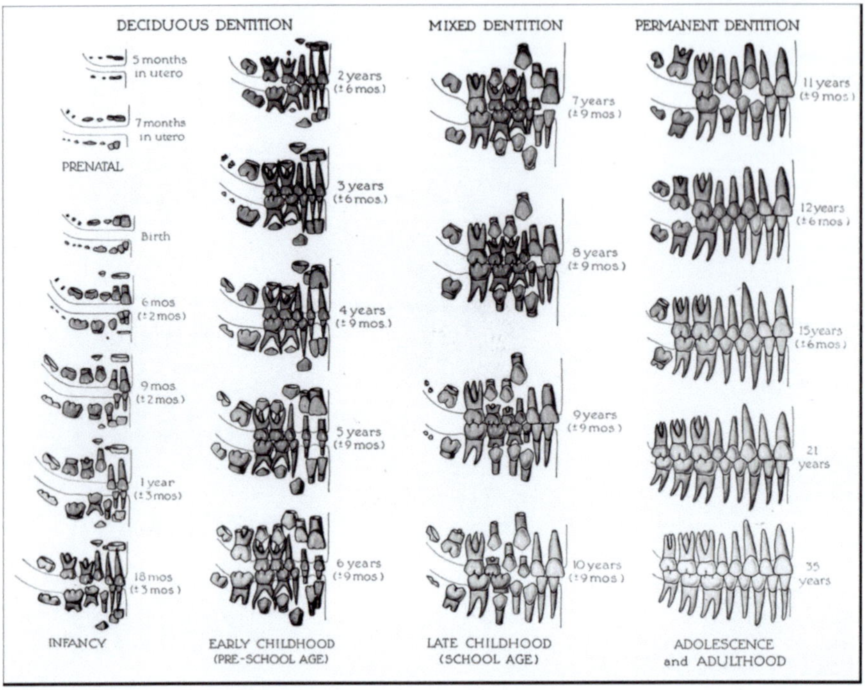

Fig. 6.4 Ubelaker's 1989 Dental Aging Chart from Human Skeletal Remains Reprinted in Buikstra and Ubelaker 1994

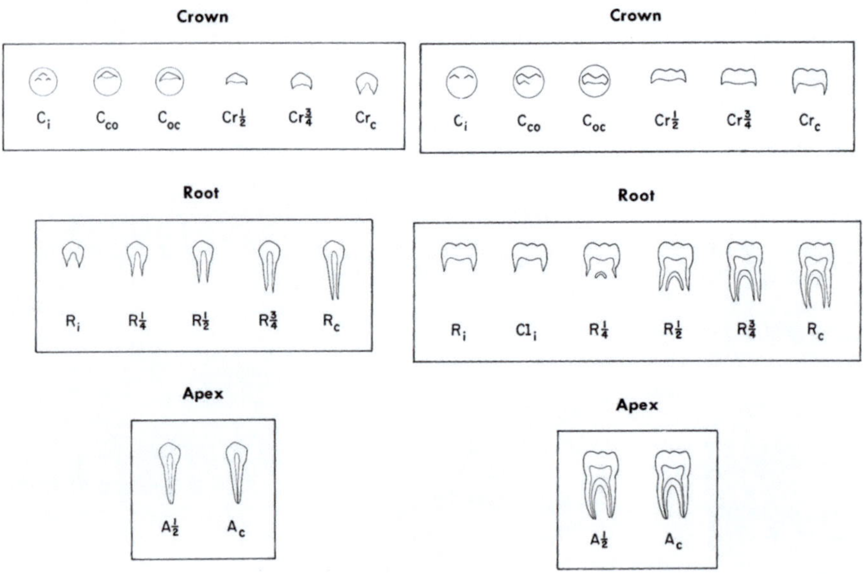

Fig. 6.5 Moorrees, Fanning and Hunt Scoring system (1963) for single root and multiroot

European and Bangladeshi population, totaling 704 panoramic radiographs. This atlas is applied on the right side and without sex discrimination. It covers all stages of dental development from 1 year to 23 years. Each drawing is the median tooth development and eruption stage for the age category but median, minimum, and maximum tooth stage and eruption level for each age category are tabulated. The main advantage of this atlas is the presence of scoring stages for the third molar. The other advantage is the drawing from the atlas refers to the eruption line relative to alveolar bone.

In 1973, Demirjian applied to seven teeth on the left side of the jaw, in which each tooth is classified into eight stages (from A to H). It is a method to be applied in the age group between 3 and 17 years [18]. This scoring system for evaluation of dental maturity only applies the concept of dental development without the concept of eruption. There are stages which must be three points which will have to be fulfilled in order to be classified as such and relate to the developmental of dental tissues. After each tooth is classified in a stage, it is converted into a table discriminated by sex to a grade. The grades of the seven teeth are added together and we obtain a degree of dental maturity that is translated into a dental age with the indication of the percentile and classified by sex.

The Haavikko method from 1970 (Fig. 6.6) is applied to the age group from 2 to 13 years with the classification in 12 stages, 6 for the crown and 6 for the root. It was a modification of Gleiser and Hunt's 1955 method. It is a method with sex discrimination. It is also applied to the third molar, with application to a higher age group, up to 23 years of age [19].[25]

Speaking about the third molar we have the Harris and Nortje method since 1984 (Fig. 6.7).[26] It does not have sex discrimination and can be applied to an age group above 14 years, with five stages (Table 6.1). For evaluation dental development of the third molar there are numerous methods. Which vary according to the scoring stages, from 4 to 15 stages. For instance, Kullman's 1992 method classifies the dental development of the third molar into seven stages and discriminates by sex. On the other hand, Mincer's 1993 method classifies the third molar into eight stages, by "race" [20, 21].[27, 28]

The above methods use tooth development as a macroscopic morphological criterion evaluated by indirect imaging, radiographic, and those results can be presented as quantitative results (measurements).

[25] Haavikko, K.: Tooth Formation Age Estimated on a Few Selected Teeth. A Simple Method for Clinical Use. Proc. Finn. Dent. Soc. 70 (1970): 15–19.

[26] M.J. Harris, C.J. Nortje, The mesial root of the third mandibular molar: a possible indicator of age, J. Forensic Odonto-Stomatol. 2 (1984) 39–43.

[27] Kullman L, Johanson G, Akesson L. Root development of the lower third molar and its relation to chronological age. Swed Dent J. 1992; 16:161–7.

[28] Other methods of assessing the stages of third molars: Gustafson and Koch 1974 with four stages; from Harris and Mckee 1990 with five stages; from Nolla 1960s with ten stages; from Moorrees of 1963 with 14 stages in the same way as the Andersen method of 1976; and the method of Gleiser and Hunt of 1955 with 15 stages.

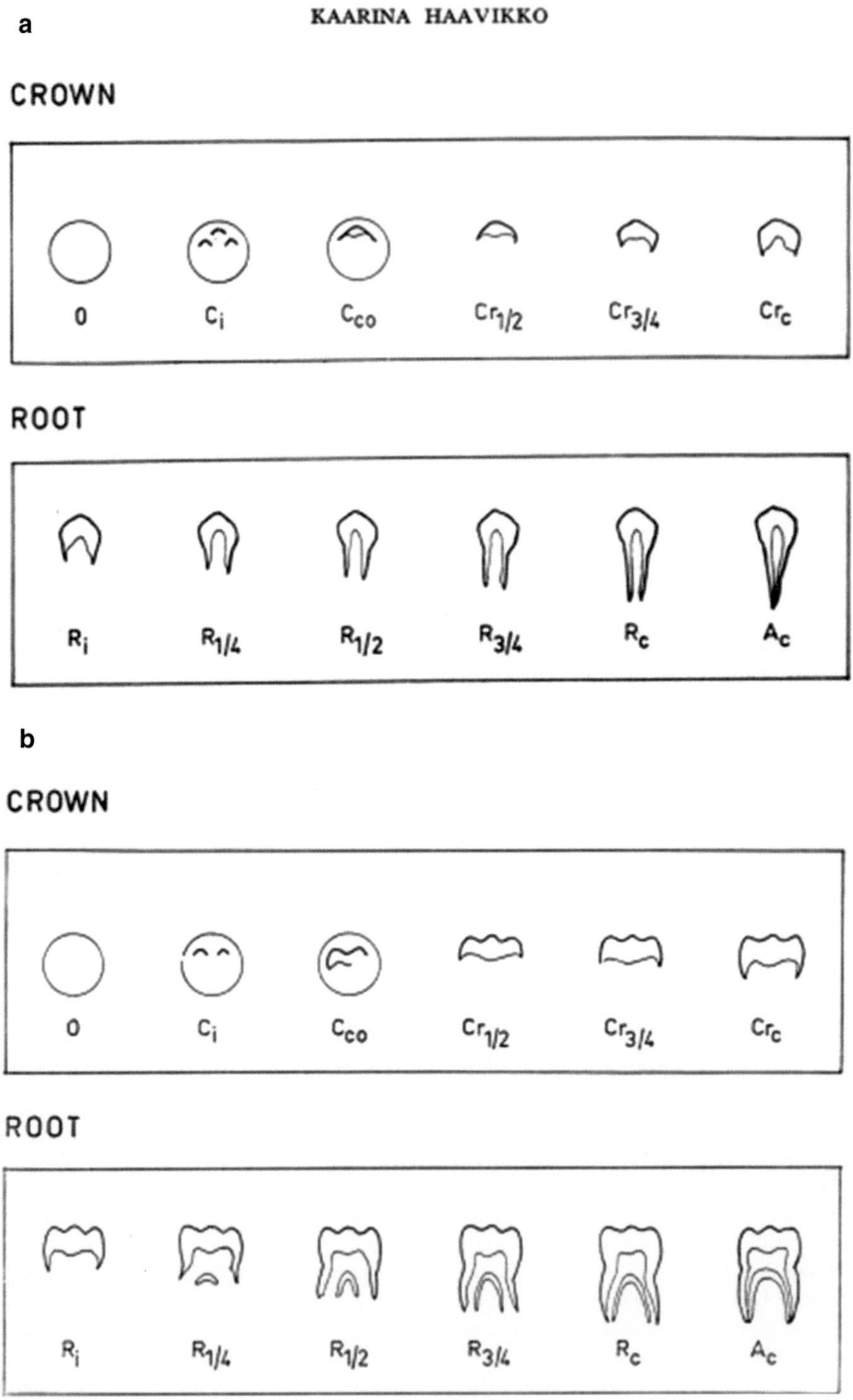

Fig. 6.6 Haavikko scoring system, 1970 for single root and multiroot

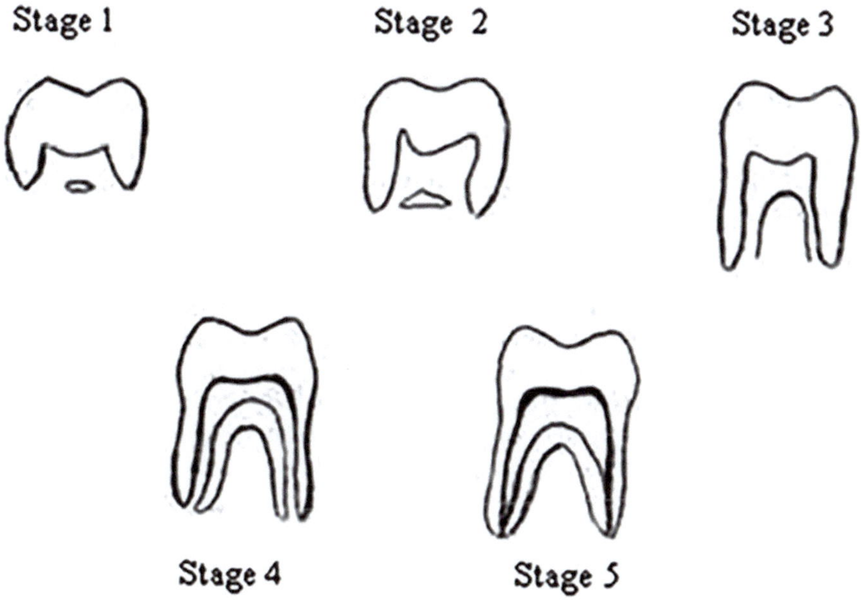

Fig. 6.7 Scoring system from Harris and Nortjé, 1984: Five stages of lower third molar root development

Table 6.1 Dental age according to the Scoring system from Harris and Nortjè 1984

Stage	Dental age
1	15,8 ± 1,4 years
2	17,2 ± 1,2 years
3	17,8 ± 1,2 years
4	18,5 ± 1,1 years
5	19,2 ± 1,2 years

One of the methods that applies a quantitative approach is the Cameriere method of 2006. It is applied to the seven mandibular teeth on the left side, excludes the third molar. Where a regression formula with discrimination by sex (European Cameriere formula) is fill with the ration given by the sum of the distances from the inner sides of the open apices and the height of the developing seven teeth [22]. The same type of method is used exclusively for a single tooth—in this case for the third molar and for the second molar from the left side. These are respectively named the third molar maturity index[29] (I3M) and second molar maturity index (I_{2M}) [23–25].[30]

[29] Cameriere R, Ferrante L, Cingolani M. Age estimation in children by measurement of open apices in teeth. *Int J Legal Med.* 2006;120 (1):49–52.

[30] The indexes were designed by Camerieri in 2008 and establish the relationship between age and maturity of second and third molars, respectively with the measurements of the openings of the apices. The I_{3M} Establishes the bridge of cut to 18 years of age. The I2M establishes the bridge of cut for 14 and 16 years of age. A new concept of *legal acts thresholds*—legal age limit.

Final Considerations and Medico-Legal Application

When estimating age using dental methods, the assessment of dental maturity is crucial. This method should be applied to individuals up to 23 years of age or older, and used in forensic cases involving living individuals or in cases of identification from corpses. Different methodologist exists. However, in examining living individuals, the most accurate methods for assessing dental age are primarily indirect radiographic methods. The most appropriate methodology should be applied to each specific forensic case, with results supported by the best available evidence.

The medical forensic examination performed for accessing the age estimation in child and adolescent consists first in the explanation of the forensic medical examination. The child or adolescent presents himself with a legal guardian, and, if necessary, a translator. The child/adolescent is asked if he/she opposes the clinical examination. A question arises about the validity of who gives the authorization for the exam, even in the presence of a minor with a legal guardian. However, it is assumed that the guardian is the legal guardian.

I present you the following situation for reflection: one situation a 6-year-old child who presents himself with his mother for a dental appointment, for example for a diagnosis for possible orthodontic treatment, and the second situation a 6-year-old child who presents himself with the legal guardian for a forensic clinical examination to perform the diagnosis of age. In the first situation, the mother is responsible for the informed consent of the dental treatment of the minor. However, the child in the dental chair will not be collaborator with the dental treatment, if the dental professionals did not explain the dental medical steps he will go through and what they are for. In fact, if a child in dental treatment does not authorize the respective treatment, he will not open his mouth.

The dental medical procedures described are probably like those performed in the medical forensic examination for age estimation. For the orthodontic diagnosis and orthodontic treatment plan, the dental medical examination consists of clinical observation of the patient, extraoral and intraoral photographs, study of biological age through radiographic examinations including radiography of the hand and left wrist, panoramic radiography, and the orthodontic study itself through radiographic examinations such as cephalometric.

In the second situation, the child has an appointed legal guardian who is responsible for him/her. The guardian is responsible for defending the best interests of the child, in this case, the performance of the medico-legal examination for the estimation of age. However, if we do not explain what will be performed during the medico-legal examination and the reason for this examination, we may be faced with a situation in which the child is not cooperative with the examination. This forensic clinical situation is the same as the first one described. The medical acts are the same: anamnesis, intraoral clinical examination, extraoral and intraoral photographs, and study of radiographic examinations.

In the clinical interview we often come across circumstances that may affect the age estimation. Including pathologies, nutritional deficiencies, medications, and congenital changes. Also, during the clinical interview, they often inform the number of siblings and their ages, the schooling they attended where they lived before, environmental factors and cultural factors that are important for age estimation accuracy. It is performed extraoral photographs of the face and intraoral photographs of intraoral status. It is performing a clinical observation with registration of several evidence. Such as the occlusion, oral hygiene, dental pathology, and dental treatments. The complementary diagnostic imaging tests requested in the scope of the examination are studied and it is verified if these belong to the examinee, for the integrity of the chain of custody.

To summarize, the forensic examination of forensic dentistry includes the clinical history (anamnesis), the clinical examination with overall estimation of dental age, and the radiographic examination with estimation of dental age. This should be carried out by methods according to the age group. In the sub-adult age group, the methodology of dental development is used (at least with the application of three different methods). The chosen methods shall be justified. The forensic report shall include the oral status of the individual, specific features of teeth according to the degree of attrition, the occlusion, the colour of the teeth, periodontal condition, dental hygiene status, dental pathology, and a minimum age, estimated age plus a measure of its uncertainty and answer to the request in the age estimation assignment.

There are several ideas and systems for controlling the quality of dental age assessment, as we have already listed some of them at the beginning of this chapter.

Regarding this quality control, IOFOS, in 2018, reviewed all existing recommendations since 2005 in all fields of forensic odontology intervention, except for bite marks [26]. The recommendations of 2018 have become more flexible due to the greater variability of methods that can be chosen for each methodology according to legal age limits.[31] However, the fact that these recommendations no longer have mandatory steps, due to the variability of methods, the choice of the method itself should consider the population, the error of the study if it is acceptable, sex among many other factors. There are essential parameters in the choice of method for a given methodology, such as the population sample used in the study of a given method, such as its size, the distribution of means of age, the sex of the reference sample; the reproducibility of the method, the scientific evaluation of the statistics presented in this method and the validation of the results. Another recommendation of IOFOS concerns the report's conclusions: include the minimum age, the estimated age and the degree of probability.

According to the Schmeling and the Study Group on Forensic Age Diagnostics (AGFAD) for age assessment, reference studies are used in which these defined developmental stages have been correlated with both the sex and the known age of the examined persons from a reference population [4, 27]. The final age assessment results of dental examination, radiological evaluation of teeth, radiological evaluation of the hand, and where appropriate, radiological evaluation of the clavicles to reach a final age estimation [28, 29]. The age-relevant variations resulting from the

[31] IOFOS (International Organization of Forensic Odonto-Stomatology) is a society equated with the American Board of Forensic Odontology (ABFO) when choosing recommendations. At present, ABFO presents recommendations more closely linked to American Dental Association (ADA) documents.

application of the reference studies for the examined person—due for instance to differences in ethnicity, socio-economic status, and possibly due to accelerated development or developmental disorder—must be discussed in the forensic report [30–39]. This forensic report should also include any effects that these parameters might have on the estimated age, and if possible, a quantitative assessment of any such effect should be given.

Depending on the issue to be addressed in the forensic evaluation, the age assessment report should indicate the most likely age and/or the minimum age of the young person examined and comment on the plausibility of the reported age. If at least one of the studied developmental characteristics (skeletal maturity, dental development) is not mature, the most likely age of the assessed person can be reported. This is determined based on the combined individual findings and a critical discussion of the specific case. If the most likely age is above the legally relevant age threshold, it is probable that the age limit has been exceeded. The report should assure age-related parameters are addressed beneficially for the affected person to give them the legal benefit of the doubt. In the case that the legally relevant age limit is surpassed with the highest standard of proof ("with probability bordering on certainty"), the minimum-age concept is applied. The minimum age is derived from the age minimum of the reference study for the determined characteristic value; this is the age of the youngest person in the reference population who had the ascertained characteristic value. If several characteristics were examined, the highest established minimum age shall prevail. The application of the minimum-age concept ensures that the forensic age of the assessed person is never overestimated but instead is almost always less than the actual age. If the determined minimum age lies over the legally relevant age limit, that age has been surpassed with probability bordering on certainty. If the determined minimum age lies over the age provided by the young person being examined, the given age can be virtually ruled out. If the given age is over the determined minimum age, the given age mentioned is compatible with the reported findings.

6.4 The Importance of Dental Age Assessment Research in the Development of More Accurate Methods for Age Estimation

The chapter concludes with a description of the importance of forensic odontology research in this field—the search for more accurate dental methods that allow greater reliability and comparability of results. This will probably be one of the areas in which scientific research in forensic odontology can produce results with high impact and applicability. Nowadays, the field of dental age assessment has enormous number of scientific publications.

Almost all scientific studies carried out in dental age assessment have as exclusion criteria for the population sample: presence of systemic pathologies. Based on these studies as references for dental age assessment examinations and in the presence of a child with systemic pathologies on the forensic examination, how can we present the results of dental age assessment? To answer this question, a study was conducted in which the method for estimating age in a sub-adult Portuguese population—already validated—was conducted with a population with systemic pathologies, with and without repercussion on dental development.[32]

In 2015, a text was published related to age estimation in 82 forensic cases of undocumented and unaccompanied children between 2009 and 2013 in Portugal. In this article was reported the absence of international consensus in the performance of these forensic examinations and the methods used to estimate age.[33] This lack of international consensus is explained in the results presented in the EASO document in the last edition of 2018.[34] The results were based on the questionnaire about the methods used to estimate age sent to 30 countries, of which 27 countries responded. It is conclusive in this document there is no consensus on how to estimate age. However, efforts have been done namely in the field of forensic odontology research [3].

The last document published related to age assessment in Europe was in December 2022 by the European Council on Refugees and Exiles and conclude "the procedures of age assessment in Europe fail to comply with the applicable legal standards in multiple ways" [3].

To conclude, the emerging direction in dental and bone age assessment research is the integration of Artificial Intelligence (AI), particularly machine learning (ML) and deep learning (DL) methodologies. These data-driven paradigms extend far beyond conventional convolutional neural networks (CNNs), encompassing hybrid and multimodal architectures capable of extracting complex morphological and radiodensity patterns from dental and skeletal imaging data. The remarkable progress in algorithmic optimization, data standardisation, and computational performance over the past decade has enabled AI systems to achieve reproducible and objective estimations of developmental stages. However, to ensure scientific robustness, reproducibility, and forensic admissibility, there is an urgent need for the establishment of validated reference standards and methodological criteria governing dataset quality, annotation protocols, model training, and performance benchmarking in both dental and bone age estimation studies.

[32] Cristiana Palmela Pereira, Lucianna Maria Russell, Maria de Pádua Fernandes, Ricardo Henrique Alves da Silva, Rui Filipe Vargas de Sousa Santos. Dental Age Estimation based on Development Dental Atlas Assessment in a Child/Adolescent Population with Systemic Diseases. *Acta stomatol Croat*. 2019;53 (3):307–317.

[33] Cristiana Palmela Pereira, Catarina Pereira Escobar, Jorge Costa Santos, Age Estimation of Unaccompanied minors: A portuguese overview. Ann Forensic Reas Anal 2 (1):1012.

[34] EASO European Asylum Support Office: EASO Practical Guide on age assessment. Second Edition, 2018. The results were obtained through a questionnaire that circulated between 2016 and 2017.

6.5 Summary and Conclusion

In summary, dental age is first estimated by observing the status of the age-related variable (for instance, matching a developing tooth to a defined stage) in an individual of unknown age. Second, age is estimated by comparing the status of the age-related variable to a reference atlas or scoring tables by reading off the estimated age value or integrating it into a mathematical model that calculates estimated age. This value is an age outcome, and should be accompanied by a measure of uncertainty, such as the interval within which the age falls. Specific calculations allow the individual to be classified into a specific age category or to predict if an individual has reached a specific age threshold with a measure of certainty.

Selecting the most appropriate method is complex, and the scientific value should be assessed using a thorough assessment of many factors, including the features of the sample, age-related variables, data type, statistical analysis, and accuracy of age estimation.

In the end, various forensic protocols for estimating age in living undocumented and unaccompanied minors asylum seekers combine dental age assessment with bone age assessment; however, no consensus on a common practice for age estimation examination has been reached internationally. In this chapter, the methodology from ABFO, IOFOS and AGFAD was presented.

6.6 Learning Outcomes

- You should be able to understand the importance of dental age assessment for children and adolescents.
- You should be able to describe the indications for dental age assessment in children and adolescents.
- You should be able to understand the different approaches for age estimation in children and adolescents.
- You should be able to understand the reasons for choosing a particular reference study to apply to forensic cases of age estimation in children and adolescents.

6.7 Self-Evaluation Questions

- What are the different types of indications for age estimation in children and adolescents?
- What is a reference study to be considered as a method for age estimation in children and adolescents?
- What is a conclusion when reporting age estimation in children and adolescents?
- Why is it important to combined teeth and bone for age estimation in children and adolescents?

6.8 Multiple Choice Questions

1. How many stages are in Demirjian's scores?
   (a) 5
   (b) 14
   (c) 8
   (d) 12
   (e) 7

Ans: c

2. How many stages are in the original Morrees, Fanning and Hunt scores?
   (a) 5
   (b) 14
   (c) 8
   (d) 12
   (e) 7

Ans: b

3. In the Demirjian's method:
   (a) The score reads the age directly
   (b) Several tables to calculate age
   (c) Use regression analysis
   (d) Use only right mandibular teeth
   (e) Use 5 teeth

Ans: b

4. The Dermirjian method includes:
   (a) As many teeth as possible
   (b) Right upper jaw
   (c) Only deciduous teeth
   (d) 7 teeth in the left mandibular jaw
   (e) 14 teeth in the mandibular jaw

Ans: d

5. The Morrees Fanning Hunt scoring:
   (a) Underestimate age
   (b) Overestimate age
   (c) Used in *The London Atlas*
   (d) Can be used in Demirjian's method
   (e) Only used in one method

Ans: c

6.9 Mind Map

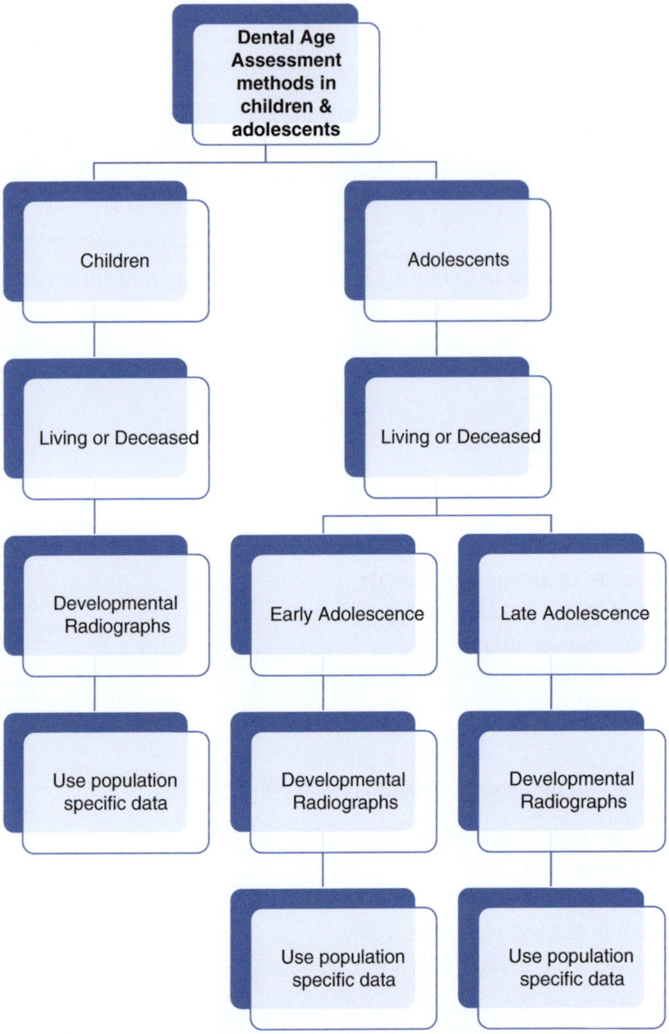

6.10 Example of Forensic Case Report of Final Age Assessment by Prof. Cristiana Palmela Pereira

1. *Case Identification Data*

   1.1 Case number: Case 1
   1.2 Referring Agency: Court
   1.3 Name of the Examiner: Cristiana Maria Palmela Pereira
   1.4 Date of examination: 2 April 2023

1.5 Setting of examination: Centre of Statistics and its Applications at University of Lisbon (CEAUL), Lisbon Portugal
1.6 Name of Subject: Must be given the full or partial name as reported by the subject or by family, witnesses, agencies, or authorities, or provided in documents. This example does not include a name
1.7 Birth Data and place of birth: The given age is 17 years, 9 months and he is from Somalia.

2. *Biographical Information of the Individual*

Sex: male

Geographic origin: Somalia

During the anamnesis no indications were found of the existence of current or past illnesses or medication use which might have impacted growth and development.

3. *Anamnesis*

During the physical examination, no indications were found of the existence of current or past illnesses or medication use which might have impacted growth and development.

Height: 167 cm

Body weight: 52 kg

3.1 Radiographs

X-ray examination of dentition (OPG)	X-ray examination of the left hand
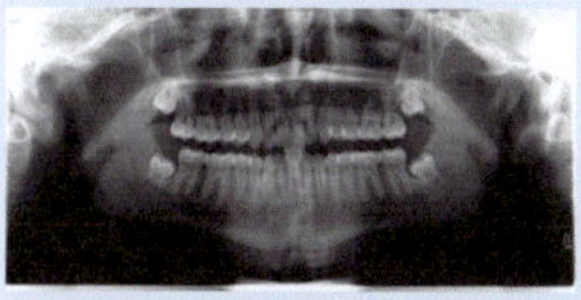	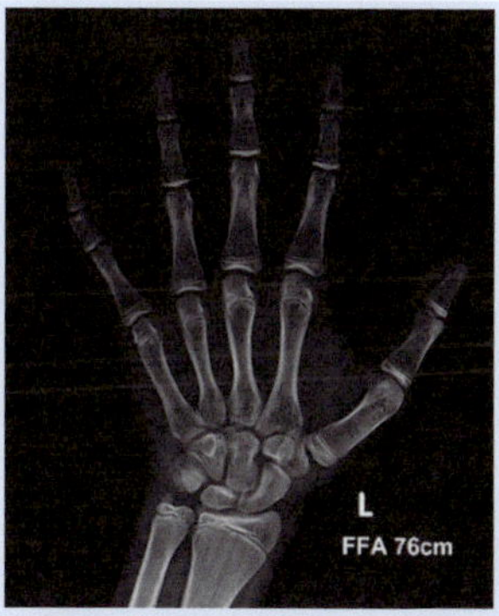

4. *Synopsis of Age Estimation Results*

In the synopsis of the findings, it was determined that the individual from Somalia stated an 17 years, 9 months, without past illnesses or medication use which might have impacted growth and development:

- Hand bone age assessment: *the mean age 14 years* (minimum 12 years and 6 months, and maximum 16 years; standard deviation of 11 months).
- Third molar dental age assessment: *The most likely dental mean age of the male is between 14 and 16 years old.* The minimum dental age is 11.5 years old, and the maximum dental age is 20.5 years old. The dental age assessment indicates the individual is beyond reasonable doubt less than 21 years old and less than 18 years old. Based on dental age assessment it *is less probable to be less than 14 years old.*

5. *Conclusion*

There is a very high probability of an age younger than the age stated by the person concerned, 17 years and 9 months. This means there is a very high probability that the given age is not correct. It is beyond reasonable doubt that the individual is younger than 21 years old and younger than 18 years old. However, it is less probable that the individual is younger than 14 years old; this means there is a very low probability that the 14th year of age has not been reached.

References

1. Wasserstein RL, Lazar NA. The ASA'S statement on p-values: context, process, and purpose. Am Stat. 2016;70:129–33. https://doi.org/10.1080/00031305.2016.1154108. ADA Technical Report No. 1077, Human Age Assessment by Dental Analysis. ADA Technical Report No. 1077_July_2020.pdf (nist.gov).
2. ADA Technical Report No. 1077, Human Age Assessment by Dental Analysis. ADA Technical Report No. 1077_July_2020.pdf (nist.gov).
3. European Asylum Support Office Practical Guide on Age Assessment. Available: https://www.easo.europa.eu/sites/default/files/easo-practical-guide-on-age-assesment-v3-2018.
4. Schmeling A, Grundmann C, Fuhrmann A, Kaatsch HJ, Knell B, Ramsthaler F, Reisinger W, Riepert T, Ritz-Timme S, Rösing FW, Rötzscher K, Geserick G. Criteria for age estimation in living individuals. Int J Legal Med. 2008;122(6):457–60.
5. Altman DG, Bland M. Absence of evidence is not evidence of absence. BMJ. 1995;311:485. https://doi.org/10.1136/bmj.311.7003.485.
6. Cohen J. Statiscal power analysis for the behavioral sciences. New York: Routledge Academic; 1988.
7. Dahlberg PS, Mosdøl A, Ding KY, Bleka Æ, Straumann GH, Rolseth V, Skjerven-Martinsen M, Delaveris GJM, Vist GE. Agreement between chronological age and bone age based on the Greulich and Pyle atlas for age estimation: a systematic review. Folkehelseinstituttet. 2017. ISBN: 978-82-8082-822-4. Available: https://www.fhi.no/en/publ/2017/samsvar-mellom-kronologisk-alder-og-skjelettalder-basert-pa-greulich-og-pyl/.
8. Greulich WW, Pyle SI. Radiographic atlas of skeletal development of the hand and wrist. Stanford: Stanford University Press; 1959.
9. Ritz-Timme S, Cattaneo C, Collins MJ, et al. Age estimation: the state of the art in relation to the specific demands of forensic practice. Int J Legal Med. 2000:29–136.
10. Schmeling A, Reisinger W, Loreck D, Vendura K, Markus W, Geserick G. Effects of ethnicity on skeletal maturation: consequences for forensic age estimations. Int J Legal Med. 2000;113(5):253–8.
11. Schmeling A, Schulz R, Reisinger W, Mühler M, Wernecke KD, Geserick G. Studies on the time frame for ossification of the medial clavicular epiphyseal cartilage in conventional radiography. Int J Legal Med. 2004 Feb;118(1):5–8.
12. Kellinghaus M, Schulz R, Vieth V, Schmidt S, Schmeling A. Forensic age estimation in living subjects based on the ossification status of the medial clavicular epiphysis as revealed by thin-slice multidetector computed tomography. Int J Legal Med. 2010;124(2):149–54.
13. Olze A, Taniguchi M, Schmeling A, Zhu BL, Yamada Y, Maeda H, Geserick G. Studies on the chronological of third molar mineralization in a Japanese population. Legal Med. 2004;6:73–9.
14. Melo M, Ata-Ali J. Accuracy of the estimation of dental age in comparison with chronological age in a Spanish sample of 2641 living subjects using the Demirjian and Nolla methods. Forensic Sci Int. 2017;270:276.e1–7. https://doi.org/10.1016/j.forsciint.2016.10.001.
15. Kahl B, Schwarze CW, Koln. Aktualisierung der Dentitionstabelle von I. Schour und M. Massler von 1941. Fortschr Kieferorthop. 1988;49:432–43.

16. AlQahtani SJ, Hector MP, Liversidge HM. Brief communication: the London atlas of human tooth development and eruption. Am J Phys Anthropol. 2010;142(3):481–90. https://doi.org/10.1002/ajpa.21258.
17. Moorees CFA, Fanning EA, Hunt EE. Age variation of formation stages for permanent teeth. J Dent Res. 1963;42(6):1490–502.
18. Demirjian A, Goldstein H, Tanner JM. A new system of dental age assessment. Hum Biol. 1973;45(2):211–27.
19. Haavikko K. The formation and the alveolar and clinical eruption of the permanent teeth. An orthopantomographic study. Disertation, Helsinfors Universitet, Finnland. 1970.
20. Cavrić J, Vodanović M, Marušić A, Galić I. Time of mineralization of permanent teeth in children and adolescents in Gaborone, Botswana. Ann Anat. 2016;203:24–32. https://doi.org/10.1016/j.aanat.2015.08.001.
21. Liversidge HM. Timing of human mandibular third molar formation. Ann Hum Biol. 2008;35(3):294–321.
22. Cameriere R, De Angelis D, Ferrante L, Scarpino F, Cingolani M. Age estimation in children by measurement of open apices in teeth: a European formula. Int J Legal Med. 2007;121(6):449–53. https://doi.org/10.1007/s00414-007-0179-1.
23. Augusto D, Pereira CP, Rodrigues A, Cameriere R, Salvado F, Santos R. Dental age assessment by I2M and I3M: Portuguese legal age thresholds of 12 and 14 year old. Acta Stomatol Croat. 2021;55(1):46–56. https://doi.org/10.15644/asc55/1/6.
24. Pereira CP, Rodrigues A, Augusto D, Santos A, Salvado F, Santos R, Cameriere R. Forensic age estimation using new models of mathematical regression formula constructed with molar indexes: dental age assessment. J Stomatol. 2021;74(2):95–100. https://doi.org/10.5114/jos.2021.106540.
25. Pereira CP, Rodrigues A, Santos A, Salvado F, Santos R, Cameriere R. Cut-off for the legal ages in the Portuguese population by third maturity index: measures of accuracy. Arch Oral Biol. 2021;125:105089. https://doi.org/10.1016/j.archoralbio.2021.105089.
26. IOFOS recommendations for quality assurance: dental age estimation, 2018. Available: http://www.iofos.eu/Quality-Ass/QA_2018_final/Age_estimation_final.pdf.
27. De Donno A, Angrisani C, Mele F, Introna F, Santoro V. Dental age estimation: Demirjian's versus the other methods in different populations. A literature review. Med Sci Law. 2021;61(1_suppl):125–9. https://doi.org/10.1177/0025802420934253.
28. Olze A, van Niekerk P, Schmidt S, Wernecke KD, Rosing FW, Geserick G, Schmeling A. Studies on the progress of third-molar mineralisation in a Black African population. Homo. 2006;57(3):209–17.
29. Olze A, Taniguchi M, Schmeling A, Zhu BL, Yamada Y, Maeda H, Geserick G. Comparative study on the chronology of third molar mineralization in a Japanese and a German population. Leg Med Tokyo. 2003;5(Suppl 1):S256–60.
30. Garamendi PM, Landa GPM, MI BJ, Solano MA (2005). Reliability of the methods applied to assess age minority in living subjects around 18 years old. A survey on a Moroccan origin population. Forensic Sci Int 154:3–12.
31. Gunst K, Mesotten K, Carbonez A, Willems G. Third molar root development in relation to chronological age: a large sample sized retrospective study. Forensic Sci Int. 2003;136:52–7.
32. Hostiuc S, Diaconescu I, Rusu MC, Negoi I. Age estimation using the Cameriere methods of open apices: a meta-analysis. Healthcare (Switzerland). 2021;9(2):237. https://doi.org/10.3390/healthcare9020237.
33. Latić-Dautović M, Nakaš E, Jelešković A, Cavrić J, Galić I. Cameriere's European formula for age estimation: a study on the children in Bosnia and Herzegovina. South Eur J Orthod Dentofacial Res. 2017;4(2):26–30. https://doi.org/10.5937/sejodr4-15528.
34. Lee SH, et al. Development of third molars in Korean juveniles and adolescents. Forensic Sci Int. 2009;188(1–3):107–11.
35. Minà G, Merelli V, Cattaneo C. Age estimation in the living: a scoping review of population data for skeletal and dental methods. Forensic Sci Int. 2021;320:110689. https://doi.org/10.1016/j.forsciint.2021.110689.

36. Mincer HH, Harris EF, Berryman HE. The A.B.F.O. study of third molar development and its use as an estimator of chronological age. J Forensic Sci. 1993;38:379–90.
37. Sousa AM d S, Jacometti V, AlQahtani S, da Silva RHA. Age estimation of Brazilian individuals using the London Atlas. Arch Oral Biol. 2020;113:104705. https://doi.org/10.1016/j.archoralbio.2020.104705.
38. Yan J, Lou X, Xie L, Yu D, Shen G, Wang Y. Assessment of dental age of children aged 3.5 to 16.9 years using Demirjian's method: a meta-analysis based on 26 studies. PLoS One. 2013;8(12):e84672. https://doi.org/10.1371/journal.pone.0084672.
39. Wolf TG, Briseño-Marroquín B, Callaway A, Patyna M, Müller VT, Willershausen I, Ehlers V, Willershausen B. Dental age assessment in 6- to 14-year old German children: comparison of Cameriere and Demirjian methods. BMC Oral Health. 2016;16(1):120. https://doi.org/10.1186/s12903-016-0315-8.

Dental Age Estimation in Adults: A Forensic Challenge

7

Ricardo Henrique Alves da Silva and Victor Jacometti

Abbreviations

CA	Chronological age
CBCT	Cone beam computed tomography
DA	Dental age
DT	Dental translucency
OPG	Orthopantomogram

Concepts and Definitions

- *Chronological Age*: the difference between the individual's date of birth and the date on which the age is being calculated.
- *Dental Age*: the assessment of the stage of dental maturity based on various factors including calcification and/or mineralization and/or eruption and/or post-eruption morphologic changes seen in teeth. Dental age can be an indication of chronological age for an individual.
- *Sub-adults*: individuals who have not reached the completion of their dental development.
- *Pulp-to-tooth ratio*: a quantitative relationship/ratio between the size or area of the pulp and the size or area of the *whole tooth* (pulp included). This ratio can be obtained by linear, area or even volume measurements.

R. H. A. da Silva (✉)
Forensic Odontology Division, Department of Stomatology, Public Health and Forensic Odontology, USP, School of Dentistry of Ribeirao Preto, Ribeirao Preto, Brazil
e-mail: ricardohenrique@usp.br

V. Jacometti
Departament of Pathology and Legal Medicine, USP, Ribeirão Preto Medical School, Ribeirao Preto, Brazil
e-mail: victor.jacometti@usp.br

© The Author(s), under exclusive license to Springer Nature Switzerland AG 2026

A. Chowdhry, P. Kapoor (eds.), *Dental Age Assessment*,
https://doi.org/10.1007/978-3-032-08788-1_7

7.1 Introduction

In Forensic Anthropology, during the biological profile establishment phase, it is of paramount importance to employ the best efforts and evidence to estimate the age of the deceased or a living individual, for criminal and/or civil reasons [31]. Dental age (DA) is basically the biological age of an individual observed through dental parameter observations, such as mineralization, development and eruption, for example, and it is a different concept from the chronological age (CA), which represents the date of birth of the same individual [26]. In this sense, dental age estimation is trivial in forensic situations of living individuals (senile people, asylum seekers, adoption purposes, etc.), dead persons (anthropological examination) and even for therapeutic purposes (puberty and growth for orthodontics), or archaeology [30].

Dental development, especially mineralization, is a constant process that presents distinct and observable stages that all teeth follow, and has less variability than other biological parameters, such as osseous development [30]. Therefore, in children or sub-adults, DA correlates well with CA, thus making dental age estimation in children a well applicable and reliable approach. Well-established methods, such as Nolla [24], Demirjian [7], Cameriere [3] and Willems [32] have already proven their efficacy, estimating DA with little to no difference from CA within several populations. Commonly, Demirjian's method [7] and its later modification including third molars [5] can be used reliably in the first two decades of life, along with skeletal assessment of the individual, achieving satisfactory results.

Nonetheless, when an individual reaches the threshold of approximately 21–23 years old, his/her last tooth has its development concluded (third molar), and if we bring in the increasingly common third molar agenesis in newer generations, this threshold might fall to the 15–16-year-old range [16]. This closes the sub-adult method applicability window and brings a new challenge to the Forensic Odontologist. Now, methods that rely on development are no longer feasible, so what should the examiner do?

In addition, forensic methods must respond to the necessities of an ageing population and to teeth resistance to taphonomic processes [16]. Like skeletal methods, when maturity is achieved, we must resort to regressive processes, that start upon adulthood, until (and in some cases after) death.

These methods, just like sub-adult ones, are currently divided into three main categories: morphological methods; radiological (or imaging) methods; and biochemical (or molecular) methods. Studied since the 1950s, these methods are mostly based on phenomena and biological processes that happen within teeth throughout life (i.e., secondary dentin deposition), somewhat synchronically with the advancement of chronological age. Each category has its advantages and disadvantages [28].

In this chapter, we will delve into these categories and their most established methods (except for the third category, which the reader should refer to in Chap. 8), to provide the forensic odontologist or anthropologist, tools to deal with forensic cases where an adult individual, living or dead, needs to have their age estimated, with robust scientific background and known data.

7.2 Morphological Methods

In 1947 and 1950, research by Gosta Gustafson [8] marked a landmark in studies on adult dental age estimation. According to this author, regressive changes such as attrition of the tooth (A); secondary dentin deposition (S); recession of periodontal ligament/periodontosis (P); cementum apposition (C); external root resorption (R) and translucency of tooth apex (T) are typical changes related to the progress of age.

Therefore, he established for each one of those six changes, four stages to be observed in ground sections of teeth, morphohistologically (n-ranging from 0 to 3). These scores then must be added, giving a total score, *Y*. This variable must then be inserted into a regression equation, described back then by Gustafson as *Estimated Age* = 11.43 + 4.56 × Y.

The error found by Gustafson was 3.6 years. This method, despite being the first to study age progression in dental parameters, had its limitations. As all morphological methods, it cannot be used in living individuals, because it requires the extraction of the tooth for the analyses. Scores are qualitative variables, hence prone to subjectivity from different examiners. In addition, all parameters were weighted equally, and the relationship between them was not considered. Further, there was no consensus on the thickness of the sections to be analyzed [20].

Several authors carried on studies on each one of those parameters. Dalitz [6] excluded root resorption and cementum apposition from the formula and increased the number of stages by 1 (0–4). He also recommended the use of up to four anterior teeth, and posterior teeth were discarded from analysis.

Bang and Ramm [1] went further with remarks found by Miles [21] and pointed out root translucency as the most important parameter in adult dental age estimation. According to the authors, translucency of the tooth apex sets in the third decade of life, advancing coronally. This is due to an alteration caused by a reduction of the diameter of the dentinal tubules, caused by increased intratubular calcification. Hence, refractive indices of dentin will be altered in a way that, basically, translucency of dentin will increase along with chronological age.

To analyze this translucency, the authors stored extracted teeth in 10% formalin, splitting multi-rooted teeth. Then, they were orientated, fixed with wax and labiolingual sections were cut into 400-μm-thick longitudinal sections, and Dental Translucency (DT) was assessed using a Vernier Caliper, in intact roots and sectioned roots. Then, measurements in several teeth and specimens were treated statistically to present two equations, one for DT length less than or equal to 9.0 mm and other for DT length greater than 9.0 mm.

- DT ≤ 9.0 mm:
  - Age $= B_0 + B_1 \times X + B_2 \times X^2$
- DT > 9.0 mm:
  - Age $= B_0 + B_1 \times X$

X: Dental translucency length. B_0, B_1 *and* B_2*: Constant term and coefficients, respectively. These values must be consulted directly in the original work.*

Johanson [10] made slight amendments to Gustafson's method, and developed seven grades and included intermediate stages (0, 0.5, 1, 1.5, 2, 2.5 and 3) for the same six criteria provided by the latter, and provided its own regression equation, as follows:

$$\text{Age} = 11.02 + (5.14 \times \text{A}) + (2.3 \times \text{S}) + (4.14 \times \text{P}) + (3.71 \times \text{C}) + (5.57 \times \text{R}) + (8.98 \times \text{T})$$

Most importantly, Johanson suggested that ground sections should be 0.25 mm thick for root translucency evaluation. This was, however, later rebutted by Metzger, Buchner and Gorsky, in the 1980s, who suggested a thickness of 1.0 mm, due to inaccuracies in the preparation and evaluation of 0.25-mm sections observed over time.

Maples [15] method also derived from Gustafson's original technique. Nevertheless, the author's findings showed that root resorption is the least dependable predictor of those suggested by Gustafson, hence this variable, along with periodontal recession (difficulty in analyzing after soft-tissue decomposition, in the dead) and attrition (dietary and occlusion variations) were discarded from the evaluation. This allowed Maples' method to be applied to teeth with destructed or no crown, archaeological samples and teeth with damaged roots and cementum.

Another important modification of Gustafson's approach was by Lamedin et al. [13]. These authors related, in a French sample, the variables periodontal recession (P) and Root translucency (T) to the overall height of the root. These measurements were taken with a Vernier Caliper, and then treated statistically via regression formula, independent to sex or ancestral affinity, as follows:

$$\text{Age} = 0.18\,\text{P} + 0.42\,\text{T} + 25.53$$

where P is Periodontosis height × 100/root height, and T is Translucency height × 100/root height.

Periodontosis is a product of degeneration of soft tissues around the tooth, going from the cervical area to the root apex. Macroscopically, it is seen as a yellowish area below the enamel that is darker than the enamel but lighter than the rest of the tooth [13]. Lamendin's method has a few shortcomings, such as the influence of extrinsic factors on periodontosis and root translucency (dental hygiene, diet, extreme thermal values, soil composition, etc.). However, its advantages over other methods, with its simplicity/reproducibility, made it a valuable method in dental age estimation in adults.

Prince and Ubelaker [27] evaluated the above technique and suggested adding sex and ancestry as predictors within Lamendin's method. In this way, they created specific formulas for different subpopulations (classified as black females, black males, white females, and white males), and managed to reduce the method's error, especially in the younger and older age groups, where Lamendin et al. [13] struggled with higher mean errors. Each of these ancestry subgroups had their own equation, which the reader should refer to in the original work, if necessary.

In Fig. 7.1, we show the measurements used by Lamendin et al. [13] and Prince and Ubelaker [27], to estimate age in adults.

Morphological methods have their value when remnants or evidence is scarce, or the Forensic Odontologist/Anthropologist is dealing with few pieces of information, such as isolated teeth. Given their incredible resistance to extreme and hazardous scenarios, these cases can become routine, and knowing the methods overviewed here is of paramount importance. Nevertheless, these methods are limited and present very high differences between estimated and real ages. Their standard errors (SEEs) can range between 5 and 12 years [29]. In addition, being

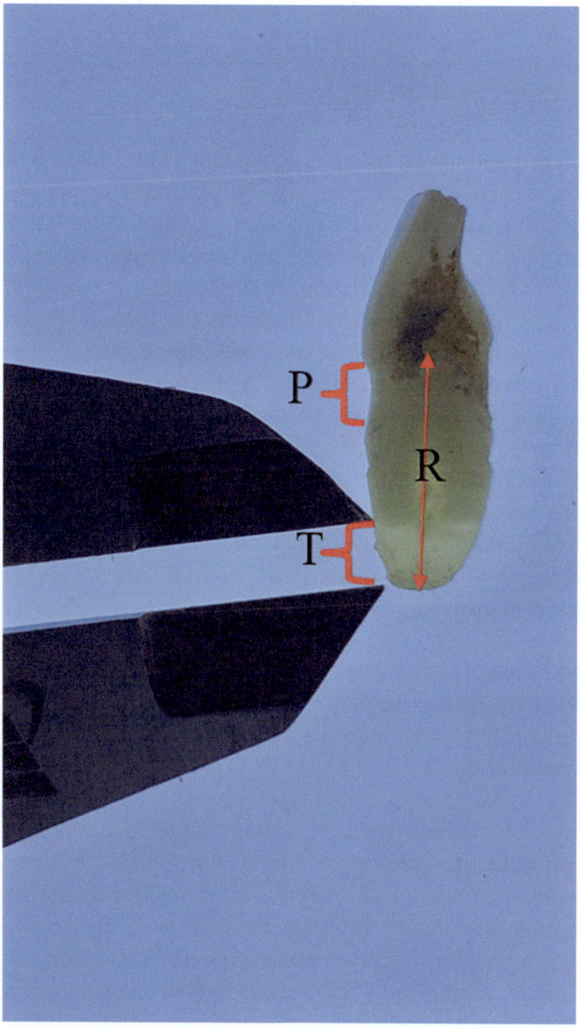

Fig. 7.1 Measurements of Lamendin et al. [13] method. P = Periodontosis height, T = Translucency height and R = Root height

destructive is a major shortcoming of these methods, in some instances, when it must deal with ethical, religious and legal issues (destruction of counterproof).

Circumventing the problem of the dental development conclusion in adults, by utilizing some of the above-described methods, other dilemmas start to rise in the horizon. As we formerly discussed, age estimation is often necessary in *living* individuals. In these cases, extracting a tooth and grinding it is not the best scientific choice, ethically speaking. On other cases, dead individuals (and their families) might have religious hurdles to provide extracted teeth for examination.

However, is the morphological approach (by the naked eye or with equipment) the only way we can observe phenomena in teeth and *inside* them? Think better: Do we have to extract teeth to observe caries, or periodontal disease?

7.3 Radiological Methods

A minimally invasive approach is utilizing imaging exams to reach dental examination. As Gustafson [9] and several other authors observed, secondary dentine deposition is a promising variable, due to its close relation to aging. In radiological examinations, dental hard tissues (greater mineral content—enamel, dentin, cementum) are seen as "whiter", clearer regions (radiopaque) and tissues that have low to no mineral content (pulp, periodontal ligament) are seen as "blacker", less clear regions (radiolucent). This means that, as secondary dentin is formed, the observable radiopaque area of a single given tooth will grow, overlapping the radiolucent area where the pulp is. This means that the pulp chamber size is diminishing as secondary dentine is forming, which leads to alterations in the *pulp-to-tooth dimensions' ratios,* an established age indicator [16].

Some dimensions (area and volume) ratios can be objectively measured in several types of imaging exams such as: Periapical x-rays, orthopantomograms (OPGs) and cone-beam computed tomography (CBCTs). All methods inside this category stem from modifications from:

- Solheim and Kvaal [11] and Kvaal et al. [12], which were based on the analysis of *linear measurements* of the pulp, tooth and root length.
- Cameriere et al. [2, 3], which were based on the analysis of the pulp and tooth *area measurements*.

Preliminarily, Solheim and Kvaal in 1994, studied age related changes in 452 single-rooted whole teeth—incisors, canines and pre-molars (both morphologically and radiologically—via periapical x-rays)—and found out interesting correlations between linear measurements of the pulp and tooth and their ratio, that could be used to assess age in adults without extracting the dental element.

Then, a year later, Kvaal et al. [12] worked further on the hypotheses above and developed a method based on standardized linear measurements from teeth in periapical x-rays from six teeth. These teeth are:

- Upper: central incisor, lateral incisor and second premolar.
- Lower: lateral incisor, canine and first premolar.

Pulp, tooth and root length along with pulp and tooth width from three different levels (A, B and C), and the ratios between them (M, W and L) were measured. The authors then reached for the best predictors amongst these variables and measurements and produced regression equations for several scenarios:

- Six teeth present.
- Three maxillary teeth present.
- Three mandibular teeth present.
- Single teeth.

Coefficient of determination [28] decreases and standard error increases as the number of teeth available diminishes. This is a notable shortcoming when estimating age from the elderly, because it is unusual to reach older ages having those six teeth present and especially sound, with no restorations or other treatments. It was not until years later when this method started being modified to orthopantomograms, due to their much higher availability in relation to periapical exams. The results, however, produced contrasting error rates in subsequent studies [14, 18, 23]. Nonetheless, using ratios to estimate age is encouraged, as it reduces the effects of tooth magnification in the x-rays and the effects of sex dimorphism related to tooth size [12].

In addition, using measurements rather than categorical scores aids in reducing subjectivity, raising inter- and intra-rater agreements. Kvaal et al. [12] method has a good and robust reproducibility in all studies that used it [16]. The use of a stereomicroscope can improve the accuracy of age estimates, in troublesome cases [33].

Another approach to pulp-to-tooth ratios would be using the *area* of the pulp and tooth and their relation, instead of linear measurements, which could be more demanding and complicated. Cameriere et al. [2] found the highest correlation coefficients and determination coefficient ($R^2 = 0.85$) in the ratio between pulp and tooth area in maxillary right canines in an Italian sample, and these measurements had a mean residual error of less than 4 years. As such, Cameriere et al. [4] looked up to reinforce this pilot study and establish the method, by measuring ratios between the areas of the pulp and tooth from both upper and lower canines. As reported by Paewinsky et al. [25], 20 points from each tooth outline and ten points for each pulp outline were identified and used to contour the pulp and tooth areas (in mm^2). The ratio between pulp and tooth areas was then calculated.

By analyzing 200 canine periapical x-rays (labio-lingual and mesio-distal) from Caucasian skeletons, and measuring ratios between pulp and tooth area within those x-rays, the authors developed, via stepwise regression, equations to age estimation, as follows:

- When the upper and lower canines are available:

$$Age = 120.737 - 337.112_{x1} - 79.709_{x2} - 364.534_{x3} - 65.655_{x4} + 1531.918_{x1x3}$$

- When only upper canines are available:

$$Age = 111.75 - 373.78_{x1} - 182.92_{x2}$$

- When only lower canines are available:

$$Age = 102.09 - 318.25_{x3} - 177.89_{x4}$$

X1: upper labio-lingual measurement.
X2: upper mesial measurement.
X3: lower labio-lingual measurement.
X4: lower mesial measurement.

Coefficients of determination for these three equations were: 0.94, 0.89 and 0.90, respectively, showing excellent adjustment of these regression models to estimate age. Mean prediction error was 2.8 years. There are roughly more than 25 scientific articles nowadays validating Cameriere et al. [4] method in several different populations [16]. Both cited studies recommend generating population-specific regression equations, in order to increase the method's accuracy and applicability.

Using the area of pulp-to-tooth ratio [4] seems slightly more advantageous than linear measurements [12], because:

1. Use of canines, especially upper canines, holds advantages due to their longer survival in comparison to other teeth, less wear, and bigger pulp chamber (which helps when contouring the pulp chamber);
2. Area measurement on digital radiographs is possible and has available software that automates this process, making it faster and less prone to observer errors (See Chap. 7);
3. Only one ratio is needed for the regression equation.

In contrast, there are studies that show a better performance of Kvaal et al. [12] in some age groups, such as 20–29 and 30–39 years old, when also evaluating canines [22]. Both methods are recommended to be used in living and dead adults and have acceptable mean error rates that, despite being considerable, are realistic for the adulthood scenario.

In CBCTs, age estimation methods for adults also derive from the pulp-to-tooth ratio concept, but, as we now are dealing with three-dimensions, it is possible to reach for the *volume* ratios. New studies are bringing insightful evidence [19] on a method that was previously discouraged due to lack of further researching, and high error rates [16]. Nevertheless, as the technology on imaging exams advances, we ought to expect also advancement in the Forensic field, with new methods and techniques being developed in order to overcome the problem of adult age estimation [29].

Biochemical methods, which will be further discussed at Chap. 8 of this book, seem to be an adequate solution to this problem [34], as it presents much lower error rates than every other age estimation method, using teeth, for adults [17].

7.4 Summary and Conclusion

Dental age estimation is well established and accurate for sub-adults, mainly because dental development is such a good and stable parameter. Hence, when dental development is done, and the person transitions from sub-adult to an adult, we need to shift our dental evaluations and start assessing regressive or involutive parameters, such as secondary dentin deposition, attrition, root translucency, etc. Morphological methods require extraction and sometimes destruction of the tooth, in order to observe each one of the used parameters, making them inapplicable to living individuals or people who have religious/ethical restrictions. In these cases, we should resort to radiological methods, which are well developed and established and have comparable error rates to morphological methods. We can use periapical x-rays, orthopantomograms or even CBCTs, although the latter is still not fully recommended in the literature. Biochemical methods emerged as a promising solution to high error rates in adult age estimation. After all this time, and published studies on the field of dental adult age estimation, it remains a challenge for any forensic practitioner and researcher.

7.5 Learning Outcomes

- You should be able to differentiate the process of dental age estimation applied to sub-adults and adults (the end of dental development and drastic shift in the analyzed parameters).
- You should be able to comprehend difficulties and limitations of age estimation in adults.
- You should be able to understand main differences between morphological and radiological methods for dental age estimation in adults, their advantages and disadvantages.

7.6 Self-Evaluation Questions

- When approximately does the end of dental development happen?
- What are we supposed to look for in teeth when no developmental parameters are available?
- How many categories are there for adult dental age estimation?
- Which category is better, and why?

7.7 Multiple Choice Questions

Q1. Which of the following categories is not for age estimation, in adults?
(a) Biochemical Methods
(b) Morphological Methods
(c) Radiological Methods
(d) Physicochemical Methods
Ans: d

Q2. Which one of these is a dental aging parameter suitable for age estimation, in adults?
(a) Dental mineralization
(b) Secondary dentin deposition
(c) Tooth eruption order
(d) Tooth decay
Ans: b

Q3. Which age estimation method below uses several morphological parameters?
(a) Nolla
(b) Kvaal
(c) Gustafson
(d) Cameriere
Ans: c

Q4. Which radiological method below is based on linear measurements?
(a) Cameriere pulp-to-tooth
(b) Kvaal
(c) Olze
(d) Demirjian
Ans: b

Q5. Which one is a shortcoming of age estimation in adults?
(a) Large error values
(b) Parameters prone to external influence i.e. grinding
(c) Lack of linearity between most variables
(d) All of the above
Ans: d

7.8 Mind Map (Fig. 7.2)

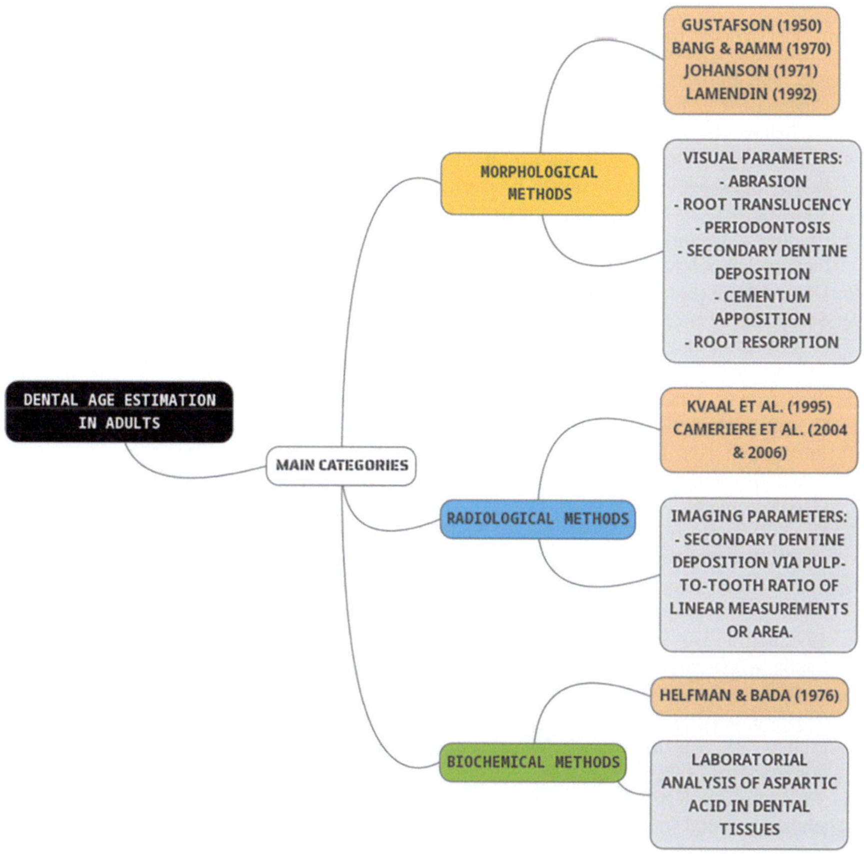

Fig. 7.2 Depicts a simplistic mind map with an overview of types and main methods for age estimation in adults by teeth

References

1. Bang G, Ramm E. Determination of age in humans from root dentin transparency. Acta Odontol Scand. 1970;28:3–5.
2. Cameriere R, Ferrante L, Cingolani M. Variations in pulp/tooth area ratio as an indicator of age: a preliminary study. J Forensic Sci. 2004;49(2):317–9.
3. Cameriere R, Ferrante L, Cingolani M. Age estimation in children by measurement of open apices in teeth. Int J Legal Med. 2006;120(1):49–52. https://doi.org/10.1007/s00414-005-0047-9.
4. Cameriere R, Ferrante L, Belcastro MG, Bonfiglioli B, Rastelli E, Cingolani M. Age estimation by pulp/tooth ratio in canines by mesial and vestibular peri-apical X-rays. J Forensic Sci. 2007;52(5):1151–5. https://doi.org/10.1111/j.1556-4029.2007.00530.x.
5. Chaillet N, Demirjian A. Dental maturity in South France: a comparison between Demirjian's method and polynomial functions. J Forensic Sci. 2004;49(5):1059–66.
6. Dalitz GD. Age determination of adult human remains by teeth examination. J Forensic Sci Soc. 1962;3:11–21.
7. Demirjian A, Goldstein H, Tanner JM. A new system of dental age assessment. Hum Biol. 1973;45:211–27.
8. Gustafson G. Åldersbestämningar på tänder. Odontol Tidskr. 1947;55:556–8.
9. Gustafson G. Age determinations on teeth. J Am Dent Assoc. 1950;41:45–54.
10. Johanson G. Age determination from teeth. Odontol Rev. 1971;22:1–126.
11. Kvaal SI, Solheim T. A non-destructive dental method for age estimation. J Forensic Odontostomatol. 1994;12(1):6–11.
12. Kvaal SI, Kollveit KM, Thompsen IO, Solheim T. Age estimation of adults from dental radiographs. Forensic Sci Int. 1995;74:175–85.
13. Lamendin H, Baccino E, Humbert JF, Tavernier JC, Nossintchouk RM, Zerilli A. A simple technique for age estimation in adult corpses: the two criteria dental method. J Forensic Sci. 1992;37(5):1373–9.
14. Landa MI, Garamendi PM, Botella MC, Alemán I. Application of the method of Kvaal et al. to digital orthopantomograms. Int J Legal Med. 2009;123(2):123–8. https://doi.org/10.1007/s00414-008-0268-9.
15. Maples WR. An improved technique using dental histology for estimation of adult age. J Forensic Sci. 1978;23:764–70.
16. Marroquin TY, Karkhanis S, Kvaal SI, Vasudavan S, Kruger E, Tennant M. Age estimation in adults by dental imaging assessment systematic review. Forensic Sci Int. 2017;275:203–11. https://doi.org/10.1016/j.forsciint.2017.03.007.
17. Matteussi GT, Jacometti V, Franco A, da Silva RHA. Age estimation in humans through the analysis of aspartic acid racemization from teeth: a scoping review of methods, outcomes, and open research questions. Forensic Sci Int. 2022;331:111154. https://doi.org/10.1016/j.forsciint.2021.111154.
18. Meinl A, Tangl S, Pernicka E, Fenes C, Watzek G. On the applicability of secondary dentin formation to radiological age estimation in young adults. J Forensic Sci. 2007;52(2):438–41. https://doi.org/10.1111/j.1556-4029.2006.00377.x.
19. Merdietio Boedi R, Shepherd S, Oscandar F, Mânica S, Franco A. Regressive changes of crown-root morphology and their volumetric segmentation for adult dental age estimation. J Forensic Sci. 2022;67:1890–8. https://doi.org/10.1111/1556-4029.15094.
20. Metzger Z, Buchner A, Gorsky M. Gustafson's method for age determination from teeth—a modification for the use of dentists in identification teams. J Forensic Sci. 1980;25(4):742–9.
21. Miles AEW. Dentition in the estimation of age. J Dent Res. 1963;42:255–63.
22. Miranda JC, Azevedo ACS, Rocha M, Michel-Crosato E, Biazevic MGH. Age estimation in Brazilian adults by Kvaal's and Cameriere's methods. Braz Oral Res. 2020;34:e051. https://doi.org/10.1590/1807-3107bor-2020.vol34.0051.

23. Nathalie BP, Medhat A, Willems AG. The application of Kvaal's dental age calculation technique on panoramic dental radiographs. Forensic Sci Int. 2005;153(2-3):208–12. https://doi.org/10.1016/j.forsciint.2004.08.017.
24. Nolla CM. The development of permanent teeth. J Dent Child. 1960;27:254–66.
25. Paewinsky E, Pfeiffer H, Brinkmann B. Quantification of secondary dentine formation from orthopantomograms: a contribution to forensic age estimation methods in adults. Int J Legal Med. 2005;119:27–30.
26. Pereira CP, Russell LM, de Pádua FM, et al. Dental age estimation based on development dental atlas assessment in a child/adolescent population with systemic diseases. Acta Stomatol Croat. 2019;53:307–17.
27. Prince DA, Ubelaker DH. Application of Lamendin's adult dental aging technique to a diverse skeletal sample. J Forensic Sci. 2002;47(1):107–16.
28. Priyadarshini C, Puranik MP, Uma SR. Dental age estimation methods: a review. Int J Adv Health Sci. 2015;12(1).
29. Ritz-Timme S, Cattaneo C, Collins MJ, Waite ER, Schütz HW, Kaatsch HJ, Borrman HI. Age estimation: the state of the art in relation to the specific demands of forensic practise. Int J Legal Med. 2000;113(3):129–36. https://doi.org/10.1007/s004140050283. PMID: 10876982.
30. Schmeling A, Geserick G, Reisinger W, Olze A. Age estimation. Forensic Sci Int. 2007;165(2-3):178–81. https://doi.org/10.1016/j.forsciint.2006.05.016.
31. Thevissen PW, Kaur J, Willems G. Human age estimation combining third molar and skeletal development. Int J Legal Med. 2012;126(2):285–92.
32. Willems G, Van Olmen A, Spiessens B, Carels C. Dental age estimation in Belgian children: Demirjian's technique revisited. J Forensic Sci. 2001;46(4):893–5.
33. Willems G, Moulin-Romsee C, Solheim T. Non-destructive dental-age calculation methods in adults: intra- and inter-observer effects. Forensic Sci Int. 2002;126(3):221–6. https://doi.org/10.1016/s0379-0738(02)00081-6.
34. Wochna K, Bonikowski R, Śmigielski J, Berent J. Aspartic acid racemization of root dentin used for dental age estimation in a Polish population sample. Forensic Sci Med Pathol. 2018;14(3):285–94. https://doi.org/10.1007/s12024-018-9984-8. Epub 2018 May 2.

Digital Methods of Dental Age Assessment

8

Jeyaseelan Augustine, Sourendra Nath Basu,
Kuldeep Singh, Priya Kumar, and Aadithya B. Urs

Abbreviations

CBCT	Cone Beam Computed Tomography
DAE	Dental Age Estimation
OPG	Orthopantomogram
PTR	Pulp to Tooth Ratio
RDT	Root Dentin Translucency
RVG	Radiovisiography

8.1 Concepts and Definitions

Dental age estimation (DAE):"The estimated mean age and the corresponding distribution of ages that result from dental age assessment" [1].

Dental age assessment: "The processes used to produce an estimation of an individual's biologic age using dental data and subsequently correlate biologic age to chronologic age" [1].

Digital imaging in dentistry (RVG, OPG, and CBCT): Digital imaging in dentistry is defined as the utilization of electronic tools/hardware to capture, view, and store the dental and orofacial anatomical structures in two-dimensional or three-dimensional plane without using traditional films.

J. Augustine (✉) · S. N. Basu · K. Singh · P. Kumar · A. B. Urs
Department of Oral Pathology, Microbiology and Forensic Odontology, Maulana Azad Institute of Dental Sciences, New Delhi, India

© The Author(s), under exclusive license to Springer Nature Switzerland AG 2026

A. Chowdhry, P. Kapoor (eds.), *Dental Age Assessment*,
https://doi.org/10.1007/978-3-032-08788-1_8

Open apex method: A technique for estimating the dental age by measuring the open apex widths and tooth lengths using panoramic radiographs. Age is estimated through a regression formula based on the sum of the ratios of the apex width and tooth length with incomplete roots and the number of teeth with closed apices [2].

Pulp-tooth ratio (PTR): A method for estimating the dental age by measuring the ratio of pulp cavity area to total tooth area, typically on periapical or panoramic radiograph, mostly in single-rooted teeth [3].

Root dentin translucency (RDT): A method for estimating the dental age by measuring the length or area of translucent dentin in tooth roots, caused by age-related dentinal sclerosis [4].

Image analysis software (ImageJ, GIMP, etc.): Image analysis software are computer programs that use digital processing techniques for the extraction of data from digital images. These data can be utilized for qualitative/quantitative analytical processes.

Artificial intelligence: "The science and technology of creating intelligent machines, especially intelligent computer programs" [5].

8.2 Learning Outcomes

After going through the chapter, the reader will

- Have a detailed understanding about digital methods of forensic DAE and their practical usage.
- Decipher the biological and technical concepts behind different DAE techniques and regression formulae.
- Learn about the steps of digital techniques employed for DAE.
- Knowledge about limitations and ethical concerns.

8.3 Introduction

The precise and accurate estimation of dental age has always been a critical aspect of forensic odontology. Dental age estimation (DAE) has also been widely used for paleo-demographic studies to establish mortality patterns and age at the time of death in ancient populations. The use of modern digital imaging technologies like radiovisiography (RVG), orthopantomogram (OPG), cone beam computed tomography (CBCT), digital photomicrography, two-dimensional flatbed scanning, and stereomicroscopy along with different computational tools for analyzing dental structures to ascertain an individual's age has revolutionized the modern approach to dental age estimation (DAE). These methods can provide a more dependable, swift, and precise alternative to traditional methods by minimizing human subjectivity with improved reproducibility. This chapter focuses on the technical aspects of digital techniques of modern dental age estimation, such as pulp-to-tooth ratio (PTR), measurement of open apex, and dentin translucency, as well as their various modifications [6].

8.4 Importance of Digital Techniques in Age Estimation

Conventional procedures for estimating dental age, including morphological and radiographic methods, have been extensively utilized for decades. Developmental changes associated with tooth formation like progressive morphological development of the tooth crown, root and apex of teeth are used as a reliable and accurate method of DAE. In adults, various post formational changes (anatomical/histological) are used for DAE such as: (i) occlusal/incisal attrition, (ii) periodontal attachment, (iii) extent of apical root resorption, (iv) pulp to tooth area ratio (associated with secondary dentin deposition), (v) cementum apposition and annulation, and (vi) dentin translucency [6]. Nonetheless, these conventional procedures frequently entail subjective interpretation and may be affected by factors such as examiner proficiency, demographic variances, and environmental influences. The increasing necessity for accuracy and consistency in age estimation has led to the implementation of digital techniques, utilizing developments in image technology and computer analysis to overcome these challenges [7].

The modern digital dental imaging modalities offer a more precise way of capturing and analyzing dental structures in both two dimensions (2D) and three dimensions (3D) [8]. The digital files acquired through these modern imaging procedures can be analyzed with the help of different image processing tools: these tools are used to evaluate various dental parameters in these images for DAE. The incorporation of these tools for digital image acquisition and analysis has improved the accuracy and reproducibility of age estimation by reducing human subjectivity. The recent introduction of artificial intelligence (AI) and machine learning algorithms has enhanced these methods further, making them more accurate, efficient, and capable of analyzing extensively larger datasets in a shorter duration.

8.4.1 Open Apices Approach for Dental Age Estimation

DAE using the open apex measurement is particularly useful in children and adolescents, where root formation is incomplete. The development of the tooth follows a chronological sequence; following crown formation from the developing tooth bud, root development starts from Hertwig's epithelial root sheath. During apexogenesis, the root apex remains open in the earlier period allowing the continuous growth of pulp tissue. The width of the root apex reduces with time as root development progresses. Usually, 2–3 years after the eruption of tooth, the root apex closes [9]. The biological basis of the open apex method is associated with the development of root apex because it has a strong correlation with human age.

In case of human deciduous teeth, apexogenesis is completed around 1–2 years after the tooth erupts into the oral cavity. Incomplete apex or open apex in human permanent teeth is generally observed in individuals under 16–18 years of age depending on the tooth type. Closed apex is generally seen in individuals with an age range of 18–25 years. However, the development and completion of root of the third molar, which is relatively more variable, can be used for age estimation in late adolescent periods. Cameriere et al. introduced a method for DAE based on the ratio between the width of the open apices and the length of the tooth along its long axis. It is a, simpler, inexpensive, faster, and non-invasive method where OPG is used to visualize the developing permanent teeth and their open apices. As OPG is a two-dimensional representation of a three-dimensional entity, distortion of recorded anatomical structures occurs. To compensate for this variation in measurement, the ratio of tooth length and width of the root apex is taken. Various open-source image processing tools are used to measure these parameters in an OPG. Methods using three-dimensional data like CBCT have also been introduced.

8.4.2 Methodology

In this method, a digital radiograph (eg: OPG) is loaded into the image processing software. For better visibility of the region of interest, the relevant areas are magnified. The most common and simple approach is to use the in-built '*Straight-Line Tool*' in the image processing software. This tool is used to measure the length of the tooth (Li). The same tool is then used for measuring the width of the apex (Ai). In the image processing software these measurements are generally recorded in pixels. Thus, the tooth length and apex width for all the permanent teeth up to the second molar present in left lower quadrant are recorded in a spreadsheet. Then the ratio (Xi) between Ai and Li is calculated (Xi = Ai/Li) for each tooth with open apices. The sum of the width of the open apices is used in case of teeth with bifurcated roots. The sum of these ratios (S) along with the count of teeth with fully formed roots (N_0) are then determined. Cameriere's formula (for European Children) is then applied to estimate age:

$$\text{Age} = 8.971 + 0.375g + 1.631X_5 + 0.674N_0 - 1.034S - 0.176S.N_0$$

where $g = 1$ for boys and 0 for girls. The acceptable estimation error margin for this method is up to 1.18 year [10].

8.4.3 Modifications

- *Region and Population Specific Calibration:*
  Cameriere's open apex method applies a more quantitative approach, and therefore is considered as one of the most reliable methods for DAE [11, 12]. While this method may be an exceptionally precise and beneficial technique for DAE in

children aged 5–15 years, it may necessitate population-specific regression formulas to preserve its accuracy. The formula introduced by Cameriere for the open apex approach was originally designed for Italian children. Later this formula was modified by incorporating different variables for European children [2]. Region-specific formulas have been derived in different areas of the world. For Indian population, Balwant Rai et al. have modified the original formula given by Cameriere [13]. Through this study Rai et al. have discovered that, except for gender and an added weight to the second premolar, all other variables such as morphological variables, the linear distance between the inner walls of the open apex of the teeth with developing roots divided by the tooth length, sum of normalized open apices, and the number of teeth with complete root development contributed significantly to the regression model. In addition, the region of the country affected the age estimation in their sample. The following linear regression formula for DAE was proposed for the Indian population:

$$\text{Age} = 9.402 - 0.879C + 0.663\,\text{N}_0 - 0.711\text{S} - 0.106\text{S.N}_0$$

where C is a variable equal to 0 for the central or North Indian and 1 for the South Indian, N_0 defines the count of teeth with fully formed roots and 'S' defines the sum of the ratios between open apex width and tooth length. Population specific regression formulas have also been introduced for Malaysian, Turkish, Egyptian, and other countries (Table 8.1) [7].

- *Open apices Method for Third Molars*
  The I3M method is a quantitative approach for DAE where the correlation between an individual's chronological age and the ratio of the width of open apices and the length of the third molar is utilized. The method consists of evaluating the apical widths of the roots of the mandibular third molars of the left quadrant. If the roots of the third molar are fully developed, it means that the apical ends of the roots are completely closed, so the value of I3M = 0.00. If the root apices are open, I3M is evaluated as (A + B)/C—the sum of the distances between the insides of two open apices (A + B) divided by the length of the tooth.
- *Open Apices Measurement from CBCT*
  A linear regression formula for DAE was developed based on the correlation between chronological age and apical surface area in CBCTs [14]. This novel and reliable method for DAE by three-dimensional surface area analysis of maxillary canine apices in Malaysian children was conducted utilizing CBCT data. The following formula was given by the authors:

$$\text{Age} = 13.897\,0.228(\text{apex surface area}) - 0.864(\text{gender}) + 0.905(\text{open / closed apex}).$$

Suggested values for the variables: Male = 0; Female = 1; Open apex = 0; Closed apex = 1.

Table 8.1 Population-specific formula that use open apex method

Authors (year)	Population	Sample size with gender-wise distribution	Age group (years)	Software used	Formula
Cugati, N et al. (2015) [16]	Malayasian	421 children (176 boys, 245 girls)	5–16	Adobe Photoshop 7	Age = 11.368–0.345 *g* + 0.553 N_0–1.096S – 0. 380S.N_0 Here, *g* is a variable; *g* = 1 for males, *g* = 2 for females
Gulsahi et al. (2015) [17]	Turkish	573 children (298 girls, 275 boys)	8–15	Mediadent V4, I ˙mage level, Nieuwkerken-Waas, Belgium	Age = 8.387 + 0.282 *g* – 1.692 × 5 + 0.835 N_0 – 0.116S – 0.139S * N_0 where *g* is a variable, with *g* = 1 for boys, and *g* = 0 for girls
Marinkovic et al. (2018) [18]	Serbian	423 children (192 boys, 231 girls	5–15	ImageJ	European formula given by Cameriere et al. [2]
El-Bakary et al. (2010) [19]	Egyptian	286 children (134 boys, 152 girls)	5–16	Image tool program for digitalized images (UTHSCS, Texas, USA)	European formula given by Cameriere et al. [2]
Rivera et al. (2017) [20]	Colombian	526 children (274 boys, 252 girls)	6–15	ImageJ, version 1.49	European formula given by Cameriere et al. [2]
Guo et al. (2015) [21]	Chinese	785 children (397 girls, 388 boys)	5–15	Adobe Photoshop	Age = 10.202 + 0.826 *g* – 4.068x_3–1.536x_4–1.959x_7 + 0.536 N_0–0.219 S.N_0 where g is a variable, 1 for boys and 0 for girls, x_3(canine)= –4.068, x_4(first premolar)= –1.536, x_7(second molar) = –1.959, S.N_0= –0.219

8.4.4 Limitations

Radiographic assessment of dental and skeletal development for DAE has been criticized as a controversial matter in recent years due to the risk–benefit ratio associated with radiation exposure: from a forensic perspective, age estimation may not be considered a reasonable justification for the use of radiation [15].

8.4.5 Steps of Age Estimation Using Digital Open Apices Method and ImageJ Software

Step 1: Click the File option in the toolbox and click on Open to select the radiograph.

Step 2: The tooth region to be measured can be zoomed with the help of Zoom option. The image may be maximized for better visibility.

Step 3: The measurements are done with the help of Straight tool (Fig. 8.1, encircled with the red color).

Step 4: Measurement of the width of the open apex *(Ai)* is done with the help of Straight tool. The inner width of the open apex is measured.

Step 5: The measurement line can be made bold by holding the ctrl + B keys. This bold option helps to make line stay permanent.

Step 6: After making it bold, ctrl + M keys are pressed simultaneously to record the measurements. Once Ctrl + M keys are pressed, a window opens as displayed in the below image. (Measured length is annotated with a blue rectangular box, Fig. 8.1).

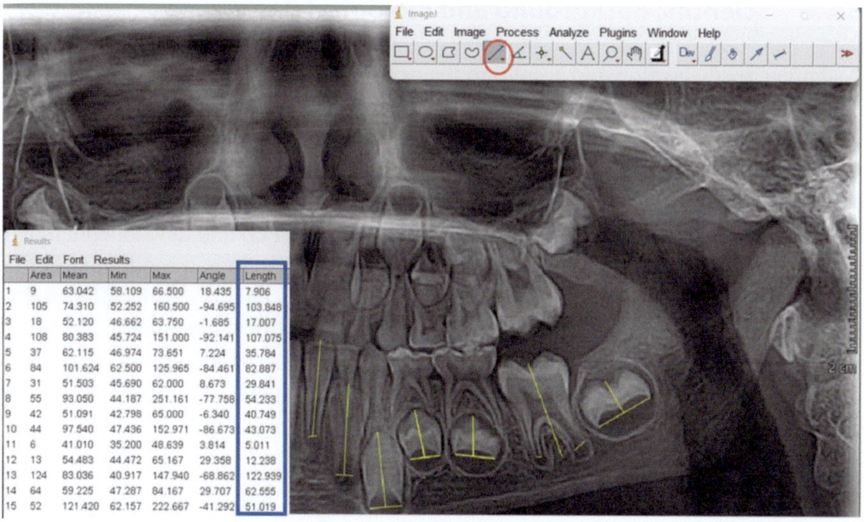

Fig. 8.1 The Image J interface after measuring the length of all the permanent teeth and tooth buds and their associated open apices. The measurement table on the left (annotated by the blue rectangular box) shows the length of each line drawn in pixels. These values are used for dental age estimation (DAE) using population-specific formula

Step 7: The same Straight tool is used to measure the length of the tooth (Li). The same bold (ctrl+B), measurement (ctrl+M) steps are followed as for the previous steps [4–6] to measure (Ai).

Step 8: The second measurement in the measurement window indicates the length of the tooth.

Step 9: The ratio can be calculated once the both measurements are done using the below formula.

$$\mathrm{Xi} = \mathrm{Ai} / \mathrm{Li}\left(where\, i\, is\ the\ tooth\ for\ which\ the\ measurement\ has\, been\ made\right).$$

Now, use the value of Xi for each of the mandibular permanent teeth on the radiograph with open apex in a population-specific formula for DAE.

8.4.5.1 PTR Technique

Age estimation is more challenging and complex in adults due to various extrinsic and intrinsic factors that affect the dental characteristics of the mature human dentition. This variability explains the larger error margin obtained with adult dental age estimation (DAE) techniques. However, the radiographic methods that analyze the regressive changes of dental characteristics provide comparatively accurate and reliable results [10].

The pulp/tooth area ratio method for DAE was proposed by Cameriere, Ferrante and Cingolani in 2004. The ratio between pulp area and tooth area in dental radiographs (OPG, IOPAR) exhibits a strong correlation with negative direction when related to chronological age.

8.4.6 Scientific Background and Biological Basis

As human teeth develop and erupt into the oral cavity, the volume of the pulp chamber regresses with time due to the deposition of secondary dentin. This physiological process occurs continuously throughout the entire life span of a human being. Thus, an inverse proportional relationship between the size of the pulp cavity and human chronological age can be established. Cameriere, Ferrante and Cingolani studied this relationship in adult orthopantomograms (OPG) and developed a linear regression formula for DAE by using the ratio between pulp and tooth area of the right maxillary canines. Later Cameriere et al. found satisfactory results after evaluating the original method on the periapical radiographs of the canine teeth of the right or the left dental arch. Finally, separate linear regression equations were developed for maxillary canines, mandibular canines and both maxillary and mandibular canines together [3, 10].

8.4.7 Methodology

According to the original method proposed by Cameriere et al., a digital orthopantomogram or a scanned conventional orthopantomogram is obtained at high resolution (e.g., 300 DPI). This image is then imported into the image analysis software such as AutoCAD/Adobe Photoshop/GIMP/ImageJ. Using the polygon/free hand selection tool, the pulp area and tooth area are demarcated and later measured in pixels. The ratio of the pulp and tooth area is calculated and substituted in the following formula given by Cameriere et al. [3]:

$$\text{Age} = 86.53 - (457.15 \times \text{PTR}) - (22.98 \times c),$$
$$\text{`}c\text{'} \text{ denotes pulp / root width at mid} - \text{root level}$$

This pulp/tooth ratio indirectly quantifies the deposition of secondary dentin. There is decrease in the size of the pulpal space (pulp chamber and root canal) due to deposition of secondary dentin.

8.4.8 Modifications and Advancements

8.4.9 DAE Using Periapical Radiographs

Cameriere et al. conducted a step-wise regression analysis on the periapical radiographs of maxillary and mandibular canine. This method exhibited the residual standard error of 4.06 years without any significant difference between females and males. Hence, the derived formula could be used for both gender groups. The authors introduced three separate formulas as follows [10]:

1. The regression formula that used pulp/tooth ratio in both maxillary (x_1) and mandibular canine (x_2):

$$\text{Age} = 114.624 - 431.183x_1 - 456.692x_2 + 1798.377x_1x_2$$

2. When only mandibular canine is considered:

$$\text{Age} = 89.456 - 461.873x_2$$

3. When only maxillary canine is considered:

$$\text{Age} = 99.937 - 532.77x_1$$

8.4.10 Population Dependent Formulas

Various published studies have reported inter-population variability when pulp/tooth ratio was used for Dental Age Estimation (DAE) in different populations. This variation is attributed to the heterogenic, population-specific nature of secondary dentin deposition. Studies have also showed that, the secondary dentin deposition varies with the type of teeth. For Indian population, Babshet et al. have developed multiple regression equations for: (i) Lateral incisor (LI), (ii) Canine (C), (iii) First premolar (PM_1) (iv) LI & C (v) LI & PM_1, (vi) C & PM_1, and (vii) Combination of all three teeth (LI + C + PM_1) [22]. The regression equation that used the combination of three teeth taken together showed the best correlation coefficient (0.438) is as follows [22]:

$$\text{Age} = 68.014 + \left(-36.743 \times \text{PTR of C}\right) + \left(-92.949 \times \text{PTR of PM}_1\right) + \left(-128.898 \times \text{PTR of LI}\right)$$

However, the mean absolute error (MAE) for the equation was 10.76 years which was slightly better than the MAE of 11.58 years exhibited by Cameriere et al.

Aguilera-Muñoz et al. developed a similar population-specific regression formula for Chilean adults using pulp/tooth ratio of lower premolars and canines. Their proposed regression formula showed a mean absolute error of 5.6–5.7 years with a 95% confidence interval. The regression equation that showed the most accurate estimate used the pulp/tooth ratio of lower left second premolar, lower left canine, lower left first premolar is as follows [23]:

$$\text{Age} = 24.455 - 0.72x$$

where x denotes the average pulp/tooth ratio of the lower left premolars and canine (Table 8.2).

8.4.10.1 Utilization of 3D Imaging

There are inherent drawbacks posed by the use of 2D radiographs and imprecise measurement due to distortion caused by projecting the 3D anatomical objects over a 2D plane. 3D volumetric imaging using CBCT has enabled researchers to overcome this limitation. Gulsahi et al. have developed a regression equation that used pulp/tooth volume from CBCTs of the Turkish population. The formula that showed the lowest standard error (83.2) was for the maxillary central incisor, which is given below:

$$\text{Age} = 68.3 - \left(837.5 \times \left(\text{PV} / \text{TV}\right)\right)$$

This study obtained a comparatively stronger correlation ($r = 0.532$ for maxillary central incisors) between PV/TV and chronological age, whereas 2D methods showed lower correlation values due to projection inconsistencies.

3D volumetric imaging of the craniofacial skeleton is achieved and saved in DICOM format. These DICOM files are then imported into 3D volume analysis software such as 3D DOCTOR, 3D Slicer, etc. Volumetric segmentation for both

Table 8.2 Population-specific formula that use PTR technique

Authors (year)	Population	Teeth studied	Software used	Formula
Aguilera-Muñoz et al. (2019) [23]	Chile	#33, #43	ImageJ	Age = 24.455–0.72x (x = average pulp /tooth ratio of the lower left premolars and canines)
Azevedo et al. (2015) [24]	Brazil	#13, #23, #33, #43	Adobe Photoshop	1. **Upper canine:** Age = 94.706–465.358 x_1 2. **Lower canine:** Age = 99.409–503.726 x_2 3. **Both canines:** Age = 122.026–471.568 x_1—486.891 x_2 + 2122.427 x_1x_2 ·x_1 = pulp/tooth area ratio for **upper canines** ·x_2 = pulp/tooth area ratio for **lower canines**
Cameriere, Ferrante et al. (2004) [3]	Italy	#13	AutoCAD	Age = 86.53–457.15 × AR − 22.98 × c AR = pulp/tooth area ratio c = pulp/root width at mid-root level
Cameriere et al. (2007) [10]	Italy	#13, #23, #33, #43	AutoCAD	Age = 114.624–431.183 x_1 - 456.692x_2 + 1798.377(x_1x_2) ·x_1 = pulp/tooth area ratio for **upper canines** ·x_2 = pulp/tooth area ratio for **lower canines**
Boyacıoğlu Doğru et al. (2017) [25]	Turkey	#13, #23, #33, #43	ImageJ	Age = 77.365–351.193 × AR (linear regression equation was developed using AR derived from maxillary canine)
Kapoor et al. (2020) [26]	India	#13	AutoCAD	Age = 6.6554 × PTR − 22.578

AR pulp tooth area ratios

tooth and pulp is done and the pulp-to-tooth volume ratio is obtained. These values are then incorporated into the regression equation for DAE. Thus, CBCT is a more practical and precise tool offering superior capabilities for DAE over conventional radiographic techniques [17].

In conclusion, the pulp/tooth ratio method is one of the most widely used and reliable techniques used for forensic DAE in adults. With the evolution of high-resolution 3D imaging technologies, the introduction of 3D volumetric segmentation software, and the integration of AI, the pulp/tooth ratio approach has become more accurate and efficient.

8.4.11 Steps of Age Estimation Using Digital Pulp-to-Tooth Ratio Method in GIMP Software

Step 1: Open GIMP software.
Step 2: Import the relevant radiographic image.
Step 3: Choose the free select tool.
Step 4: Mark the tooth area with the free select tool. Select the outline of the tooth by clicking the left mouse button on every curvature or sharp bend (Fig. 8.2a).

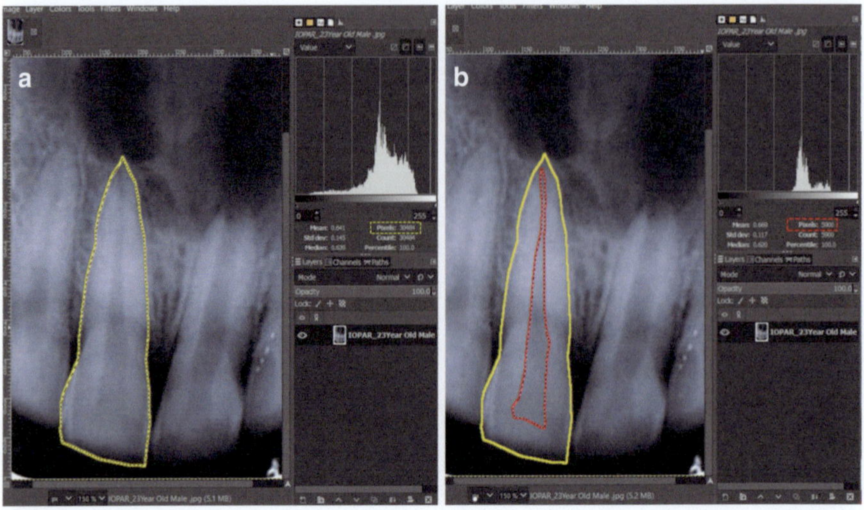

Fig. 8.2 (**a**) The whole tooth area is selected using the “free select tool” and segmented in yellow color using the “stroke selection” option. The selected tooth area in this case measures 30,484 pixels (yellow dotted rectangular box); (**b**) the pulp area is then selected using the “free select tool” and segmented in red color using the “stroke selection” option. The selected pulp area in this case measures 5900 pixels (red dotted rectangular box)

Step 5: Optionally, after completion of selection, select a color from the toolbox, choose stroke selection, and apply strokes to segment the selected area for proper visualization (Fig. 8.2a).

Step 6: Note the pixels in the histogram after marking the tooth area (Fig. 8.2a, yellow dotted rectangular box). If the histogram is not visible on the default screen, click Windows>Dockable Dialogs>Histogram.

Step 7: Mark the pulp outline with the free select tool in a similar manner. Optionally use stroke selection to apply a different segment for the pulp area (Fig. 8.2b).

Step 8: Note the pixels in the histogram after marking the pulp area (Fig. 8.2b, red dotted rectangular box).

Step 9: Calculate the ratio of the pulp area to the tooth area. The ratio is substituted in the relevant formula to estimate the age of the individual.

8.4.12 Root Dentin Translucency (RDT) Method

Gustafson in 1950 had first described a method for DAE using dentin translucency. The translucency of dentin is least affected by external factors; thus, it makes the method more reliable when correlated with chronological age [27]. For forensic DAE, the dentin translucency method often reported a very strong correlation with human chronological age.

8.4.13 Biological Basis

Dentin translucency is a physiological process that occurs due to the accumulation of hydroxyapatite crystals inside the dentinal tubules as a result of dentin degeneration. With increasing age, dentinal translucency increases due to gradual deposition of minerals that occlude the microscopic dentinal tubules. Unoccluded dentinal tubules have different intertubular and intratubular refractive indices, and this causes scattering of transmitted light. As a result, dentin appears opaque when seen in a ground section. On the other hand, the occluded dentinal tubules and the intertubular matrix show a similar refractive index; this allows the light to pass without scattering and produces the appearance of translucency [27]. Translucent dentin becomes visible around the third decade of life. It starts from the apex of the root and progresses towards the crown. The longitudinal extent of the transparent dentin relative to root length is used as an indicator for DAE. Bang and Ram studied the Norwegian population and developed a linear regression equation for age estimation using dentin translucency [4].

8.4.14 Methodology

According to the method proposed by Bang and Ramm, extracted teeth were preserved in 10% neutral-buffered formalin after removal of soft tissue from the root surface. For multirooted teeth, each root was measured separately following splitting. Labio-lingual sections of 400 micrometres in thickness are prepared from these teeth using hard-tissue microtomes. The tooth section is placed over a lightbox with a constant light source to illuminate the translucent root dentin. A sliding caliper is used to measure the extent of translucent dentin from the root apex till the borderline between translucent and opaque dentin towards the coronal aspect. In case the borderline was not horizontal, then the average of the maximum and minimum length of the translucent dentin with respect to the root apex is measured. The recorded measurements are then incorporated in the linear regression formula to estimate the dental age. For the dentin translucency measuring less than 9 millimetres, Bang and Ramm proposed the following second-degree polynomial equation for DAE:

$$A = B_0 + B_1 \cdot X + B_2 \cdot X^2$$

where A = estimated dental age, X = measured length of root dentin translucency, and B_0, B_1, B_2 are coefficients specific to different types of teeth [4].

For dentin translucency measuring greater than 9 mm, the following first-degree polynomial equation was proposed by the same authors:

$$A = B_0 + B_1 \cdot X$$

With the advent of digital technologies for image acquisition and analysis, the measurement of dentin translucency has become easier with enhanced reproducibility, limiting inter- and intra-observer variability [28]. The tooth section is scanned using a flatbed scanner at a resolution of 600 dpi. An ABFO scale is also placed near the tooth to ensure proper life-sizing of the scanned teeth section. The scanned image is imported into image editing software (e.g., ImageJ, Adobe Photoshop, GIMP, etc.) to measure root dentin translucency using the inbuilt measuring tools. For measuring the length of translucent dentin, the similar methodology explained by Bang and Ramm is followed. Various population-specific regression formulae have also been developed and have proven to have better performance for DAE [29].

8.4.15 Modifications

8.4.15.1 Enhanced Correlation with Age and Development of Population-Specific Formula

Though root dentin translucency seems to be least affected by external stimuli, various taphonomic, gender, and age-related factors may affect dentin translucency. Thus, the estimated age can be different if the same formula is used for different populations (Table 8.3). Acharya, AB, et al. used raw data developed from multiple population-specific studies and applied them to the Indian population. From this study they have generated a linear and a quadratic regression formula for DAE in the Indian population and compared its performance with the formula given by Bang and Ramm. The quadratic regression formula showed a better correlation coefficient in comparison to the linear regression formula and the original formula given by Bang and Ramm [29]. For uneven height of translucent root dentin, the authors used the average of the maximum and minimum height of RDT as proposed by Bang and Ramm.

Also, Ashith B. Acharya proposed a separate formula for uneven height of RDT, where the maximum RDT length was utilized to develop a regression equation for DAE in Indian population [30]. Instead of taking the average of the maximum and minimum height of RDT, only the maximum height from the apical extent was measured, and DAE was conducted using the following formula:

$$\text{Age} = 40.0391 + \left(2.1063 \times \text{maximum translucency length}\right)$$

Despite being least affected by external factors, age seems to be overestimated for the individuals aged between 20 and 49 years old. For the individuals of age group 60–89 years, the estimated dental age seems to be underestimated [27].

8.4.15.2 Use of Root Dentin Translucency Area for Dental Age Estimation

Acharya AB proposed a formula that utilized digital measurement of the root dentin translucency (RDT) areas as an alternative to root dentin length for DAE. The inbuilt 'magic wand tool' in Adobe Photoshop is used to select the root dentin translucency zone over the image of the tooth section. The RDT area is calculated in mm^2 using the following formula:

Table 8.3 Population-specific formula that uses root dentin translucency for DAE

Authors (year)	Population	Sample size (no. of teeth)	Age group	Method used for tooth section scanning	Software used for measurement	Formula
Acharya AB et al. (2008) [29]	Indian	100	19–82	Flat-bed scanner	Adobe Photoshop	Linear regression equation: $Age = 35.5619 + (3.4828 \times T)$ Quadratic regression equation: $Age = 29.9074 + (7.4507 \times T) + (-0.4369 \times T^2)$
Nancy Tang (2014) [27]	British	666	21–81	All teeth were photographed with a Nikon Coolpix 4500 digital camera	ImageJ	Original formula given by Bang and Ramm was used.
Munoz and Calla (2023) [31]	Peru	248	30–70	Flat-bed scanner	Adobe Photoshop software	Linear regression equation: $Age = 32.294 + 4.323 \times T$ Quadratic regression equation: $Age = 24.028 + (9.090 \times T) + (-0.516 \times T^2)$
Drusini et al. (1991) [32]	Italy	152	22–76	Black and white video camera fixed at 512 x 512 pixels	image analysis system, the IBAS 2000	For anterior teeth: $Y = 31.6800 + 0.5104X$ Premolar: $Y = 15.0315 + 0.7207X$

T transparency length, *Y* estimated dental age, *X* root dentin translucency

$$\text{RDT Area}\left(\text{in mm}^2\right) = \left(\left[\text{Image area in mm}^2 \div \text{Image area in pixels}\right]\right) \times \left(\text{RDT in pixels}\right)$$

Using this measurement the following regression equation was proposed:

Linear regression equation:

$$\text{Age} = 38.86 + \left(1.06 \times \text{RDT area}\right)$$

Quadratic regression equation:

$$\text{Age} = 31.75 + \left(2.97 \times \text{RDT}\right) + \left\{-0.07 \times \left(\text{RDT Area}\right)^2\right\}$$

Both equations showed comparable results with the conventional DAE using maximum RDT length in terms of correlation coefficient and standard errors of estimate [33]:

8.4.16 Steps of Age Estimation Using Digital Root Dentin Translucency Method and GIMP Software

8.4.16.1 Steps to Measure Dentin Translucency with GIMP Software

Step 1: Open the scanned tooth section image in the GIMP software (Fig. 8.3a).

Step 2: To measure root dentin translucency length (RDT), a guiding ruler is taken by dragging from the pointer present in the measuring scale of the image (Fig. 8.3b). For uneven height of the RDT, the maximum height is marked using one guide (Fig. 8.3b, Guide 01). Another guiding ruler is used to mark the minimum height of the RDT (Fig. 8.3b, Guide 02). (To drag the guiding ruler, the move tool in the toolbox should be used).

Step 3: Another guiding ruler is placed in the apical part of the RDT.

Step 4: The measurement units should be changed from pixels (px) to mm (Fig. 8.3b).

Step 5: Measuring tool is used to measure the dentin translucency. The measuring tool is dragged from the upper guideline to the lower guideline to find out the length of the RDT. This calculated value will be substituted in the population-specific formula to find the age. For uneven height of RDT, the average of maximum (Fig. 8.3c) and minimum (Fig. 8.3d) RDT length is calculated [4].

Step 6: The average length of the RDT is then applied to a population-specific regression equation for DAE.

8.4.16.2 Steps for Measuring RDT Area Using GIMP for DAE

Step 1: Open the scanned tooth section image in the GIMP software (Fig. 8.3a).

Step 2: The translucency area can be selected by clicking the fuzzy select tool in the dark area of the radicular dentin. Additional translucent areas may be selected by keeping the shift key pressed while the additional selection of translucent dentin is made.

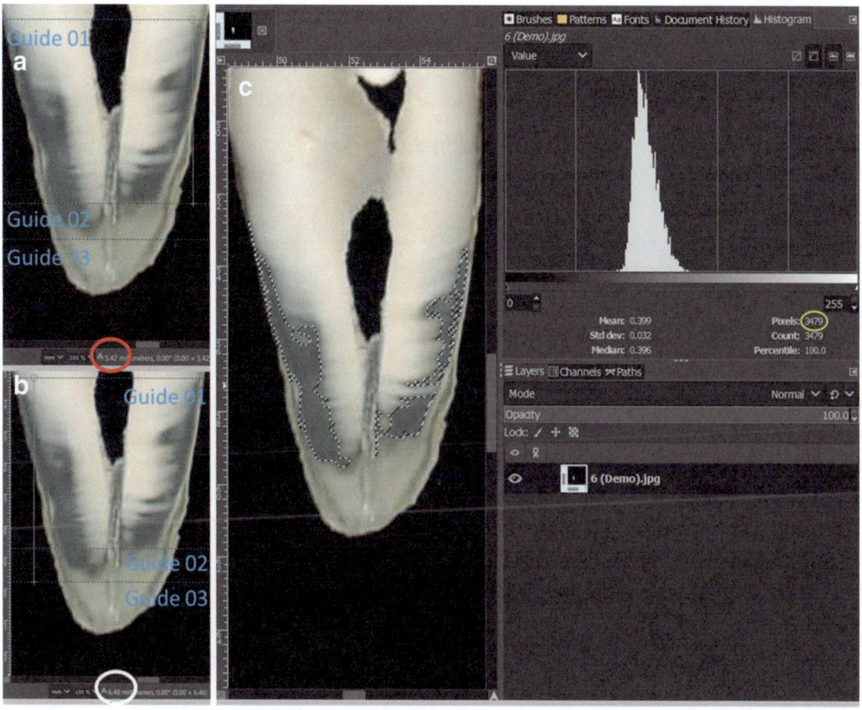

Fig. 8.3 (**a**) The distance between Guide 01 and Guide 02 indicates the length height (5.42 mm in this scenario, value encircled in red color) of RDT; (**b**). The distance between Guide 01 and Guide 03 indicates the maximum length (6.48 mm in this case, value encircled in white color) of the RDT. (**c**) RDT area after being annotated with the "fuzzy select" tool; on the right the pixel value indicate the RDT area (value encircled with yellow color)

After marking the translucent area with the fuzzy select tool, the pixels in the histogram should be noted. The noted value is the translucency area in pixels.

Step 3: The measurement of RDT area requires the following parameters:

(i). *Image area in pixels:* When the image is imported and opened in GIMP, the total area of the imported image is shown in pixels below the histogram on the right.

(ii). *Image area in square millimeters:* The operator needs to click on the 'image" tab in GIMP, following which a drop-down list will appear; from this list "canvas size" is selected. A new window titled "Canvas Size" now opens; here the pixel value is changed to mm. Thus, the width and height of the image are obtained in mm, and the area is now calculated after multiplying them.

(iii). TA in mm is now calculated from the two above components using the following equation:

$$TA = \text{image area in sq.mm} / \text{image area in pixels} \times \text{translucency area in pixels}$$

The value for TA is applied to a population-specific regression equation for DAE.

8.5 Conclusion

Though various taphonomic, geographical, and other parameters seem to cause underestimation or overestimation of dental age, the integration of digital imaging tools for scanning and analysis has greatly improved the conventional procedures of forensic DAE in terms of usability, precision, reliability, and reproducibility. Future research endeavors should focus on generating larger, diverse dental databases across different populations across the globe. As artificial intelligence and automation technology continue to evolve, the digital methods will likely play an increasingly vital role in forensic odontology, archeology, and dentistry, offering new possibilities for DAE with a reduced margin of error.

8.6 Multiple Choice Questions

Q1. What are the various post-formational changes that are used for DAE?
- (a) Incisal attrition, internal resorption, external resorption
- (b) Dental caries, abfraction, abrasion
- (c) Dentin translucency, apical root resorption, incisal wear
- (d) Periodontal attachment loss, change in tooth color, degree of melanin deposition over attached gingiva

Ans: c

Q2. Which one of the following can capture dental images in both two- and three-dimensional planes?
- (a) RVG
- (b) CBCT
- (c) IOPAR
- (d) OPG

Ans: b

Q3. What is the value of "g" for European children as given in the original formula by Cameriere?
- (a) g = 1 for boys, g = 0 for girls
- (b) g = 0 for boys, g = 1 for girls
- (c) g = 0 for boy, g = 0 for girls
- (d) g = 1 for boy, g = 1 for girls

Ans: a

Q4. As human teeth develop and erupt into the oral cavity the volume of the pulp chamber
   (a) Increases with time
   (b) Regresses with time
   (c) Stays constant
   (d) None of the above

Ans: b

Q5. Dentin translucency occurs due to the accumulation of which of the following inside the dentinal tubules?
   (a) Silicate crystals
   (b) Calcium oxalate crystals
   (c) Air bubbles
   (d) Calcium hydroxyapatite crystals

Ans: d

Q6. As per the original method proposed by Bang and Ramm, if the tooth has translucency area with different height, the measurement is taken as follows:
   (a) For uneven height of translucent root dentin, the authors used the maximum height
   (b) For uneven height of translucent root dentin, the authors used the average of the minimum height
   (c) For uneven height of translucent root dentin, the authors used the summation of the maximum and minimum height
   (d) For uneven height of translucent root dentin, the authors used the average of the maximum and minimum height

Ans: d

8.7 Self-Evaluation Questions

1. What are the major limitations of conventional techniques of dental imaging for age estimation methods?
2. How can digital imaging methods overcome the limitations of conventional techniques in DAE?
3. Explain the biological basis behind the open apices method for DAE.
4. How does the pulp-to-tooth ratio change with age, and why is it considered reliable for adult age estimation?
5. Why does root dentin become translucent with age and how can it be used for DAE?
6. Discuss the limitations of using 2D radiographic methods (like OPG) for DAE and explain how 3D imaging (CBCT) overcomes these limitations.
7. Describe how root dentin translucency is measured using digital tools, and how this measurement is used to estimate age.
8. Why are population-specific regression formulas important in DAE? Give examples of how regional variations affect age estimation accuracy.

9. What are the specific roles of various images processing software in the digital workflow of age estimation?

References

1. American Dental Association Technical Report No. 1077 For human age human age assessment by dental analysis. ABFO Standards and Guidelines for Dental Age Assessment—ADA Technical Report No. 1077–2020. https://abfo.org/wp-content/uploads/2021/02/ADA-Technical-Report-No.-1077_July_2020.-02-2021.pdf; 2020.
2. Cameriere R, Ferrante L, Cingolani M. Age estimation in children by measurement of open apices in teeth. Int J Legal Med. 2006;120(1):49–53.
3. Cameriere R, Ferrante L, Cingolani M. Variations in pulp/tooth area ratio as an indicator of age: a preliminary study. J Forensic Sci. 2004;49(2):317–9.
4. Bang G, Ramm E. Determination of age in humans from root dentin transparency. Acta Odontol Scand. 1970;28(1):3–35.
5. Weber F. Artificial Intelligence. In: Artificial intelligence for business analytics. Wiesbaden: Springer Fachmedien Wiesbaden; 2023. p. 33–64.
6. David TJ, Lewis J. Forensic odontology: principles and practice—Thomas J. David, Jim Lewis; n.d.
7. Rodríguez-Niklitschek C, Oporto GH, Chuhuaicura P, Alemán I, Fonseca GM. Cameriere's open apices methodology for dental age estimation in children: a scoping review from a Latin American perspective. Forensic Sci Med Pathol. 2023;20(3):1049–57.
8. Mallya SM, Diplomate P. In: Mallya S, Lam E, editors. White and Pharoah's oral radiology: principles and interpretation. 8th ed. ISBN: 9780323543842; 2018. p. 1608.
9. Nanci A, Causa H. Ten Cate's oral histology development, structure, and function 9th ed. [Internet]. n.d.. Available from: www.konkur.in
10. Cameriere, R., Ferrante, L., & Cingolani, M. Age estimation in children by measurement of open apices in teeth. Int J of Legal Med.2006;120(1):49–52.
11. Galić I, Pacifici A, Carbone D, Pacifici L, Jerončić A, Cameriere R. Age estimation by the Cameriere's normalized measurements (CNM) of the single permanent mandibular tooth on a panoramic radiograph. Legal Med. 2017;26:65–72.
12. AlShahrani I, Yassin SM, Togoo RA, Tikare S, Khader MA, Alkahtani ZM. Age estimation by measurement of open apices in tooth roots: study using Saudi Arabian samples. J Forensic Leg Med. 2019;62:63–8.
13. Rai B, Kaur J, Cingolani M, Ferrante L, Cameriere R. Age estimation in children by measurement of open apices in teeth: an Indian formula. Int J Legal Med. 2010;124(3):237–41.
14. Asif MK, Ibrahim N, Al-Amery SM, Muhammad AMA, Khan AA, Nambiar P. A novel method of age estimation in children using three-dimensional surface area analyses of maxillary canine apices. Legal Med. 2020 May;1:44.
15. Machado MA, Daruge Júnior E, Fernandes MM, Lima IFP, Cericato GO, Franco A, et al. Effectiveness of three age estimation methods based on dental and skeletal development in a sample of young Brazilians. Arch Oral Biol. 2018;85:166–71.
16. Cugati N, Kumaresan R, Srinivasan B, Karthikeyan P. Dental age estimation of growing children by measurement of open apices: A Malaysian formula. J Forensic Dent Sci. 2015;7(3):227.
17. Gulsahi A, Kulah CK, Bakirarar B, Gulen O, Kamburoglu K. Age estimation based on pulp/tooth volume ratio measured on cone-beam CT images. Dentomaxillofacial Radiol. 2018;47(1):20170239.
18. Marinkovic N, Milovanovic P, Djuric M, Nedeljkovic N, Zelic K. Dental maturity assessment in Serbian population: A comparison of Cameriere's European formula and Willems' method. Forensic Sci Int. 2018;288:331.e1–5.

19. El-Bakary AA, Hammad SM, Mohammed F. Dental age estimation in Egyptian children, comparison between two methods. J Forensic Leg Med. 2010;17(7):363–7.
20. Rivera M, De Luca S, Aguilar L, Velandia Palacio LA, Galić I, Cameriere R. Measurement of open apices in tooth roots in Colombian children as a tool for human identification in asylum and criminal proceedings. J Forensic Leg Med. 2017;48:9–14,
21. Cheng GY, Han M, Chi Y, Long H, Zhang D, Yang J, et al. Accurate age classification using manual method and deep convolutional neural network based on orthopantomogram images. Int J Legal Med. 2021 Jul 1;135(4):1589–97.
22. Babshet M, Acharya AB, Naikmasur VG. Age estimation from pulp/tooth area ratio (PTR) in an Indian sample: a preliminary comparison of three mandibular teeth used alone and in combination. J Forensic Leg Med. 2011 Nov;18(8):350–4.
23. Aguilera-Muñoz F, López-Lázaro S, De Luca S, Navarro-Cáceres P, Fonseca GM. Dental age estimation in adults by pulp/tooth ratio in lower premolars and canines by orthopantomographs, in a Chilean sample. Int J Morphol. 2019;37
24. de Azevedo ACS, Alves NZ, Michel-Crosato E, Rocha M, Cameriere R, Biazevic MGH. Dental age estimation in a Brazilian adult population using Cameriere's method. Braz Oral Res. 2015;29(1):1–9.
25. Hatice BD, Nihal A, Nursel A, Humeyra Ozge Y, Goksuluk D. Applicability of Cameriere's and Drusini's age estimation methods to a sample of Turkish adults. Dentomaxillofac Radiol. 2017;46(7):20170026.
26. Kapoor N, Kothari P, Shukla RK, Mishra SD, Badiye A. Age estimation from tooth-pulp area ratio: A preliminary study. La Revue de MédecineLégale. 2020;11(1):11–4.
27. Tang N, Antoine D, Hillson S. Application of the Bang and Ramm age at death estimation method to two known-age archaeological assemblages. Am J Phys Anthropol. 2014;155(3):332–51.
28. Shah J, Ranghani A, Limdiwala P. Age estimation by assessment of dentin translucency in permanent teeth. Indian J Dent Res. 2020;31(1):31.
29. Acharya AB, Vimi S. Effectiveness of Bang and Ramm's formulae in age assessment of Indians from dentin translucency length. Int J Legal Med. 2009 Nov;123(6):483–8.
30. Acharya AB. A new digital approach for measuring dentin translucency in forensic age estimation. Am J Forensic Med Pathol. 2010 Jun;31(2):133–7.
31. Alvarado Muñoz E, Requena Calla SR. Accuracy of age estimation using root dentin translucency in Peruvian adults. A pilot study. J Forensic Odontostomatol. 2023;41(1):19–26.
32. Drusini A, Calliari I, Volpe A. Root dentine transparency: age determination of human teeth using computerized densitometric analysis. Am J Phys Anthropol. 1991;85
33. Acharya AB. Forensic dental age estimation by measuring root dentin translucency area using a new digital technique. J Forensic Sci. 2014;59(3):763–8.

9 Aspartic Acid Racemization and Radiocarbon Dating: Advanced Biochemical Techniques for Dental Age Assessment

Jyotirmoy Roy and Abraham Johnson

> *"The tragedy of old age*
> *Is not that one is old,*
> *But that one is young"*
> *—Oscar Wilde*

9.1 Introduction

Dental age estimation is one of the most efficient methods of age assessment, in the absence of an official birth record. Historically teeth have been used for age estimation and human identification due to its individualistic and resilient nature [65]. England is where the very first studies on the use of teeth as a trustworthy age assessment technique were conducted. In 1837, with the introduction of the "Factory Act", many underaged children were forbidden to work. Among them was an individual who was restricted from working as he was missing a premolar, rendering him a juvenile. Until this time height was used as a reliable parameter for age estimation. Driven by the prevailing disarray, Dr. Edwin Saunders conducted his study on 1049 people and testified before Congress that teeth are a more reliable indicator of age than height [57]. In the year 1894, Dr. E'mile Magitot was summoned to assess the age of an unmarked body who was believed to be the son and heir of King Louis XVI and his wife Queen Marie Antoinette of France. The absence of deciduous teeth and partially erupted third molars, as noted in Dr. Magitot's report,

J. Roy
Department of Oral & Maxillofacial Pathology and Microbiology, Guru Nanak Institute of Dental Sciences and Research, Khardaha, West Bengal, India

A. Johnson (✉)
School of Medico-Legal Studies, National Forensic Sciences University, Gandhinagar, Gujarat, India
e-mail: abraham.johnson@nfsu.ac.in

© The Author(s), under exclusive license to Springer Nature Switzerland AG 2026

A. Chowdhry, P. Kapoor (eds.), *Dental Age Assessment*,
https://doi.org/10.1007/978-3-032-08788-1_9

suggested that the person was between 18 and 20 years old at the time of death and so could not be the lost heir [17]. Groundbreaking progress was made with the advent of radiographic imaging in the field of forensic odontology. In the year 1944, using radiographic images of developing jaw, Schour and Massler published their research regarding the chronological stages of tooth development. A chart that shows the 21 phases of tooth development was created and used as a tool for determining age. They updated their chart in 1944, establishing the foundation for current dental age estimation, by adding one more stage of tooth development from birth to age 35 [22].

The biochemical approach that primarily uses the chronological changes in biomarkers is one of the most reliable methods of estimating dental age. All amino acids, with the exception of glycine, contain a stereocenter at their -C atom, which makes them optically active; that means the amino acid can take one of two forms: "D" or "L," which are mirror images. All organisms preserve their amino acids in the "L" form, with a few notable exceptions. Slow ageing produces modest but discernible alteration, and the "L" shape eventually transforms to the "D" form. The pace of this progressive conversion is known as racemization, and it is determined by the type of amino acid, average temperature, humidity, acidity (pH), and other environmental factors [42]. Racemization occurs more swiftly in warm, damp environments than in cold, dry conditions. Strong acidity and mild to severe alkalinity both cause significantly increased racemization rates [53]. Amino acid sequencing has traditionally been employed in paleobiology, molecular palaeontology, archaeology, forensic science, taphonomy, sedimentary geology, and other domains. Abelson was the first to report on the amino acid composition of early-aged fossil shell, bone, and tooth samples [53]. According to Hare and Abelson, D- amino acids were discovered in fossils as a result of protein L- amino acid conversion [29]. The older the fossil, the higher the D/L ratio, and beyond a certain age, amino acids formed in racemic form. Ever since this development, amino acid racemization was used to assess the age of different protein-containing materials. Since L-isoleucine can be easily separated from D-alloisoleucine using an amino acid analyzer, and aspartic acid, the most acidic of amino acids, is the first to depart the ion exchange column, they were given special attention [18]. Aspartic acid is now the amino acid of choice for conducting dental age assessment and is widely utilized for both legal and scientific objectives.

Another biochemical method that can be used for effective age estimation is the radiocarbon dating, often known as carbon dating or ^{14}C dating, and it is a technique for determining the age of organic material by utilizing the properties of radioactive carbon isotopes [33]. Willard Libby developed the method at the University of Chicago in the late 1940s, based on the fact that cosmic rays continually interact with atmospheric nitrogen to form radiocarbon (^{14}C) in the Earth's atmosphere [33]. The resultant ^{14}C combines with oxygen in the air to produce radioactive carbon dioxide, which plants absorb through photosynthesis and animals ingest. As an animal or plant dies, it ceases to exchange carbon with its environment, and the amount of ^{14}C it holds begins to decrease as the ^{14}C decays. By measuring the amount of ^{14}C in a sample from a dead plant or animal, such as a piece of wood or a fragment of bone, the amount of ^{14}C in the sample can be used to calculate when the animal or plant died. Scientists have been striving to determine the fraction of ^{14}C in the atmosphere during the past 50,000 years since the 1960s [6]. Using a calibration curve, the collected data is now used to transform a specific measurement of radiocarbon in a sample into an estimate of the sample's calendar age. Other changes are required to account for the varied proportions of ^{14}C in different types of animals (fractionation) and the variable quantities of ^{14}C across the biosphere (reservoir effects) [64].

9.2 Dental Age Estimation Through Aspartic Acid Racemization

Prior to the advent of life, only L-amino acids are assumed to have been chosen for protein creation. As a result, survival necessitates homochirality [39]. In contrast, Kuhn hypothesized in 1936 that the accumulation of erroneous stereoisomers could be the cause of ageing by providing kinetic considerations for the inevitable racemization of optically active substances inside biological systems [36]. Racemization is a spontaneous post-translational process that leads to the production of an optically active racemic mixture. Amino acids are converted from their natural L-form to their unusual D-form mirror twin [37]. Racemization should occur in any metabolically stable protein that has not been turned over during the life of a long-lived organism, and these proteins will have altered conformations as a result of racemization, which will most likely result in changes in their biological activities or chemical properties. As a result of these alterations, changes in the physicochemical properties of implicated proteins may contribute to the progressive changes associated with ageing [27]. The first studies of amino acid racemization assumed that amino acids produced abiotically would adopt an amino acid pool with equal amounts of L and D forms, whereas biological processes would produce an excess of L-forms; these methods were developed to search for evidence of extraterrestrial life in meteorites also [30, 31, 2]. Racemization of amino acids was initially utilized to date various fossil materials, such as marine sediments and fossil bones [63]. Kuhn's basic hypothesis about the inevitability of racemization in live mammals was confirmed in humans in 1975 by the work conducted by Helfman and Bada, who examined aspartic acid racemization in human tooth enamel and discovered that D/L ratios rise with age [1]. Furthermore, they established that, because hemoglobin is a rapidly turned-over protein, the fraction of D-aspartic acid in human hemoglobin does not rise with age. Following that, a relationship was discovered between racemization, aging, and illness.

9.2.1 Chemistry of D- Aspartic Acid Formation

All amino acids (excluding glycine) have two optical isomer forms, L and D based on their ability to spin polarised light. L-amino acids are found in biological systems because ribosomal subunits prefer the L-enantiomer [37]. Racemization is a process

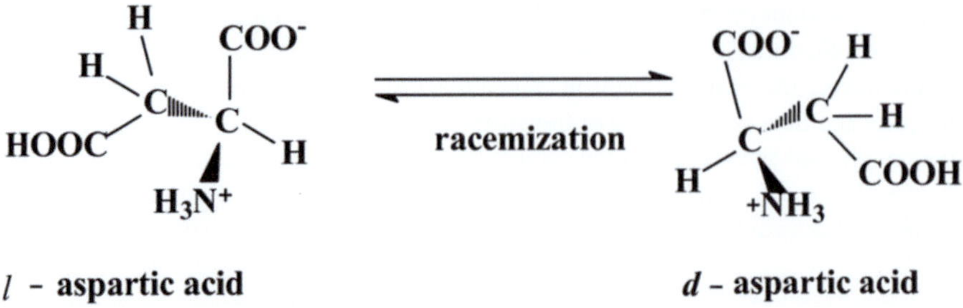

Fig. 9.1 Racemization chemistry

that results in the production of D-amino acids, which increase with age. All amino acids go through this process, but aspartic acid racemizes the quickest, making it the subject of the greatest interest. D-Asp is produced by transitional succinimide intermediates coming from Asx (Asn) residues. These processes start with the peptide-bond nitrogen's nucleophilic attack on the side-chain carbonyl group, which leads to the formation of an unstable five-membered L-succinimide ring [11]. The isomerization and racemization that ensue from the hydrolysis of this ring give rise to peptides and -Asp in both D and L configurations [Fig. 9.1].D-Asp is produced via Asn deamidation. During this process, the functional amine group of Asn is removed, which could lead to the formation of a succinimide intermediate that can racemize or isomerize [66]. Due to changes in the carbon chain, isomerization involves a change in the shape of the peptide backbone from to. A succinimide intermediate is required for this technique. The succinimide ring can hydrolyze to produce two different conformations: L-Asp (native conformation) and L-Asp (L-isoAsp) [20].

9.2.2 Application of Aspartic Acid Racemization

The application of the aspartic acid racemization study ageing has led to the main topic of this chapter. Its connection to ailments has also been researched, considering how it accumulates with age. Aspartic acid racemization has been used to calculate the turnover rates of long-lived proteins in addition to these mechanisms. The rate of D-amino acid buildup in a tissue where the protein has almost no turnover, such as collagen in tooth dentin, is measured using a first-order kinetic equation, where k_T = protein turnover rate and k_1 = inversion rate and D and L are the optical isomers [3].

$$k_T = k_1\left[1-\left(D/\left(D+L\right)\right)\right]/\left[D/\left(D+L\right)\right]$$

9.2.3 Methods of Quantifying Aspartic Acid Racemization

The process of quantifying aspartic acid in a biological sample especially a tooth in this context involves multiple steps such as—Sampling strategy, Sample handling, Fraction analysis, Demineralization, Hydrolysis, and Chromatographic separation.

9.2.3.1 Sampling Strategy

Numerous studies have analyzed racemization in various regions of dentin, including primary and secondary dentine [51], as well as root and crown, and vertical sections of the crown (lingual vs. labial regions, vertical sections, vertical and horizontal sections) [21, 40, 45]. According to the common consensus, inconsistent findings are caused by variations inside each tooth's dentine, particularly in the secondary dentine, which is formed more recently. This is due to the fact that dentine age is not the same as chronological age and that the age of the tooth upon extraction must be adjusted for the time it takes for the tooth to form [21]. Ohtani advises utilizing entire longitudinal sections rather than transverse ones taken from the center of the tooth since racemization differs from labial to lingual sides ([46] [49]). Researchers, like Mornstad et al.., concluded that root dentine supplied accurate age estimates because it has been proved to give a faster racemization rate than crowns [38]. This dentine is less prone to dental disease, the development of reparative dentine, and/or dental therapy since it is younger than the crown dentine.

9.2.3.2 Sample Handling

Tissue Fixation

Tooth samples that have been preserved in fixatives like formaldehyde have been used [43] in many investigations. Proteins are known to be crosslinked by formaldehyde, particularly at amino, amide, and guanidino side chains. As a result, soluble proteins can be bound to the insoluble (collagen-rich) matrix. Formalin fixatives are not advised since the amount of racemization produced by acid hydrolysis varies in the acid-soluble extract of formaldehyde-stored dentine [19].

Other researchers have removed any adhering soft tissue from the teeth using sodium hypochlorite rather than formalin. It is possible to sterilize and remove soft tissue by immersing all of the teeth in undiluted bleach for a whole night. Conversely, hypochlorite will penetrate the dentine, and if oxidation is selective, prolonged exposure could alter the D&L Asx ratio, making it technique-dependent.

Tissue Washing

Washing is an equally crucial phase as fixation. The acetone wash and 0.2 M HCl are the two basic methods for washing samples. Acetone is preferred over phosphophoryns (PPs)because an acid wash can eliminate low molecular weight amino acids from the sample. Additionally, it has been noted that components involved in quick racemization disappear higher PP concentrations, which ultimately affects the aspartic acid enantiomer ratio [26].

Pulverization

Pulverizing calcified tissues before demineralization and protein extraction is widely used in sample preparation when a chelating agent like ethylenediaminetetraacetic acid (EDTA) is used in place of a mineral acid [10]. Although this might speed up the extraction process, it has been suggested that the severe mechanical breakdown of calcified tissues could lead to the degradation of artifactual proteins. Possible causes of deterioration include mechanical shearing of collagen or a mechanochemical effect, in which chemical reactions are triggered by mechanical movements like fracture and deformation [34]. It is advised that pulverization by grinding be carried out in liquid nitrogen (−18 °C; heating rate of 15 °C/min, SPEX Mill) for 3 min, as heat production may play a role in protein breakdown [55].

9.2.3.3 Fraction Analyzed

The total protein proportion of dentine has been the most frequently reported racemization in earlier investigations, and it seems to be adequately trustworthy for determining age [41]. The operational terms for these components are the soluble and insoluble fractions, and the extraction technique affects how they are prepared. The insoluble fraction has the slowest rate of racemization because triple-helical collagen makes up the majority of its composition [58]. The component that racemizes the quickest is the soluble protein fraction, making it the most precise for estimating age. However, it's critical to restrict acid exposure and keep the extraction temperature as low as possible to prevent harming the labile proteins in this fraction, particularly the Asx-rich PPs [44].

9.2.3.4 Demineralization

To isolate a portion of the total dentine protein, demineralization is required; this is commonly done using mineral acid (HCl) or, less frequently, a chelating agent (typically EDTA). Dentine must be ground into powder prior to the EDTA treatment in order to shorten the extraction period (2 weeks with solution changes). To stop the action of native dentine proteolytic enzymes, protease inhibitors (PIs) must also be included. Without the use of PIs, HCl demineralization is substantially quicker and simpler and can be applied to dentine. The recommended method for demineralization utilizes 0.6 N HCl with continuous agitation at -4C. It is essential that low temperature is used throughout preparation, otherwise peptide bond hydrolysis and racemization will occur [12].

9.2.3.5 Hydrolysis

The dentine sample is typically hydrolyzed with 6 M HCl at 100 °C for 6 h [54]. There are variations, though (Shimoyama and Harada: 108 °C for 20 h; Carolan et al.: 110 °C for 9 h) [9]. When comparing rates amongst investigations, racemization is a factor that must be taken into account due to longer hydrolysis times. According to Csapo' et al., shorter hydrolysis times at higher temperatures will lead to less racemization for the same amount of peptide bond hydrolysis because hydrolysis has a larger activation energy (28 kcal/mol) than racemization (22 kcal/mol) [15].

9.2.3.6 Chromatographic Separation

Separating and quantifying D- and L-Asp enantiomers in dentine have been performed using both HPLC and GC techniques. Both strategies have advantages and disadvantages, and one is not always superior to the other.

High-Performance Liquid Chromatography (HPLC)

The downside of the initial ion-exchange HPLC technique, used by Gillard et al. and Masters, is that it only allows the analysis of Asp and requires a lengthy elution period. Reverse-phase liquid chromatography using precolumn o-phthaldehyde (OPA) derivatization is a more effective HPLC technique [21]. Recently, modifications to this HPLC strategy have been employed with encouraging outcomes. Proline and Hyp, two crucial signs of collagen presence, do not cause an OPA reagent reaction, on the other hand [28].

Gas Chromatography (GC)

Research using GC is preferred in the field of forensic science [51]. All of the amino acids can be separated and quantified in one chromatographic run using a chiral capillary column. The amino acids are commonly derivatized as N-trifluoroacetic acid isopropyl esters [62]. The stationary phase's sensitivity to oxygen and the coelution of a Hyp derivative with L-Asp are two downsides of GC, though. No specific chromatography method is recommended, despite the fact that some of the authors have encountered difficulties with the widely used GC methodology due to interference with Hyp. The calibration standards for the method should be carefully selected and appropriate for the approach. Ideally, these should be processed simultaneously with the test samples from pools of dentine samples with known D/L ratios [62] (Fig. 9.2).

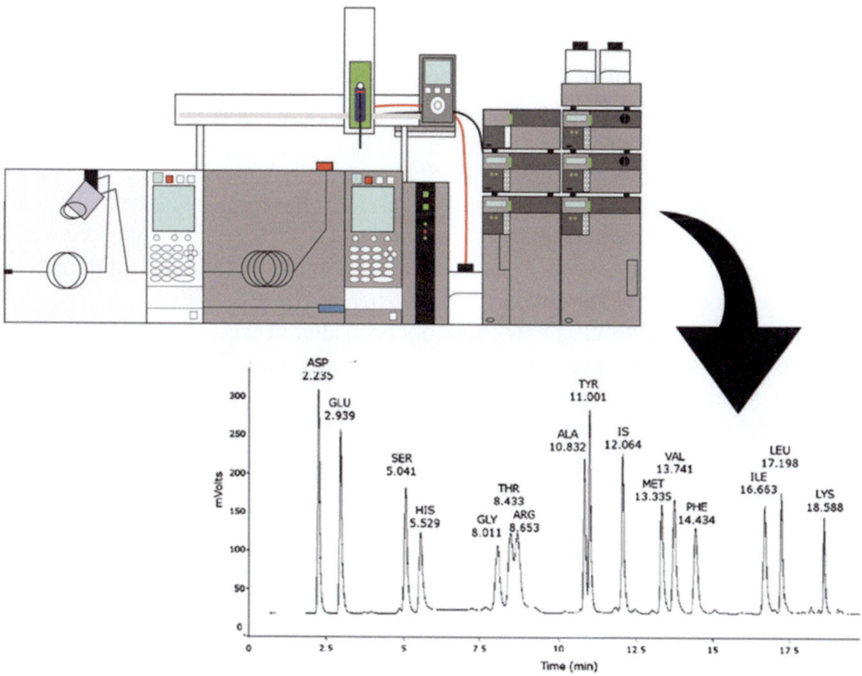

Fig. 9.2 Result page of the software analysis of HPLC & GC

9.3 Dental Age Estimation Through Radiocarbon Dating

Various kinds of carbon-containing compounds can be discovered in various environments around the world. These materials are cycled through various carbon reservoirs using solar energy over a range of timescales. The photosynthetic cycle—which includes the fixation of atmospheric carbon dioxide in plant materials, the incorporation of a small amount of this carbon into animal tissues, and subsequent decomposition, and the cycling of different chemical species in the oceans, atmosphere, and major lake systems (carbon dioxide, carbonate, bicarbonate), are the two major systems that interact to produce this process. Numerous geologic occurrences, such as the deposition of carbonates in sediments and volcanic activity, have an impact on the carbon cycle. There are three naturally existing isotopes of carbon: two stable (12C and 13C) and one unstable or radioactive (^{14}C). With a half-life of roughly 5700 years, ^{14}C is a naturally occurring radioactive isotope of carbon. One unintended effect of cosmic ray bombardment is the natural creation of ^{14}C in the high atmosphere. After being produced, it undergoes oxidation to produce $^{14}Co2$, which spreads ^{14}C throughout the atmosphere of the globe. Only a small amount enters the terrestrial ecology; the vast majority is absorbed by the oceans [13].

9.4 General Consideration for Radiocarbon Dating

Radiocarbon dating requires several specific assumptions to be true for the result to be precise relatively limited boundaries for a radiocarbon age to be equal to its real or calendar age at a satisfactory degree of precision [59]. These assumptions can be summarized as follows:

1. The concentration of ^{14}C in each carbon reservoir has remained essentially constant over the ^{14}C time scale.
2. On a global scale, there has been complete and rapid mixing of ^{14}C throughout the various carbon reservoirs.
3. Carbon isotope ratios in samples have not been altered except by ^{14}C decay since these sample materials ceased to be an active part of one of the carbon reservoirs (as at the death of an organism).
4. The half-life of^{14}C is accurately known.
5. Natural levels of ^{14}C can be measured to appropriate levels of accuracy and precision.

For the technique to be used critically there must also be a known connection or association between the material to be researched and some particular event or phenomenon to be dated. Experts in radiocarbon are still looking into the five suppositions listed above. The contextual requirement is typically met by the field archaeologist, geologist, or historical specialist who collects and submits materials for investigations.

9.5 Production and Distribution of Radiocarbon

A variety of nuclear processes can result in the generation of ^{14}C. However, the most common natural process involves the bombardment of ^{14}N by cosmic-ray-produced neutrons in a rather restricted energy range [35]. The proton component of cosmic rays collides with gaseous components of the atmosphere, resulting in the production of neutrons in a spallation process. In laboratory research, other products of neutron reactions with ^{14}N have been discovered, however ^{14}C will occur in over 90% of these collisions [8]. It's worth noting that, due to the availability of atmospheric nitrogen, modest variations in nitrogen concentration in the atmosphere have little influence on ^{14}C synthesis, which is governed solely by neutron supply. It is widely assumed that practically all ^{14}C atoms will have been oxidized to generate carbon dioxide within a few minutes or at most many hours. The precise mechanisms involved, however, remain unknown. Natural ^{14}C makes its first appearance in the terrestrial carbon cycle as $^{14}Co_2$ [4]. Several researchers have suggested that cosmic-ray-produced neutrons (or neutrons produced by lightning strikes) could produce ^{14}C in situ in plant structures (particularly wood) at relatively high altitudes. Even under the most ideal circumstances, the effect on wood from high altitude locales would be minimal over the Holocene and probably over the last 50,000 years, according to Harkness and Burleigh [24]; Radnell et al. [48, 16]. Geographic location affects the rate at which the atmosphere naturally produces ^{14}C. Any change in this quantity will immediately affect how quickly ^{14}C is created because the amount of ^{14}C produced is dependent on neutron intensity. Cosmic-ray neutron intensity in the geomagnetic poles is approximately five times more than at the equator. Fortunately, this gradient in ^{14}C concentration mostly disappears after individual $^{14}CO_2$ molecules are mixed by air turbulence, especially in the lower portions of the earth's atmosphere.

9.6 Decay of Radiocarbon

Radiocarbon decays into ^{14}N and a neutrino by producing a beta particle. Beta particles are a type of high-speed electron that is released from nuclei and has a wide range of energy. The highest energy of ^{14}C beta emissions is roughly 0.156 MeV (1 MeV = 106 electron volts), putting it in the weak beta emitter category [6].

9.7 Methodology of Radiocarbon Dating

Radiocarbon dating can be conducted with a wide range of samples but in this context only calcified organic samples will be discussed. The goal is to explore the challenges surrounding the use of various types of organics as samples for ^{14}C analysis in terms of physical and chemical features. When assessing the integrity of sample materials, contamination and fractionation effects must be considered.

9.7.1 Contamination

Contamination is the process of non-indigenous organics being incorporated into a sample matrix. The impacts of foreign carbon on ^{14}C readings are determined by the type and condition of the sample material, the characteristics of the geochemical environments in which the sample has been immersed, and the time period over which such actions took place. Because each circumstance is different, the measures taken to avoid contaminating consequences may need to be tailored to each one [47].

9.7.2 Fractionation

Natural fluctuations in carbon isotope levels can cause fractionation, it can also happen during the processing of samples in the laboratory if specific safeguards are not taken. Variations in stable carbon ratios ($^{13}C/^{12}C$) have been shown to have a predictable influence on the $^{14}C/^{12}C$ ratio [14]. This discovery contradicted one of the ^{14}C method's basic assumptions, namely that there were no other influences on the $^{14}C/^{12}C$ ratio beyond ^{14}C decay. Following $^{13}C/^{12}C$ measurements (usually represented as $\delta^{13}C$), it was discovered that organic compounds contain a wide range of $\delta^{13}C$ values. The differences in $\delta^{13}C$ levels between terrestrial and marine animals are particularly noticeable. A broad agreement has emerged on a set of criteria and processes for converting samples with varied $\delta^{13}C$ levels to a single scale [14].

9.8 Sample Pretreatment Strategies

The goal of sample pretreatment is to get rid of any carbon-containing compounds that could have differing ^{14}C activity than the native sample material. Major contaminants can be grouped into four broad categories (i) physically removable, (ii) acid soluble, (iii) base soluble, and (iv) solvent soluble. A careful visual assessment of the sample and manual removal of visible surface and/or invasive non-sample material, such as rootlets and microorganisms, are the initial steps in any laboratory preparation. Cutting the surface layer off of somewhat solid macro sample materials may be helpful. In order to document the physical characteristics of the sample material, a close visual examination is required. The type of carbon-containing chemicals that make up the sample should be carefully identified as a first priority [52].

The most common pretreatment is the use of acidic solutions, such as hydrochloric acid (HCl), to eliminate absorbed carbonates. Because the ^{14}C activities of dissolved $CaCo_3$ are often substantially lower than current values, such pretreatment is required. Because of the likelihood of exchange with ambient CO_2, while a sample is being pretreated, extractions with NaOH or other base solutions must be carefully carried out. This difficulty is usually avoided by reacidifying the sample once the base solution has been removed by filtering and washing [52].

9.9 Preparation of Calcified Organic Samples

Aliquots of the samples are placed in culture tubes for pre-treatment between sample generation and analysis in order to remove any surface carbon that might have contaminated the hard tissue. Since tooth material has a carbon concentration of 0.5–0.6%, full-sized samples for 14C analysis are typically prepared using aliquots of 80–150 mg. The samples are first soaked in 1.0 N HCl for 1.5 h at room temperature, followed by three washes in 18.2 M DDH_2O and an overnight drying period at 95 ° C on a heating block. The goal of the acid pre-treatment is to etch, rather than fully dissolve, the outer surface that has previously been subjected to a harsh alkali environment [56]. The base always contains some carbonate throughout this preparation stage, which may interact with tooth structure. Alkali solutions also precipitate carbonate and bicarbonate in solution while absorbing CO_2 from the atmosphere. Each dried sample is divided into 5–10 pieces and placed in a single-use reactor before being once more weighed to the nearest 0.1 mg. The stronger acid etching method removes a few milligrams of the outer enamel surface from a 100 mg sample. Sample splits are hydrolyzed to CO_2 in separate reaction chambers, then evacuated, heated, and acidified at 90 ° C with concentrated orthophosphoric acid. In separate reactors, the evolved CO_2 is filtered, trapped, and reduced to graphite in the presence of an iron catalyst. When aliquots are used, almost all CO_2 samples are greater than 500 g C. CO_2 is split using stable isotope ratio mass spectrometry, and 13C is found. For samples that are too small to establish a CO_2 split, a 13C correction of 15 +/2 is commonly utilized. Background values are kept under control by sticking to protocols, baking sample tubes and CuO oxidizer on a regular basis, and keeping the lab clean [25].

9.10 Accelerator Mass Spectrometry (AMS) Analysis

The measurement of graphite targets is carried out by the 10-MV HVEE FN-class tandem electrostatic AMS equipment. The method was utilized to obtain highly accurate readings of secondary standards for turbidities that were 18,000 years old [5]. The device makes use of a high-output negative ion solid graphite Cs-sputter source developed by LLNL that can sputter 250–350 g of $^{12}C^-$ from a full-sized sample, or roughly 900 counts of ^{14}C per second from a current sample. The overall system efficiency of the FN AMS system is about 15%. Timeframes for analysis are brief, usually less than 5 min, because dental samples are commonly full-sized and recent. By calculating the contributions from present and fossil carbon, Brown and Southon explain how to account for background contamination created during AMS sample processing. All data are standardized using six identically produced NIST SRM 4990B (Oxalic Acid I) primary standards. Oxalic acid II, IAEA-C6, and TIRI wood are secondary standards and quality controls for spectrometer performance [7].

9.11 From ^{14}C Measurement to Age Estimation

Based on the particular tooth and the person's sex, the typical age at which tooth development is complete has previously been determined. When the sex is unknown, the typical tooth-development time for boys and girls can be calculated. The ^{14}C content recorded in the tooth is compared to Levin and Kromer's or Calibomb's reference data (http://calib.qub.ac.uk/CALIBomb) to establish a person's year of tooth development. The average development time for each type of tooth can be subtracted to approximate the person's birthdate. If it's not clear whether a person was born before or after the peak of atmospheric ^{14}C levels caused by the bomb testing, two teeth with differing formation periods can be examined to see if the ^{14}C measurement corresponds to the rising or decreasing section of the curve [32].

9.12 Limitation of the Histochemical Method of Dental Age Estimation

In comparison to radiographic or histological approaches, the histochemical approach to determining dental age is more precise. These tactics concentrate on procedural facts as opposed to subjective assessments. The primary drawback of the aspartic acid racemization rate technique for determining dental age is that it heavily depends on the ratio of D & L aspartic isotopes. The rate of aspartic acid racemization in the oral cavity has been researched in relation to dental caries, dietary practices, and the placement of each type of tooth [50]. Teeth with caries and dentin involvement demonstrated a higher prevalence of aspartic acid racemization as compared to healthy teeth. This may be viewed as a drawback of this approach of age calculation, as an examination of such teeth would result in a misleading chronological age estimate. Teeth that are located deeper in the mouth, such as molars, particularly the third molar, have a greater incidence of amino acid racemization than teeth that are located more anteriorly.

Radiocarbon dating, on the other hand, is based on the concentration of ^{14}C carbon in a sample. This concentration varies depending on the sample type; calcified structures keep roughly the same amount of ^{14}C, but soft tissue such as blood, nail, and hair may have a varied amount of radioactive carbon due to tissue turnover [60]. The approach is based on the fact that ambient levels of radiocarbon have been greatly influenced by above-ground nuclear weapons testing in the mid-twentieth-century during the previous 60 years. Before the nuclear age, there was minimal variation in the amount of radiocarbon in the environment over a century. Between 1955 and 1963, however, atmospheric radiocarbon levels nearly quadrupled. They've been gradually returning to natural levels since then. The quantity of radiocarbon in humans or their remains has changed dramatically over the last six decades, depending on when they were born or, more specifically, when their tissues were developed. Because the quantity of ^{14}C in the atmosphere is progressively reverting to its original level, this suggests a limited duration of value [61]. This approach should continue to be helpful for year-of-birth calculations for anyone born in the next 10 or 20 years, barring any new nuclear detonations. After then, everyone born would be anticipated to have the same level of carbon-14 as before the nuclear testing era [23].

9.13 Future Prospective of Dental Age Estimation Through Histochemical Methods

Despite the fact that the aspartic acid racemization approach for estimating dental age is accurate and dependable, further inter-laboratory study is needed. As previously said, numerous important factors must be investigated, and a uniform SOP must be constructed. Because the degree of racemization varies with regional and demographic variables, population-specific algorithms are also necessary. To provide scientifically better results, improvements in sample handling methods are also necessary.

Modern bomb-pulse radiocarbon dating was most precise during the 1960s and 1970s, when atmospheric radiocarbon levels peaked. However, this accuracy has gradually declined since then as atmospheric radiocarbon concentrations have approached pre-bomb levels. Within the next few decades, atmospheric radiocarbon concentrations are anticipated to fall below pre-1950 levels [23]. Samples will have the same amounts of ^{14}C as artifacts from the previous several centuries until atmospheric radiocarbon activity falls below that of 1950 AD. A sample from 2050 AD, for example, may have the same radiocarbon date as one from 1050 AD, while a sample from 2100 AD could have the same date as one from 100 AD [23]. To clarify this issue and ensure that a sample is from the twenty-first century rather than a historical relic, investigators will at the very least require additional contextual and taphonomic evidence which leads us to the challenging future of age estimation through radiocarbon dating.

9.14 Multiple Choice Questions

Q1. Which of the following types enantiomer is favored by the ribosomal subunit?
- (a) L—enantiomer
- (b) D—enantiomer
- (c) Both of them
- (d) None of them

Ans: a

Q2. Concentration of which enantiomer increases with age?
- (a) L—enantiomer
- (b) D—enantiomer
- (c) Both of them
- (d) None of them

Ans: b

Q3. Which is the more accurate method for dental age estimation?
(a) Analysis of aspartic acid racemization
(b) Radio carbon dating
(c) Both of them
(d) None of them

Ans: b

Q4. Major drawback of dental age estimation through radiocarbon dating?
(a) Sample preparation
(b) High cost of analysis
(c) Gradual normalization of ^{14}C isotope in the atmosphere
(d) Technique sensitivity

Ans: c

Q5. Major drawback of dental age estimation through analysis of aspartic acid racemization?
(a) Sample preparation
(b) High cost of analysis
(c) Effect on the rate of racemization due to presence of any pathology
(d) Technique sensitivity

Ans: c

References

1. Bada JL, Helfman PM. Amino acid racemization dating of fossil bones. World Archaeol. 1975;7(2):160–73.
2. Bada JL, McDonald GD. Peer reviewed: detecting amino acids on Mars. Anal Chem. 1996;68(21):668A–73A.
3. Bank RA, Bayliss MT, Lafeber FP, Maroudas A, Tekoppele JM. Ageing and zonal variation in post-translational modification of collagen in normal human articular cartilage: the age-related increase in non-enzymatic glycation affects biomechanical properties of cartilage. Biochem J. 1998;330(1):345–51.
4. Baxter MS, Farmer JG. Radiocarbon: short-term variations. Earth Planet Sci Lett. 1973;20(3):295–9.
5. Brock F, Higham T, Ditchfield P, Ramsey CB. Current pretreatment methods for AMS radiocarbon dating at the Oxford radiocarbon accelerator unit (ORAU). Radiocarbon. 2010;52(1):103–12.
6. Bronk RC. Radiocarbon dating: revolutions in understanding. Archaeometry. 2008;50(2):249–75.
7. Brown TA, Nelson DE, Vogel JS, Southon JR. Improved collagen extraction by modified Longin method. Radiocarbon. 1988;30(2):171–7.
8. Campbell JA. Past variations of natural radiocarbon as recorded in UK wood. University of Glasgow (United Kingdom); 1977.
9. Carolan VA, Gardner ML, Lucy D, Pollard AM. Some considerations regarding the use of amino acid racemization in human dentine as an indicator of age at death. J Forensic Sci. 1997;42(1):10–6.
10. Cloos P. Age related changes of proteins in human dentin. Konservatorskolen; 1995.
11. Cloos PA, Fledelius C. Collagen fragments in urine derived from bone resorption are highly racemized and isomerized: a biological clock of protein aging with clinical potential. Biochem J. 2000;345(3):473–80.

12. Collins MJ, Galley P. Towards an optimal method of archaeological collagen extraction: the influence of pH and grinding. Anc Biomol. 1998;2(2/3):209–23.
13. Craig H. Mass-spectrometer analyses of radiocarbon standards. Radiocarbon. 1961;3:1–3.
14. Craig H. The geochemistry of the stable carbon isotopes. Geochim Cosmochim Acta. 1953;3(2–3):53–92.
15. Csapó J, Csapó-Kiss Z, Wágner L, Tálos T, Martin TG, Folestad S, Tivesten A, Némethy S. Hydrolysis of proteins performed at high temperatures and for short times with reduced racemization, in order to determine the enantiomers of D-and L-amino acids. Anal Chim Acta. 1997;339(1–2):99–107.
16. Damon PE, Sternberg RS, Radnell CJ. Modeling of atmospheric radiocarbon fluctuations for the past three centuries. Radiocarbon. 1983;25(2):249–58.
17. David RS, Richard AW. Manual of forensnic odontology: 5th ed. American society of forensic odontology. CRC Press; 2013. p. 34.
18. Fountoulakis M, Lahm HW. Hydrolysis and amino acid composition analysis of proteins. J Chromatogr A. 1998;826(2):109–34.
19. French D, Edsall JT. The reactions of formaldehyde with amino acids and proteins. Adv Protein Chem. 1945;2:277–335.
20. Geiger T, Clarke S. Deamidation, isomerization, and racemization at asparaginyl and aspartyl residues in peptides. Succinimide-linked reactions that contribute to protein degradation. J Biol Chem. 1987;262(2):785–94.
21. Gillard RD, Pollard AM, Sutton PA, Whittaker DK. An improved method for age at death determination from the measurement of D-aspartic acid in dental collagen. Archaeometry. 1990;32(1):61–70.
22. Goodman AH, Allen LH, Hernandez GP, Amador A, Arriola LV, Chávez A, Pelto GH. Prevalence and age at development of enamel hypoplasias in Mexican children. American Journal of Physical Anthropology. 1987;72(1):7–19.
23. Graven HD. Impact of fossil fuel emissions on atmospheric radiocarbon and various applications of radiocarbon over this century. Proc Natl Acad Sci. 2015;112(31):9542–5.
24. Harkness DD, Burleigh AR. Possible carbon-14 enrichment in high altitude wood. Archaeometry. 1974;16(2):121–7.
25. Hedges RE, Lee-Thorp JA, Tuross NC. Is tooth enamel carbonate a suitable material for radiocarbon dating? Radiocarbon. 1995;37(2):285–90.
26. Helfman PM, Bada JL. Aspartic acid racemisation in dentine as a measure of ageing. Nature. 1976;262(5566):279–81.
27. Helfman PM, Bada JL. Aspartic acid racemization in tooth enamel from living humans. Proc Natl Acad Sci. 1975;72(8):2891–4.
28. Jones BN, Pääbo S, Stein S. Amino acid analysis and enzymatic sequence determination of peptides by an improved o-phthaldialdehyde precolumn labeling procedure. J Liq Chromatogr. 1981;4(4):565–86.
29. Kimber RW, Hare PE. Wide range of racemization of amino acids in peptides from human fossil bone and its implications for amino acid racemization dating. Geochim Cosmochim Acta. 1992;56(2):739–43.
30. Kvenvolden K, Lawless J, Pering K, Peterson E, Flores J, Ponnamperuma C, Kaplan IR, Moore C. Evidence for extraterrestrial amino-acids and hydrocarbons in the Murchison meteorite. Nature. 1970;228(5275):923–6.
31. Kvenvolden KA, Lawless JG, Ponnamperuma C. Nonprotein amino acids in the Murchison meteorite. Proc Natl Acad Sci. 1971;68(2):486–90.
32. Levin IN, Kromer BE, Hammer SA. Atmospheric Δ14CO2 trend in Western European background air from 2000 to 2012. Tellus B: Chemical and Physical Meteorology. 2013;65(1):20092.
33. Libby WF. Radiocarbon dating. Science. 1961;133(3453):621–9.
34. Linde A, Bhown M, Butler WT. Noncollagenous proteins of dentin. A re-examination of proteins from rat incisor dentin utilizing techniques to avoid artifacts. J Biol Chem. 1980;255(12):5931–42.

35. Lingenfelter RE. Production of carbon 14 by cosmic-ray neutrons. Rev Geophys. 1963;1(1):35–55.
36. Masters PM, Bada JL, Zigler JS. Aspartic acid racemisation in the human lens during ageing and in cataract formation. Nature. 1977;268(5615):71–3.
37. McCudden CR, Kraus VB. Biochemistry of amino acid racemization and clinical application to musculoskeletal disease. Clin Biochem. 2006;39(12):1112–30.
38. Mörnstad H, Pfeiffer H, Teivens A. Estimation of dental age using HPLC-technique to determine the degree of aspartic acid racemization. J Forensic Sci. 1994;39(6):1425–31.
39. Motoie R, Fujii N, Tsunoda S, Nagata K, Shimo-oka T, Kinouchi T, Fujii N, Saito T, Ono K. Localization of d-β-aspartyl residue-containing proteins in various tissues. Int J Mol Sci. 2009;10(5):1999–2009.
40. Ogino T, Ogino H, Nagy B. Application of aspartic acid racemization to forensic odontology: post mortem designation of age at death. Forensic Sci Int. 1985;29(3–4):259–67.
41. Ohtani S, Kato S, Sugeno H, Sugimoto H, Marumo T, Yamazaki M, Yamamoto K. A study on the use of the amino-acid racemization method to estimate the ages of unidentified cadavers from their teeth. Bull Kanagawa Dent Coll. 1988;16(1):11–21.
42. Ohtani S, Ohhira H, Watanabe A, Ogasawara A, Sugimoto H. Estimation of age from teeth by amino acid racemization: influence of fixative. J Forensic Sci. 1997;42(1):137–9.
43. Ohtani S, Yamamoto K. Age estimation using the racemization of amino acid in human dentin. J Forensic Sci. 1991;36(3):792–800.
44. Ohtani S, Yamamoto K. Estimating age through the amino acid racemization of acid-soluble dentinal peptides. Nihon hoigaku zasshi= The Japanese journal of legal medicine. 1990;44(4):342–5.
45. Ohtani S. Different racemization ratios in dentin from different locations within a tooth. Growth, development, and aging: GDA. 1997;61(2):93–9.
46. Ohtani S. Estimation of age from dentin by using the racemization reaction of aspartic acid. Am J Forensic Med Pathol. 1995;16(2):158–61.
47. Olson EA. The problem of sample contamination in radiocarbon dating. Columbia University; 1963.
48. Radnell CJ, Aitken MJ, Otlet RL. In situ 14C production in wood. In: Berger, R, Suess, HE, editors. Radiocarbon Dating. Proceedings of the Ninth International Conference. Los Angeles and La Jolla 1976. University of California Press; 1979. p. 643–57.
49. Ritz S, Schütz HW, Peper C. Postmortem estimation of age at death based on aspartic acid racemization in dentin: its applicability for root dentin. Int J Legal Med. 1993;105(5):289–93.
50. Ritz-Timme S, Collins MJ. Racemization of aspartic acid in human proteins. Ageing Res Rev. 2002;1(1):43–59.
51. Saleh N, Deutsch D, Gil-Av E. Racemization of aspartic acid in the extracellular matrix proteins of primary and secondary dentin. Calcif Tissue Int. 1993;53(2):103–10.
52. Sava TB, Simion CA, Gâza O, Stanciu IM, Păceşilă DG, Sava GO, Wacker L, Ştefan B, Moşu VD, Ghiță DG, Vasiliu A. Status report on the sample preparation laboratory for radiocarbon dating at the new Bucharest RoAMS center. Radiocarbon. 2019;61(2):649–58.
53. Schroeder RA, Bada JL. A review of the geochemical applications of the amino acid racemization reaction. Earth Sci Rev. 1976;12(4):347–91.
54. Shimoyama A, Harada K. An age determination of an ancient burial mound man by apparent racemization reaction of aspartic acid in tooth dentin. Chem Lett. 1984;13(10):1661–4.
55. Sohma J. Mechanochemistry of polymers. Prog Polym Sci. 1989;14(4):451–596.
56. Stafford TW, Jull AT, Brendel K, Duhamel RC, Donahue D. Study of bone radiocarbon dating accuracy at the University of Arizona NSF accelerator facility for radioisotope analysis. Radiocarbon. 1987;29(1):24–44.
57. Stavrianos CH, Mastagas D, Stavrianou I, Karaiskou O. Dental age estimation of adults: a review of methods and principals. Res J Med Sci. 2008;2(5):258–68.
58. Takagi Y, Veis A. Isolation of phosphophoryn from human dentin organic matrix. Calcif Tissue Int. 1984;36(1):259–65.

59. Taylor R. Radiocarbon dating of Pleistocene bone: toward criteria for the selection of samples. Radiocarbon. 1980;22(3):969–79.
60. Ubelaker DH. Radiocarbon analysis of human remains: a review of forensic applications. J Forensic Sci. 2014;59(6):1466–72.
61. Vogel JC, Fuls A, Visser E. Accurate dating with radiocarbon from the atom bomb tests: research in action. S Afr J Sci. 2002;98(9):437–8.
62. Waite ER, Collins MJ, Van Duin AC. Hydroxyproline interference during the gas chromatographic analysis of D/L aspartic acid in human dentine. Int J Legal Med. 1999;112(2):124–31.
63. Wehmiller J, Hare PE. Racemization of amino acids in marine sediments. Science. 1971;173(4000):907–11.
64. Wigley TM, Muller A. Fractionation corrections in radiocarbon dating. Radiocarbon. 1981;23(2):173–90.
65. Willems G. A review of the most commonly used dental age estimation techniques. J Forensic Odontostomatol. 2001;19(1):9–17.
66. Zello GA, Menendez CE, Rafii M, Clarke R, Wykes LJ, Ball RO, Pencharz PB. Minimum protein intake for the preterm neonate determined by protein and amino acid kinetics. Pediatr Res. 2003;53(2):338–44.

Lesser-Known Methods for Dental Age Estimation

10

Ivan Bedek and Ivana Čuković-Bagić

Abbreviations

AaA	Age of attainment
ASA	Average stage of attrition
DARLInG	Dental Age Research London Information Group
RDS	Reference data sheet
TDS	Tooth developmental stage

10.1 Introduction

There are numerous methods for dental age estimation that have been seldom used and are mentioned only rarely, even though they blazed the trail for those methods commonly used today. Some methods have been introduced recently and await detailed verification of their accuracy and applicability. Although it is difficult to recount all the methods for dental age estimation mentioned in the literature, the most important lesser-known methods have been selected for discussion in this chapter.

I. Bedek (✉)
Bedek Dental Clinic, Zagreb, Croatia
e-mail: ivanbedek@bedek.hr

I. Čuković-Bagić
Department of Paediatric and Preventive Dentistry, University of Zagreb, School of Dental Medicine, University Hospital Centre Zagreb, Zagreb, Croatia
e-mail: cukovic-bagic@sfzg.hr

© The Author(s), under exclusive license to Springer Nature Switzerland AG 2026

A. Chowdhry, P. Kapoor (eds.), *Dental Age Assessment*,
https://doi.org/10.1007/978-3-032-08788-1_10

10.2 The Gustafson Method

In 1950, Gösta Gustafson [1] introduced a new method for age estimation using six age-related changes observed in teeth after eruption. These changes included attrition, change of the level of periodontal attachment, secondary dentin deposition, resorption of the root, cementum apposition, and root translucency. Translucency was rated on a 1 mm ground section and the other five changes on a 0.25 mm thick ground section. All observed changes were rated with values 0 to 3 (Fig. 10.1). Age was estimated according to the equation '$Age = 11.43 + 4.56x$' where 'x' represents the sum of the values (0–3) pertaining to the six parameters observed.

The teeth used by Gustafson were extracted from individuals of determined age. Their age combined with the sum of the values derived from observed changes in the teeth enabled the construction of a regression line with an average error in age estimation of 3.63 years. Gustafson observed that the accuracy of age estimation increases if more than one tooth is used in the estimation process.

The method is limited in scope. Apart from age, other factors can and do exert an influence on the six observed changes that Gustafson used. These factors must be considered. Bruxism, diet, morphology of the teeth, the direction and force of masticatory movements as well as the number of teeth present in the mouth can affect the amount of dental hard tissue loss. Deposition of secondary dentine can be influenced by attrition, abrasion, periodontal disease as well as by caries and dental treatment. Periodontal disease changes the periodontal attachment level. Cementum apposition can be influenced by periapical pathology. Root resorption can be induced by dental trauma, periapical periodontitis, excessive force, hormonal imbalances and pressure from impacted teeth. Translucency can be affected by periodontal infection and different pathologies of the pulp [2].

Despite these limitations, Gustafson's method has been tested in numerous populations, and it should be stated that the methodology used has given rise to the development of other methods for dental age estimation among adults.

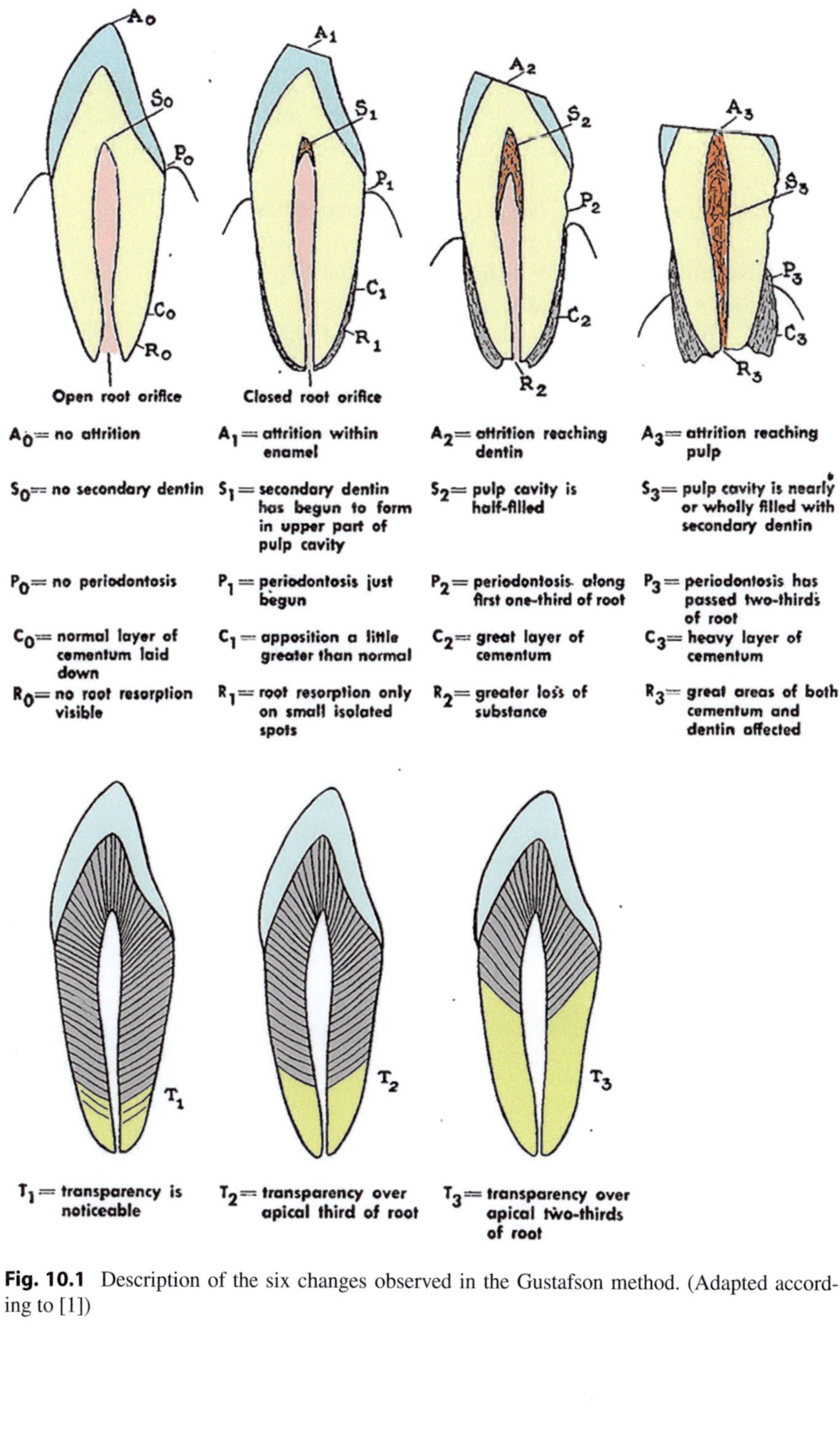

Fig. 10.1 Description of the six changes observed in the Gustafson method. (Adapted according to [1])

10.3 The Li and Ji Method

A method for age estimation based on the average stage of molar attrition was presented in 1995 by Li and Ji [3]. The sample originated from 57 cadavers and 54 modern dry skulls in north-eastern China; this enabled 633 molars to be analysed.

The ten stages of attrition (Fig. 10.2) were described as follows:

Stage 0: No attrition. The cusp is sharp. Gullies and ridges are clear.
Stage 1: Slight attrition on the top and ridges of the cusp.
Stage 2: Cusp appears obtuse, or a limited oblique facet appears on the surface.
Stage 3: The greater part of the cusp is worn away. The wear facet is depressed slightly or obviously and may connect with one or more other facets.
Stage 4: Dentine appears as a spot in which the average diameter is <1 mm.
Stage 5: Dentine appears as a spot in which the average diameter is >1 mm and the attrition plane is level or sunk deeply.
Stage 6: One exposed dentine spot coalesces with another and/or the cusp is almost entirely worn away.
Stage 7: One exposed dentine spot coalesces with two others and/or the cusp is entirely worn away.
Stage 8: Exposed dentine appears as a circle and there is a small starlike island of enamel within; the secondary dentine may also be exposed.
Stage 9: Dentine is exposed on the entire occlusal surface and the secondary dentine has been exposed.

Based on regression analysis, six linear equations were obtained that enabled age estimation based on the attrition condition of the first and second mandibular and maxillary molars, taking into consideration the average wear of all cusps named ASA (average stage of attrition). The ASA is calculated by dividing the sum of the

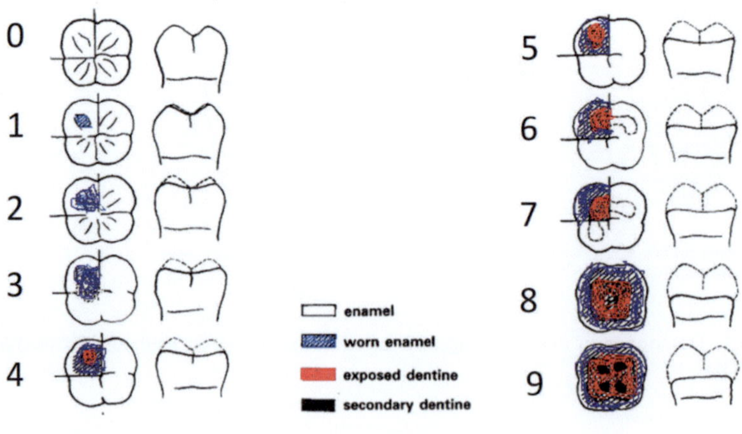

Fig. 10.2 Li and Ji stages of attrition. (Adapted according to [3])

Table 10.1 Equations for age estimation in the Li and Ji method

Jaw	No.	Equation
Maxilla	1	$Y = 11.42 + 6.32\ M_1$
	2	$Y = 14.44 + 7.44\ M_2$
	3	$Y = 12.23 + 4.11\ M_1 + 2.75\ M_2$
Mandible	1	$Y = 12.76 + 6.30\ M_1$
	2	$Y = 15.31 + 7.27\ M_2$
	3	$Y = 13.63 + 3.98\ M_1 + 2.83\ M_2$

Y is the estimated age, M_1 is ASA of the first molar and M_2 is ASA of the second molar

attrition stages of all the cusps by four. The equations for the age estimation are presented in Table 10.1.

As the authors claimed that there is no significant difference in attrition among men and women, the equations pertain to both sexes. The maximum error in age estimation was 4.53 years.

In 2000, a new scoring system for tooth wear in the service of age estimation was presented [4]. The authors noticed higher tooth wear scores among males; therefore, it was apparent that the equations for age estimation differed among sexes. Kim's scoring system provided an estimation of an individual's age within ±3 years in 42.4% of males and 49.4% of females, and within ±5 years in 61.8% of males and 63.3% of females.

Seven years later, Yun et al. modified Kim's scoring system, obtaining an increase in the accuracy of the age estimation [5]. They used 1092 pairs of full arch casts originating from the Korean population. New calculating tables for age estimation were designed by multiple linear regression analysis. According to the authors, the method is considered reliable and accurate for age estimation of the Korean population at any age above 20 years.

The above-mentioned methods were also tested in the American population [6]. The authors concluded that Kim's and Yun's methods can offer a seriation into 'older' and 'younger' adult categories and provide more reliable age interval estimates than cranial sutures in cases where only the skull is available. However, the application of these methodologies resulted in inaccurate age estimates. Approximately 60% of age estimates fell within ±10 years of the chronological age, which is a marked decline from the achieved accuracy in the original studies of Kim and Yun [4, 5].

Dental age estimation based solely on attrition was critiqued by Ball, who highlighted the weaknesses and limitations of this approach. Apart from physiological tooth wear linked to aging, multiple factors such as bruxism, diet, environment and medication significantly contribute to dental hard tissue loss resulting in uncertain and inaccurate age estimation [7].

10.4 The Moorreess-Fanning-Hunt Method

One of the most interesting studies based on context was published in 1963 by Coenraad F. A. Moorrees, Elisabeth A. Fanning and Edward E. Hunt Jr. [8]. The aim of the study was to "provide norms of the formation of ten permanent teeth"—all mandibular teeth and maxillary incisors. For this purpose, part of the sample was

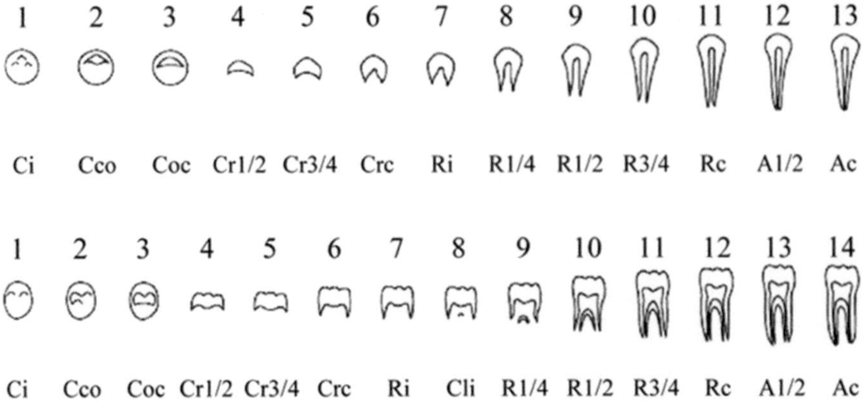

Fig. 10.3 Moorrees-Fanning-Hunt stages of development. (Adapted according to [8])

collected from a longitudinal study conducted at the School of Public Health, Harvard University. A larger part of the sample originated from the longitudinal data of the famous Fels program started in 1929—a longitudinal study in Yellow Springs, Ohio that followed children's development from birth to adulthood. The participants were Caucasian American children of middle socio-economic status. Dental health was excellent among these children and the development of their teeth was followed by lateral or oblique jaw radiographs that were taken at birth, at one, three, six, nine and twelve months and then continued at half-yearly intervals well into early adulthood.

A study of the depicted design would be unimaginable today; therefore, due to ethical issues, the data obtained can no longer be collected. Despite the significant ethical issues with regard to sample collection, the valuable data pertaining to dental development in early age is irreplaceable.

Morreesse, Fanning and Hunt used a thirteen-stage developmental scale for incisors and premolars and a fourteen-stage scale for molars (Fig. 10.3). As noted, this scale was previously used in Fanning's thesis [9] and represents a slight modification of the developmental stages used in previously published studies [10–12].

The results were presented in a graphical format that omitted the summary statistics, which is recognized as the main limitation of the study. However, this study is the only published longitudinal study to date that focuses on the development of permanent teeth in very young children from birth [13]. Moreover, its influence is clearly visible in the later studies that presented new methods for dental age estimation [14, 15].

10.5 The DARLInG Method

DARLInG is an acronym for Dental Age Research London Information Group. The webpage at www.dentalage.co.uk includes a direct mission statement: "an assembly of pages, diagrams, numerical explanations and statistics has been written to provide a detailed and understandable explanation of the theory and practice of dental age estimation". The goal of the project is to provide clear scientific information regarding dental age estimation for legal and clinical use.

In practice, this age estimation is based on determining the developmental stages of permanent teeth according to Demirjian's scale [15], which consists of eight developmental stages. The aim of the authors is to ensure that dental age estimation is always sex and ethnically specific. For that purpose, the process of age estimation is conducted using a prepared Excel file into which the developmental stages of permanent teeth are entered. After selecting a proper Reference Data Set (RDS), the calculation is carried out automatically.

The Reference Data Sets (RDS) are sex and ethnically specific tables that clearly show the Age at Attainment (AaA) for each Tooth Development Stage (TDS) for every permanent tooth. The information in the tables includes the average age of attainment (AaA) for certain TDS, standard deviation, minimal and maximal age for the TDS as well as age for the developmental stage of every permanent tooth within percentiles. "The DARLInG group" offers reference datasets for several populations, including British Caucasians, Hong Kong Chinese, Afro-Caribbean, Maltese, Israeli, South Korean and Western Saudi populations [16–19].

Since the DARLInG method closely refers to Demirjian's, both methods were tested and compared in the western Indian population [20]. The DARLInG method that used the British Caucasian RDS provided a relatively higher level of accuracy in age estimation compared to the Demirjian method. However, the difference between chronological and dental age was significant for both methods. This clearly indicates the link between the Demirjian and DARLInG methods. The similarity in the accuracy of age estimation derives from the origin of the sample used by Demirjian (French Canadian) and the British Caucasian RDS of the DARLInG method. Should the specific RDS for the chosen population be used, the DARLInG method would show similar results to the modified Demirjian method for the specific population.

The main advantage of the DARLInG method is the possibility to extract the data from each study that uses Demirjian's developmental scale to create population specific Reference Data Sheets (RDS). This information would represent a good reference, which is sex and ethnically specific for an accurate age estimation in the specific population.

10.6 Bedek et al. Models

A recent study published by Bedek et al. [21] questioned the possibility of an accurate and reliable age estimation method considering fewer than seven mandibular permanent teeth. Simply phrased, the greatest disadvantage of the Demirjian and Willems methods that are commonly used for dental age estimation in children is patent: it is impossible to estimate age if all seven mandibular permanent teeth are not present. This refers to cases of hypodontia and incomplete human remains as well as cases with early extracted permanent teeth. Based on Demirjian's developmental stages, the authors developed new models with new coefficients that enable age estimation using one to seven mandibular teeth (Table 10.2) on a representative sample of the Croatian population. Apart from the model with one tooth, all other models were found to be more accurate than the Willems method. Unlike most studies, the results of the age estimation were presented as a percentage of correct estimations within intervals of ±0.5, ±1, ±1.5 and ± 2 years. This method of presenting the results prevents misunderstanding in individual age estimation, which may occur when only the average mistake is presented as the measure of the accuracy.

Table 10.2 Coefficients and intercepts for different models with one to seven teeth. Age is to be calculated by formula: dental age = intercept + coefficients assigned to the stages of teeth in the model [21]

Model		Stage							
31–37	Tooth	A	B	C	D	E	F	G	H
	31	…	…	…	…	…	0.047	−0.108	0.737
Boys	32	…	…	…	…	…	0.408	0.134	0.624
	33	…	…	…	0.974	1598	2275	2484	3162
	34	…	…	…	−0.794	−0.375	0.295	0.502	1260
	35	…	…	2459	2159	2724	3038	3144	3258
	36	…	…	…	…	…	1416	1001	1263
	37	…	…	−1740	−2155	−1859	−1666	−1090	0.000
Intercept = 4.396									
Model		Stage							
31–37	Tooth	A	B	C	D	E	F	G	H
	31	…	…	…	…	…	1065	0.579	0.945
Girls	32	…	…	…	…	…	0.735	1163	1646
	33	…	…	…	0.415	0.189	0.479	0.784	1574
	34	…	…	…	1055	1202	1777	1983	2901
	35	…	…	…	−0.226	−0.264	0.052	−0.376	0.106
	36	…	…	…	…	…	−1090	−0.455	0.000
	37	…	…	…	−0.155	0.076	0.496	1014	2331
Intercept = 5.095									
Model		Stage							
31 33 34 35 36 37	Tooth	A	B	C	D	E	F	G	H
	31	…	…	…	…	…	0.139	0.048	0.938
Boys	33	…	…	…	0.826	1517	2381	2589	3268
	34	…	…	…	−0.865	−0.401	0.312	0.533	1292
	35	…	…	2365	2174	2712	3020	3130	3243
	36	…	…	…	…	…	1526	1006	1414
	37	…	…	−1653	−2144	−1846	−1662	−1090	0.000
Intercept = 4.544									
Model		Stage							
32 33 34 35 36 37	Tooth	A	B	C	D	E	F	G	H
	32	…	…	…	…	…	0.385	1022	1569
Girls	33	…	…	…	0.433	0.227	0.584	0.886	1676
	34	…	…	…	1037	1118	1676	1881	2799
	35	…	…	…	−0.202	−0.169	0.145	−0.283	0.199
	36	…	…	…	…	…	−1090	0.494	0.954
	37	…	…	…	−0.159	0.071	0.488	1007	2324

(continued)

Table 10.2 (continued)

Intercept = 5.077									
Model		Stage							
31 33 34 36 37	Tooth	A	B	C	D	E	F	G	H
	31	...	...	...	...	...	0.137	0.039	1049
Boys	33	...	...	...	0.706	1359	2249	2479	3183
	34	...	...	...	−0.835	−0.246	0.596	0.905	1713
	36	...	...	...	...	...	1410	0.902	1332
	37	...	...	0.717	0.171	0.712	0.980	1604	2754
Intercept = 4.664									
Model		Stage							
32 33 34 36 37	Tooth	A	B	C	D	E	F	G	H
	32	...	...	...	...	...	0.396	1067	1615
Girls	33	...	...	...	0.431	0.222	0.577	0.872	1700
	34	...	...	...	1039	1047	1742	1905	2907
	36	...	...	...	...	...	−1090	0.419	0.872
	37	...	...	...	−0.230	0.010	0.471	0.893	2416
Intercept = 5.079									
Model		Stage							
31 33 34 37	Tooth	A	B	C	D	E	F	G	H
	31	...	...	...	...	...	0.708	0.63	1715
Boys	33	...	...	...	−0.081	−0.150	0.858	1092	1796
	34	...	...	...	0.047	0.757	1740	2055	2858
	37	...	...	0.749	0.279	0.809	1105	1720	2874
Intercept = 5.451									
Model		Stage							
32 33 34 37	Tooth	A	B	C	D	E	F	G	H
	32	...	...	...	...	...	0.879	1384	2130
Girls	33	...	...	...	0.388	0.135	0.565	0.85	1679
	34	...	...	...	0.656	0.786	1613	1772	2774
	37	...	...	...	0.232	0.474	0.937	1359	2881
Intercept = 5.122									
Model		Stage							
33 34 37	Tooth	A	B	C	D	E	F	G	H
Boys	33	...	...	...	−0.699	−0.530	0.721	0.985	1688
	34	...	...	...	0.144	1274	2282	2583	3381
	37	...	...	0.761	0.467	1497	1797	2402	3556
Intercept = 6.069									
Model		Stage							
32 34 37	Tooth	A	B	C	D	E	F	G	H
Girls	32	...	...	...	...	...	0.859	1401	2330
	34	...	...	...	0.564	0.701	1773	2164	3551
	37	...	...	...	0.226	0.548	1171	1752	3356
Intercept = 5.350									

A year later, now being referred to as Bedek et al. models, the method was tested in the South Indian population [22]. The Bedek et al. models were found to be accurate and suitable, and their use was recommended, especially in cases of hypodontia and incomplete human remains. Moreover, it was concluded that a maximum accuracy of age estimation was obtained using fewer teeth and that all models surpassed the accuracy of the Willems method.

Bedek et al. models were also tested in the northwestern Turkish population on a representative sample [23]. The authors concluded that all models apart from the model with one tooth were more accurate than the Willems method. On consideration of the simplicity of usage and the proven accuracy to date, these Bedek et al. models represent a promising new method for age estimation. However, as they have yet to be tested across more expansive populations, it is perhaps too early to verify their long-term applicability. It is worth noting, however, that in forensic scenarios time can be a crucial factor in the determination of age and identity. A method that is simple, user friendly, applicable in various forensic cases and that can produce accurate results in a short timeframe will often prove to be the method of choice over time.

10.7 Learning Outcomes

- You should have become familiar with the lesser-known methods for dental age estimation, some of which preceded the commonly used methods today.
- You should be able to comprehend applicability and notice the potential of the new methods for dental age estimation among adults and children in different forensic scenarios.

10.8 Self-Evaluation Questions

- Which are the six age-related changes Gustafson uses in his method?
- What is the main advantage of the Bedek et al. models when compared to the Willems and Demirjian methods?
- What is the Fels study?
- What is the value of Reference Data Sets—sex and ethnically specific tables in the DARLInG method?
- What is the main concern regarding the dental age estimation methods that are based solely on attrition?

10.9 Multiple Choice Questions

Q1: Which kind of dental age estimation method is the Gustafson method?

(a) Histological method
(b) Radiological method
(c) Biochemical method
(d) None of the above

Ans: a

Q2: Which statement is true?

(a) The Li and Ji method uses the same equation for both genders
(b) The Li and Ji method is based solely on an average stage of molar attrition
(c) The Li and Ji method recognizes ten different stages of attrition
(d) All of the above

Ans: d

Q3: What is not true about the Fels study?

(a) It was conducted in the American population
(b) It is the longest longitudinal study of growth and development
(c) It focuses only on tooth development
(d) The information regarding teeth development was used by Moorrees, Fanning and Hunt

Ans: c

Q4: The DARLInG method:

(a) Uses Demirijan developmental stages
(b) Is not sex specific
(c) Is not ethnically specific
(d) Is a method of dental age estimation among adults

Ans: a

Q5: Bedek et al. models:

(a) Use the Demirjian developmental scale
(b) Are developed on a sample from the Croatian population
(c) Can be used in cases of mandibular hypodontia
(d) All of the above

Ans: d

10.10 Mind Map

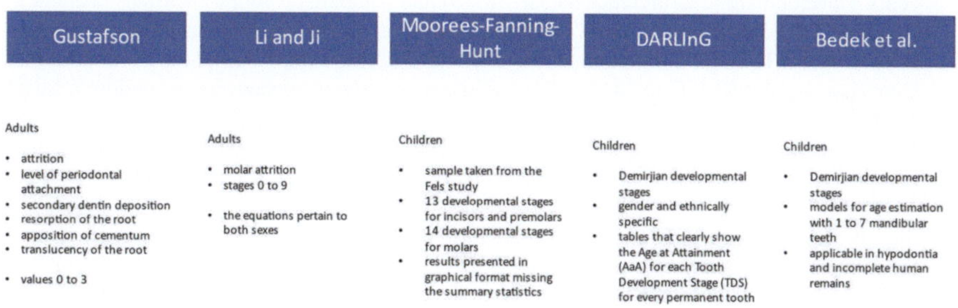

References

1. Gustafson G. Age determination on teeth. J Am Dent Assoc. 1950;41(1):45–54.
2. Chandler S, Phillips V. Testing Gustafson's dental age estimation method on a sample of Western Cape adults. S Afr Dent J. 2018;73(9)
3. Li C, Ji G. Age estimation from the permanent molar in Northeast China by the method of average stage of attrition. Forensic Sci Int. 1995;75
4. Kim YK, Kho HS, Lee KH. Age estimation by occlusal tooth wear. J Forensic Sci. 2000;45(2):303–9.
5. Yun JI, Lee JY, Chung JW, Kho HS, Kim YK. Age estimation of Korean adults by occlusal tooth wear. J Forensic Sci. 2007;52(3):678–83.
6. Faillace KE, Bethard JD, Marks MK. The applicability of dental wear in age estimation for a modern American population. Am J Phys Anthropol. 2017;164(4):776–87.
7. Ball J. A critique of age estimation using attrition as the sole indicator. J Forensic Odontostomatol. 2002;20(2):38–42.
8. Moorrees CFA, Fanning EA, Hunt EE. Age variation of formation stages for ten permanent teeth. J Dent Res. 1963;42(6):1490–502.
9. Fanning EA. A longitudinal study of tooth formation and root resorption from birth to preadolescence. 1960.
10. Gleiser I, Hunt EE. The permanent mandibular first molar: its calcification, eruption and decay. Am J Phys Anthropol. 1955;13(2):253–83.
11. Garn SM, Lewis AB, Polacheck DL. Variability of tooth formation. J Dent Res. 38:135.
12. Nolla CM. The development of the permanent teeth. J Dent Child. 1960;27:254–66.
13. Šešelj M, Sherwood RJ, Konigsberg LW. Timing of development of the permanent mandibular dentition: new reference values from the Fels longitudinal study. Anat Rec. 2019;302(10):1733–53.
14. Haavikko K. Tooth formation age estimated on a few selected teeth. A simple method for clinical use. Proc Finn Dent Soc. 1974;70(1):15–9.
15. Demirjian A, Goldstein H, Tanner JM. Demirjian, a., a new system of dental age assessment. Hum Biol. 1973;45(2):211–27.
16. Roberts GJ, Parekh S, Petrie A, Lucas VS. Dental age assessment (DAA): a simple method for children and emerging adults. Br Dent J. 2008;204(4):1–4.
17. Mitchell JC, Roberts GJ, Donaldson ANA, Lucas VS. Dental age assessment (DAA): reference data for British caucasians at the 16 year threshold. Forensic Sci Int. 2009;189(1–3):19–23.
18. Elshehawi W, Alsaffar H, Roberts G, Lucas V, McDonald F, Camilleri S. Dental age assessment of Maltese children and adolescents. Development of a reference dataset and comparison with a United Kingdom Caucasian reference dataset. J Forensic Leg Med. 2016;39:27–33.
19. Moze K, Roberts G. Dental age assessment (DAA) of afro-Trinidadian children and adolescents. Development of a reference dataset (RDS) and comparison with Caucasians resident in London, UK. J Forensic Leg Med. 2012;19(5):272–9.
20. Balgi P, Katge F, Singh S, Jayaraman J. Comparative assessment to determine the accuracy of Demirjian and DARLInG methods of dental age estimation in western Indian children. Legal Med. 2020;1:42.
21. Bedek I, Dumančić J, Lauc T, Marušić M, Čuković-Bagić I. New model for dental age estimation: Willems method applied on fewer than seven mandibular teeth. Int J Legal Med. 2019;134(2):735–43.
22. Sheriff SO, Medapati RHR, Ankisetti SA, Gurrala VRR, Haritha K, Pulijala S, et al. Testing the accuracy of Bedek et al's new models based on 1-to-7 mandibular teeth for age estimation in 7-15 year old south Indian children. J Forensic Odontostomatol. 2020;38(2):22–39.
23. Çarıkçıoğlu B, Sezer B. Dental age estimation with fewer than mandibular seven teeth: an accuracy study of Bedek models in Turkish children. Clin Oral Investig. 2022;13

11 Evaluation of Dental Age Estimation in Individuals with Craniofacial Disorders

Ayse Tuba Altug

11.1 Introduction

Dental age is a method of estimating an individual's chronological age based on the developmental processes of their teeth. It is a common method used in anthropology and forensic sciences. Wisdom teeth, which begin to erupt as an individual approaches the age of 20, are considered an indicator that the person is of a certain age to have legal capacity [1]. However, knowing the individual's dental age during dental applications is important for clinical success. From a similar perspective, a good understanding of the dental developmental process is also useful in the treatment of individuals with craniofacial disorders.

Many studies have been conducted on the scientific platform on dental age, forensic odontology, identification of human remains, age estimation, and legal capacity. These studies have been able to give statistically average values for physically healthy individuals. However, it should not be forgotten that both in syndromes that concern the whole body and in craniofacial anomalies, the growth and development process has been interrupted during the embryological period. This situation may also be valid for teeth that give their first buds in the prenatal period. In one study, it was reported that the same gene region may be effective in cleft lip and alveolus and congenital maxillary lateral incisor agenesis [2]. Based on this perspective, we can consider that there is a close connection between craniofacial anomalies and the developmental processes of teeth. In summary, regardless of the purpose for which they will be evaluated, it should not be forgotten that individuals with craniofacial anomalies may have different dental age ranges and dental developmental anomalies than healthy individuals.

A. T. Altug (✉)
Ankara University, Faculty of Dentistry, Department of Orthodontics, Ankara, Türkiye
e-mail: aysealtug@ankara.edu.tr

© The Author(s), under exclusive license to Springer Nature Switzerland AG 2026

A. Chowdhry, P. Kapoor (eds.), *Dental Age Assessment*,
https://doi.org/10.1007/978-3-032-08788-1_11

In order to understand what we may expect regarding dental age estimation in individuals with craniofacial anomalies, let us first summarize how a human face and dentition develop during the embryological period.

11.2 Developmental Process of Craniofacial Disorders in the Embryological Period

Embryological life in humans is an amazing period that lasts an average of 9 months and includes differentiation at the cellular level, physical growth, and development.

The first 3 months of embryological life, also called the first trimester, encloses countless miracles such as the differentiation of cells on a precise timeline to form organs, the expression and silencing of genetic material at the right time and location for the organism to function perfectly, the early differentiation of embryonic cells into any type of cell in the body, and many more.

It would be appropriate to briefly summarize the developmental stages of maxillomandibular structures that form the face in the embryological period and to mention the stages of dental development in prenatal life prior to discussing the dental age development of individuals with craniofacial disorders [3].

The face originates from the first pharyngeal arch, and the processes that will form the face become apparent between the fourth and fifth weeks of prenatal life. These processes are the frontal nasal process (processus frontonasalis) that forms the forehead, the root of the nose, and the middle part of the upper lip (prolabium); the maxillary processes (processus maxillaris) that form the cheeks, the lateral part of the upper lip, and the maxilla; and the mandibular processes (processus mandibularis) that form the mandible and the lower lip. The nasal placodes develop on the sides of the frontonasal process and form the nostrils. The stomodeum, which is the outline of the oral cavity, is formed between the mandibular and maxillary processes. The formation and fusion of the structures that make up the face are completed in the tenth week of prenatal life. If these processes fail to unite respectively, various facial clefts may occur. Cleft lip and palate, which is the most common craniofacial disorder, occur as a result of the failure of these processes to fuse. In addition, unilateral or bilateral microsomia may occur as a result of the inadequate development of these tissues forming the face due to genetic, environmental, or vascular reasons.

It is obvious that our face, which begins and completes its development in the very early period of prenatal life, goes through a very delicate and sensitive process. Any factor that affects this process causes various craniofacial disorders to occur. It is also a fact that the same factors will have different developmental effects on maxillary and mandibular dentoalveolar structures and teeth.

11.3 Evaluation of Dental Age Estimation in Individuals with Cleft Lip and Palate

Cleft lip and palate deformities are the most common craniofacial disorders that develop between the sixth and tenth weeks of prenatal life due to genetic and/or environmental factors. Although it is thought of as the failure of the lip and maxillary segments to fuse, it is a developmental anomaly that also has different effects on craniomaxillofacial and dentoalveolar structures. For example, it has been reported that the posterior and total cranial base, which are in a region far from the cleft region, are shorter in these individuals compared to noncleft individuals [4].

- *What can we observe in terms of dental development in individuals with cleft lip and palate?*

Many studies reported several dental abnormalities in number, size, shape, timing of formation, and eruption in individuals with cleft lip and palate—CL(P). These differences can be observed adjacent to the cleft deformity or distant from the cleft area. In addition, it has been reported that three-dimensional (3D) crown size differences may occur in the cleft and noncleft segments [5]. Moreover, these differences occur not only in the maxillary but also in the mandibular dental arch. Based on this, it should not be forgotten that when determining the dental age of individuals with cleft lip and palate, significant differences may occur compared to noncleft individuals. It would be useful to reinforce this view with different perspectives.

It is an expected phenomenon that individuals with cleft lip and palate, whether unilateral or bilateral, will experience eruption delays due to local factors such as scar tissue in the maxillary lateral incisors or maxillary canines [6]. It has also been evaluated in various articles that there may be delays in the eruption of the deciduous teeth of individuals with cleft lip and palate due to factors such as gender, race, nutrition, general growth, premature birth, or additional syndromes [7]. The development of the germs of deciduous teeth in prenatal life may be effective in the occurrence of such problems in deciduous dentition. However, the topic of dental age estimation focuses on the permanent dentition period.

Ranta [8] mentioned that the timing of tooth formation in the permanent dentition is delayed in children with CL(P) compared to noncleft children. The delay lengthens, with increasing severity of cleft, from 0.3 to 0.7 years and is similar in all permanent teeth in both jaws [8]. Markovic et al. [9] reported the dental age estimation in individuals with CL(P) by comparing different methods. Although different methods evaluated in the study gave different results, dental ages in individuals with CL(P) were found to be delayed compared to the noncleft individuals [9].

de Carvalho Carrara et al. [10], in their study conducted on individuals with unilateral cleft lip and palate, showed that both maxillary and mandibular teeth erupted later in males than in females. They also emphasized that lateral incisors and canines in the cleft region may tend to erupt later than all other teeth, as expected [10].

- *What could be the reasons for the delay in tooth formation and/or tooth eruption age in individuals with cleft lip and palate?*

11.3.1 Surgical Scar Tissue

When considering the reasons for delayed dental age in individuals with CL(P), the first explanation would be the surgical scar tissue in the cleft area. In their systematic review, Van Dyck et al. [11] reported that although the maxillary lateral incisor in the cleft region is the most late-erupting tooth. However, they also reported delays in the distant regions [11]. Another finding highlighted by the majority of included studies in this systematic review was an increased risk of asymmetrical tooth development in CL(P) patients.

11.3.2 Presence of Supernumerary Teeth

Another reason for the delay in the eruption of teeth in the cleft area may be the presence of supernumerary teeth in that area. Supernumerary teeth or malalignment in the cleft area can create physical barriers to the eruption of normal teeth, further delaying the process. Although congenitally missing maxillary lateral incisors are frequently encountered in CL(P) individuals, supernumerary teeth can also be frequently encountered in the cleft region or in distant regions. Fonseca-Souza et al. [12] reported in their systematic review and meta-analysis study that the rate of dental anomalies was higher in individuals with orofacial clefts compared to non-cleft individuals and that supernumerary teeth were the most common anomaly after missing lateral incisors [12].

11.3.3 Similar Genetic Background

MSX1 and MSX2 genes, members of the muscle segment homeobox gene family, are of critical importance especially in the formation of teeth, skeleton, and skin. MSX1, besides its crucial effects on prenatal craniofacial development, is also expressed in the developing tooth bud during morphogenesis [13]. In addition, *MSX2* controls both physiological and pathological tissue mineralization. Amri et al. [14] showed the effects of the MSX2 gene on bone remodeling and tooth growth in their study on mice by indirectly affecting the signaling network effective in osteoclastic activity and tooth eruption [14].

Genetic variabilities should also be considered when evaluating the delay in tooth eruption in individuals with cleft lip and palate. Although the etiology of cleft lip and palate is considered multifactorial, many candidate genes have been identified in the development of this condition. Most of these genes play a role in the development of teeth as well as maxillofacial development. In a study, the MSX1 gene, which was identified as a candidate gene in both CL(P) and congenitally missing maxillary lateral incisors in noncleft individuals, was evaluated. In both anomalies, the presence of the same single-nucleotide polymorphism (c. *6C>T, rs 8670) in this gene was reported. This result suggests that both cleft lip and palate and dental development are under the influence of similar genes [2]. These data suggest that Msx2 may act indirectly on dentinogenesis by controlling osteoclast activity and the signaling network related to eruption, supporting and further extending the concept that Msx2 controls formation of mineralized tissues by inhibition of the Wnt/b-catenin pathway, Sost in dentin and Dkk1 in bone, as previously demonstrated [14].

11.3.4 Nutritional Factors and Number of Early Surgeries

Another issue to consider in cleft lip and palate individuals is whether the neonatal nutritional difficulties and a large number of surgeries experienced by these individuals will cause delays in their general growth and dental development. Cesur et al. [15] compared the sella turcica areas *(on the lateral cephalometric radiographs)* and skeletal maturity of unilateral CL(P) and noncleft individuals using hand-wrist radiographs [15]. The researchers reported that sella turcica areas were similar in both groups, but there was a significant delay in growth in CL(P) individuals compared to noncleft individuals in the early period (ages between 7 and 11 years). It has also been emphasized that this delay is more pronounced in males than in females. The good news is that no difference was found between individuals with cleft lip and palate and noncleft individuals in the other two groups, ages 11–14 and 14–18. This result shows that the developmental delay seen in individuals with CL(P) at an early age can be compensated for at an older age.

11.4 Dental Age Evaluation of Individuals with Cleft Palate Only

It is important to note that the embryological developmental processes and etiological factors of cleft lip and palate (CL(P)) and cleft palate only (CP) are different from each other. For this reason, in studies on dental development and dental age determination, the results are different for both situations. Fonseca-Souza et al. [12] reported in a systematic review study that the frequency of dental anomalies in individuals with CP only was lower than in individuals with CL(P) [12].

11.5 Evaluation of Dental Age Estimation in Hemifacial Microsomia

Hemifacial microsomia (HFM) is a condition in which one side of the face does not grow normally. Along with the underdevelopment of the face on the side with microsomia, ear deformities are often seen on this side. Since this disorder is caused by developmental problems of the first and/or second branchial arches during the embryological period, the mandible, maxilla, temporomandibular joint, orbit, external and internal ear, cranial nerves, and associated soft tissues developing from these arches are affected to varying degrees. The size and shape of teeth can also be affected, often resulting in smaller or irregularly shaped teeth due to developmental anomalies. Furthermore, eruption patterns may be delayed or altered, leading to misalignments and malocclusion.

In individuals with HFM, it is anticipated that tooth eruption issues and occlusal canting will arise on the affected side, primarily due to skeletal retardation [16].

Studies on dental development in HFM cases used different methods to assess tooth development, such as Nolla's stages, Demirjian's Dental Age, and Demirjian and Goldstein's tooth maturation assessment. These studies reported that the prevalence of delayed dental development ranged from 20.5% to 54.3% [17–21].

A systematic review by Elsten et al. in [17] reported that individuals with craniofacial microsomia have a tendency to have dental anomalies compared to unaffected individuals. They also suggested that these dental developmental anomalies might be related to how the condition develops [17].

Ahiko et al. [18] investigated the dental development of HFM patients with Nolla's stages of tooth calcification. The study suggested that the mandibular molars on the affected side showed delayed calcification compared with the unaffected side [18]. A study by Ongkosuwito and colleagues in [19] looked at dental age in children with HFM. They compared tooth development on the affected side of the face to the unaffected side [19]. The study found that children with more severe types of HFM (types IIb and III) tended to have delayed tooth development, especially when they were younger. The fact that tooth development was temporarily delayed in these children and that some teeth were missing suggests that the development of the mandible and the teeth are connected. Ongkosuwito et al. [19] also found that children who initially experienced delays in tooth development quickly caught up to the normal pace of tooth growth [19].

Unlike many studies on this subject, Loevy et al. [20] observed that 45.7% of the individuals included in the study showed symmetry of tooth maturation on the affected and non-affected sides, regardless of the severity of the mandibular anomaly [20]. They recorded asymmetric tooth maturation between the two sides in 54.3% of the cases. Of these cases with asymmetric development, 54.4% showed more advanced dental maturation on the affected side and 45.5% showed more advanced dental development on the non-affected side. Although this study presents contradictory and different results from other studies, when all studies are evaluated together, we should always expect deviations from normal in the dental development of individuals with HFM [21].

11.6 Dental Development in Down Syndrome Patients

Down syndrome patients have a chromosomal abnormality which is caused by 21st chromosome trisomy. Most commonly, it is associated with non-disjunction during gametogenesis (meiosis). It is characterized by a range of signs and symptoms that indicate developmental delay of motor and cognitive functions, systemic alterations, maxillary and mandibular growth, and dental development. Santos [22] found a delay in canine and second molar development in Down syndrome patients upon studying the mineralization chronology using panoramic radiographs [22]. Moraes [22] however found that two-thirds of 102 Down syndrome patients were within normal standards of mineralization chronology when comparing their dental age with chronological age [22]. A contrasting study by Diz P [23] studied dental and chronological age in 155 (3–17 years old) white Spanish children with cerebral palsy, mental retardation, and Down syndrome [23]. Although they did not report any significant difference in boys, they found a significant delay in dental age compared with chronological age in girls with Down syndrome and cerebral palsy. Thus, further research is warranted to evaluate the dental age in syndromic patients including Down syndrome, to be used further for anthropology, forensics, medico-legal studies, and dentistry applications.

11.7 Summary and Conclusion

Studies on the mineralization chronology or development of permanent teeth in individuals with craniofacial abnormalities have shown that these individuals have some aberrations in dental development and eruption of teeth compared with normal individuals.. This may also result from the use of various orthopedic or expansion appliances used for the correction of maxillary or mandibular growth including Quad-Helix or maxillary protraction appliances.

Similar to individuals with cleft lip and palate, in cases of hemifacial microsomia resulting from the disturbances of the first and second pharyngeal arches, there is a delay in the development and eruption times of the teeth on the affected side. This incident may be effective in further exacerbating the occlusal cant and increasing asymmetry that occurs due to inadequate mandibular development. With this additional factor, orthodontic and orthopedic treatments of individuals with HFM may become more challenging. Further, syndromic patients including Down syndrome, Turner syndrome, Crouzon syndrome, Cleidocranial dysplasia, Anchondroplasia, Progeria, Williams syndrome, etc. present with conditions where there may be a significant delay in dental development compared with chronological age. This may be explored further for its significance in forensic and medicolegal scenarios where assessment of dental age is a necessity.

References

1. Scheurer E, Quehenberger F, Mund MT, Merkens H, Yen K. Validation of reference data on wisdom tooth mineralization and eruption for forensic age estimation in living persons. Int J Legal Med. 2011;125(5):707–15.
2. Altug AT, Senol A, Ozkepir ON, Dogan H, Ceylaner S, Ozdiler E. Evaluation of MSX1 gene as the common candidate gene of nonsyndromic congenital hypodontia and cleft lip and palate. J Cleft Lip Palate Craniofac Anom. 2017;4(Suppl 1):S31–7.
3. Avery JK, Chiego DJ Jr. Essentials of oral histology and embryology—a clinical approach. 3rd ed. Elsevier: Mosby; 2006.
4. Abuhijleh E, Aydemir H, Toygar-Memikoğlu U. Three-dimensional craniofacial morphology in unilateral cleft lip and palate. J Oral Sci. 2014;56(2):165–72.
5. Kaplan M, Gorgulu S, Cesur E, Arslan C, Altug AT. 3D evaluation of tooth crown size ın unilateral cleft lip and palate patients. Niger J Clin Pract. 2020;23(5):596–602.
6. Peterka M, Tvrdek M, Müllerová Z. Tooth eruption in patients with cleft lip and palate. Acta Chir Plast. 1993;35(3–4):154–8.
7. Kobayashi TY, Gomide MR, Carrara CF. Timing and sequence of primary tooth eruption in children with cleft lip and palate. J Appl Oral Sci. 2010;18(3):220–4.
8. Ranta R. A review of tooth formation in children with cleft lip/palate. Am J Orthod Dentofacial Orthop. 1986;90(1):11–8.
9. Markovic E, Marinkovic N, Zelic K, Milovanovic P, Djuric M, Nedeljkovic N. Dental age estimation according to European formula and Willems method: comparison between children with and without cleft lip and palate. Cleft Palate Craniofac J. 2021;58(5):612–8.
10. de Carvalho Carrara CF, de Oliveira Lima JE, Carrara CE, Gonzalez Vono B. Chronology and sequence of eruption of the permanent teeth in patients with complete unilateral cleft lip and palate. Cleft Palate Craniofac J. 2004;41(6):642–5.
11. Van Dyck J, Cadenas de Llano-Pérula M, Willems G, Verdonck A. Dental development in cleft lip and palate patients: a systematic review. Forensic Sci Int. 2019;300:63–74.
12. Fonseca-Souza G, de Oliveira LB, Wambier LM, Scariot R, Feltrin-Souza J. Tooth abnormalities associated with non-syndromic cleft lip and palate: systematic review and meta-analysis. Clin Oral Investig. 2022;26(8):5089–103.
13. MacKenzie A, Leeming GL, Jowett AK, Ferguson MWJ, Sharpe PT. The homeobox gene Hox 7.1 has specific regional and temporal expression patterns during early murine craniofacial embryogenesis, especially tooth development in vivo and in vitro. Development. 1991;111:269–85.
14. Amri N, Djolé SX, Petit S, Babajko S, Coudert AE, Castaneda B, Simon S, Berdal A. Distorted patterns of Dentinogenesis and eruption in Msx2 null mutants: involvement of Sost/Sclerostin. Am J Pathol. 2016;186(10):2577–87.
15. Cesur E, Altug AT, Toygar-Memikoglu U, Gumru-Celikel D, Tagrikulu B, Erbay E. Assessment of Sella turcica area and skeletal maturation patterns of children with unilateral cleft lip and palate. Orthod Craniofac Res. 2018;21(2):78–83.
16. Altug-Atac AT, Grayson BH, McCarthy JG. Comparison of skeletal and soft-tissue changes following unilateral mandibular distraction osteogenesis. Plast Reconstr Surg. 2008;121(5):1751–9.
17. Elsten EECM, Caron CJJM, Dunaway DJ, Padwa BL, Forrest C, Koudstaal MJ. Dental anomalies in craniofacial microsomia: a systematic review. Orthod Craniofac Res. 2020;23(1):16–26.
18. Ahiko N, Baba Y, Tsuji M, Suzuki S, Kaneko T, Kindaichi J, Moriyama K. Investigation of maxillofacial morphology and dental development in hemifacial microsomia. Cleft Palate Craniofac J. 2015;52(2):203–9.
19. Ongkosuwito EM, de Gijt P, Wattel E, Carels CE, Kuijpers-Jagtman AM. Dental development in hemifacial microsomia. J Dent Res. 2010;89(12):1368–72.
20. Loevy HT, Shore SW. Dental maturation in hemifacial microsomia. J Craniofac Genet Dev Biol Suppl. 1985;1:267–72.

21. Farias M, Vargervik K. Dental development in hemifacial microsomia. I. Eruption and agenesis. Pediatr Dent. 1988;10(2):140–3.
22. Moraes ME, Bastos MS, Santos LR, Castilho JC, Moraes LC, Medici Filho E. Dental age in patients with down syndrome. Braz Oral Res. 2007;21(3):259–64.
23. Diz P, Limeres J, Salgado AFP, Tomás I, Delgado LF, Vázquez E, Feijoo JF. Correlation between dental maturation and chronological age in patients with cerebral palsy, mental retardation, and down syndrome. Res Dev Disabil. 2011;32(2):808–17.

12 Dental Age Assessment: Report Writing Guidelines

Jayasankar P. Pillai and Deepika Bablani Popli

Abbreviations

DAA	Dental age assessment
IOFOS	International Organization for Forensic Odonto-Stomatology
ABFO	American Board of Forensic Odontology
SAI	Sports Authority of India
MLC	Medicolegal case

12.1 Introduction

Dental age assessment (DAA) is widely regarded as one of the most reliable techniques in forensic science for determining an individual's age. It is a highly specialized area within forensic science that leverages the developmental stages of dentition to estimate an individual's chronological age. This chapter documents the DAA process for the subject in question, outlining the purpose and importance of report writing in DAA, the selection of effective age estimation techniques, and the standards and guidelines for writing a clear and evidence-based report [1, 2].

This chapter aims to serve as a comprehensive guide for anyone involved in estimating age from human dentition, offering the latest information and insights on writing DAA reports. It provides a clear and scientifically supported explanation of the age assessment process, including examples of forensic report writing to ensure that the findings are reliable and relevant to the intended legal context. This chapter

J. P. Pillai (✉)
Department of Oral Pathology, Government Dental College and Hospital, Ahmedabad, India

D. Bablani Popli
Oral Pathology & Microbiology, Faculty of Dentistry, Jamia Millia Islamia, New Delhi, India

© The Author(s), under exclusive license to Springer Nature Switzerland AG 2026

A. Chowdhry, P. Kapoor (eds.), *Dental Age Assessment*,
https://doi.org/10.1007/978-3-032-08788-1_12

is designed for private practitioners conducting dental age assessments, as well as for individuals, organizations, or agencies that utilize age assessment data for academic and medicolegal purposes.

12.2 Purpose and Importance of Report Writing in DAA

Accurate age estimation is crucial, particularly in legal contexts where determining an individual's age can influence decisions related to criminal responsibility, the age of majority, or eligibility for various licenses. Dental age assessment (DAA) involves the precise, scientifically-based analysis of teeth and surrounding structures to estimate a person's age, requiring specialized knowledge and experience in forensic odontology. Forensic odontologists utilize DAA techniques to assess the most likely dental age in both deceased and living individuals.

In the case of deceased individuals, DAA helps narrow search parameters and plays a vital role in identifying missing or unidentified persons. For living individuals, DAA provides answers to a wide range of legal inquiries, such as confirming the age of majority, determining legal responsibility for crimes, and verifying eligibility for licenses, immigration, or participation in specific sports [3].

DAA enables authorities to estimate an individual's chronological age or age range through the methodical evaluation of dental and surrounding structures. Age estimation methods commonly involve assessing mineralization levels, eruption stages, and root formation in developing teeth. In adults, regressive changes, including morphological, histological, and biochemical alterations in teeth, also contribute valuable insights for age estimation.

12.3 Guidelines for Choosing an Effective Age Estimation Technique

The selection of an appropriate age estimation method depends on the type of forensic evidence available to the forensic odontologist and the specific circumstances of the case. According to guidelines by Ritz-Timme et al. [4], age estimation methods must meet certain criteria to ensure their validity and reliability:

1. The methods should be presented to the scientific community, generally through peer-reviewed publications.
2. Clear information regarding the accuracy of the age estimation method should be accessible.
3. The methods must demonstrate a sufficient level of accuracy.
4. For age estimation in living individuals, medical ethics and relevant legal regulations must be observed [5].

Additionally, according to the Daubert Standard [6–8], which govern the admissibility of evidence in trial courts, forensic methodologies used for age estimation must address the following key questions:

1. Has the method been tested through population-based studies?
2. Has the method undergone peer review and been published in scientific journals?
3. What is the known or potential error rate of the method?
4. Are there established standards for controlling the technique's operation?
5. Has the method been widely accepted within the relevant scientific community?

The *Daubert Standard* provides a framework for trial court judges to evaluate the reliability and relevance of expert testimony before it is presented to a jury. This standard is equally applicable in forensic odontology, particularly in age estimation cases, and it emphasizes the need for population-specific age estimation regression equations. As a result, dental age estimation research has expanded globally, with new methodologies and validation studies being conducted across diverse populations.

12.4 Standards and Guidelines for DAA Report Writing

Despite the availability of various resources on age estimation methodologies, there remains a lack of comprehensive scientific literature specifically focused on guidelines for reporting age estimation cases. Forensic experts conducting medicolegal age assessments should adhere to the standards and guidelines established by professional forensic odontology organizations, such as the International Organization for Forensic Odonto-Stomatology (IOFOS), the American Board of Forensic Odontology (ABFO), and the Scientific Working Group for Forensic Anthropology (SWGANTH) [9, 10]. It is also essential to note that the results of age assessment methods typically provide an estimated age range rather than an exact calendrical age, emphasizing the probabilistic nature of age determination in forensic contexts.

The findings from a global survey on age estimation report writing [1, 11] revealed notable inconsistencies in the way these reports are structured and the information they include. Despite the high frequency of using multiple methods for age estimation (90%), there was a lack of standardization in report formats, even within the same country. The survey, which involved forensic experts from 14 countries, showed that 95% of participants included details of the methods used, but other aspects of reporting, such as the inclusion of population-based references (70%) or limitations of the methods (80%), were less consistent. Furthermore, while key demographic data like sex and date of examination were almost universally included, factors such as the mental and cognitive state of the individual were often omitted. The absence of a standardized format and variable content in age estimation reports could potentially impact the legal interpretation of the findings, highlighting the need for clearer, universally accepted guidelines in forensic odontology report writing.

An age assessment report is an essential medicolegal case (MLC) document prepared by a forensic expert at the request of an investigating officer. This report serves as a key link between the investigator and judicial authority, conveying both the facts observed during the examination and the expert's conclusions. The report is presented as evidence for the jury and is subject to scrutiny by the defense during cross-examination. Therefore, it is vital that the report is clear, concise, and free of unnecessary technical jargon to ensure it is accessible and understandable to the legal authorities.

Age estimation reports should outline the specific methods applied, citing relevant sources, such as guidelines, textbooks, or peer-reviewed studies [2, 12, 13]. Given that dental and skeletal development can vary based on sex and ancestry, it is crucial to adopt population-specific methodologies when estimating dental age. In cases where such standards are not available, broader, more inclusive standards should be used, with these choices clearly documented in the report. Additionally, factors such as the examinee's ethnic background, nutritional status, socioeconomic conditions, and mental and cognitive behavior should also be included in the report. Furthermore, to provide a complete picture, photographs of the dentition—both clinically and radiographically—may be included to support the findings.

The format for age estimation reports is often provided as proformas or annexures by authorities overseeing age estimation cases. For instance, the Sports Authority of India (SAI) includes Annexure-II, which serves as a standardized format for such reports. It is crucial that dental age estimation is conducted by qualified forensic odontologists, not only skilled in the analytical procedures but also proficient in report writing, ensuring both ethical and legal standards are met.

Some fundamental guidelines to follow when reporting an age estimation case include the following:

1. The report should be neatly handwritten or typed on official letterhead.
2. Include the full details of the reporting forensic odontologist (name, degree, affiliations, contact details).
3. Mention the name, designation, and address of the requesting authority.
4. Include consent from the examinee or guardian, especially for minors.
5. Describe the materials used in the analysis, such as radiographs, software, etc.
6. Document the dentition status, both clinically and radiographically.
7. Provide a detailed description of the methodology used for age estimation.
8. Cite sources for the methodologies used.
9. Include relevant digital images, such as radiographs or clinical photographs, if necessary.
10. Ensuring accuracy and consistency in findings.
11. Maintaining objectivity and avoiding bias.
12. Add a disclaimer regarding the report's findings and limitations.

The age estimation report must be signed and sealed by the forensic odontologist to ensure its authenticity. Upon completing the analysis, the expert should submit the report in a sealed envelope to the requesting authority, with each page signed and the total page count noted to prevent tampering. Forensic exhibits, such as teeth, jawbones, or radiographs, should be dried, packed, and sealed in a container with individual seals and signatures from the forensic odontologist. Additionally, the forensic odontologist and the relevant institution should each retain a copy of the report for record-keeping purposes.

12.5 Challenges for DAA Report Writing

Writing a dental age assessment report comes with several challenges. These include the lack of standardized reporting formats across different jurisdictions, which leads to inconsistencies. The technical complexity of age estimation methods, influenced by factors like mineralization stages and socioeconomic conditions, complicates the process. Ethical and legal considerations are especially critical when working with living individuals, requiring reports to be both scientifically accurate and easily understandable to legal professionals. Ensuring the reliability of findings and clearly acknowledging any limitations are essential for maintaining the credibility of the report. These challenges underscore the importance of well-trained forensic odontologists and adherence to standardized practices to ensure the reliability, clarity, and legal integrity of DAA reports [14].

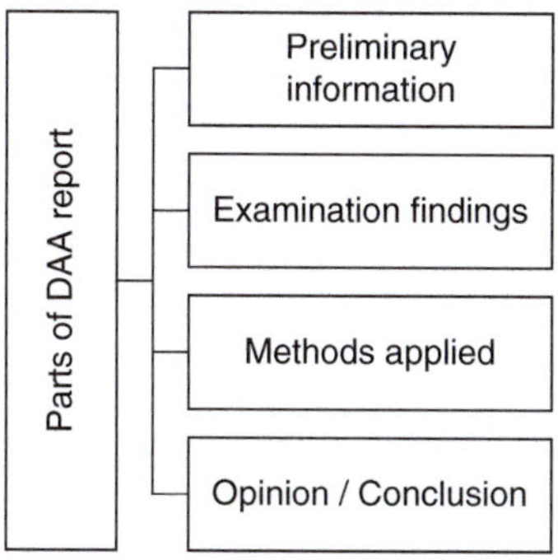

12.6 Samples for DAA Report Writing

The following is a sample copy of the label on the sealed envelope/container while returning the sample after analysis.

FORENSIC SAMPLE FOR DENTAL AGE ASSESSMENT

Sample / Exhibit / Specimen No.______
Nature of Sample: __________ (tooth, jaw bone, X-ray….)
Investigation required: Age assessment from dental structures
Sample received from: ____________ (Police station/ Institute/ FSL) on date: ________
Name of the Forensic Odontologist conducting the investigation:
Institute/ Hospital Name:
Date of Investigation:
Name and mobile number of the person receiving the sample: ______on date: ______ and time: _____

Signature of the Forensic Odontologist with office seal.

SAMPLE LABEL

Sample copy of the label on the envelope containing the age estimation report done on a live person (accused/victim/survivor).

DENTAL AGE ASSESSMENT REPORT

Name of the person:
Sex: Male/ Female
MLC No: _____________
Investigation required: Age assessment
Requisition from: __________(Police station/ institute) Vide letter no.:____ dated: ___
Name of the Forensic Odontologist conducting the investigation:
Institute/ Hospital Name:
Date of Investigation:
Name of the police person receiving the report: ________ buckle no.______on date: ______ and time: _____
Total number of pages in the report:________

Signature of the Forensic Odontologist with office seal.

SAMPLE LABEL

INSTITUTE'S NAME & LOGO
DENTAL AGE ASSESSMENT REPORT

Date:

To
The name and address of the person who sent the request letter.

Sir/ Madam,
Sub:

1. PRELIMINARY INFORMATION:

Case Identification Number:
Case Referring authority/ agency: ________________________Vide letter no.:_________ dated: ________
Name and address of the Subject referred for age estimation:
Sex: Male/ Female Date of Birth (if declared):
ML Case No: ____________ EPR No.: _________
Requisition from: __________(Police station/ institute)
Name of the Forensic Odontologist conducting the investigation:
Institute/ Hospital Name: Date of Investigation:

Consent:

I,_____________ hereby voluntarily consent and agree to the following:

1. Clinical examination of the oral cavity for the age assessment procedure.
2. Radiological examination for the purpose of age estimation.
3. Photography of my upper and lower dentition in different views as part of investigation.
4. Allow impressions of my upper and lower dentition for making dental models, if required.
5. The age estimation report may be used for legal evidence, research and academic purposes.
6. I have also been informed that I can refuse the examination at any stage and also refuse information to be given to the police. In this event I understand that I will be responsible for any problem arising in the process of crime investigation and court trial.
7. The investigating officer has explained to me all the above points in my mother tongue (..........) language / or in the language which I can understand.

Name and Signature of the person
Name and signature of the Guardian in case of minor and below age 12 years
Name and signature of the witness / female Nurse (if the examinee is a girl/woman)

Biographical Information of the subject:
Ethnicity/ ancestry (if known):
Height: ___Cm.
Weight:____Kg.
Nutritional status:
Socioeconomic status:
Mental state:
Cognitive ability:

2. EXAMINATION

Clinical Examination:
Teeth visible:

(Insert the image of the radiographs / OPG used for age assessment)

Radiographical examination:
Teeth present:

3. METHODS

Dental Age estimation method(s) of analysis:

4. Opinion/ conclusion:

Disclaimer:

Name, Address, Contact details and signature of the Forensic Odontologist:
Official seal of the Institute.

References:

Total number of pages in the report: _________

12.7 Conclusion

In conclusion, it is essential for forensic odontologists to follow established guidelines, such as those from ABFO, IOFOS, and relevant national standards, when conducting age estimation procedures and report writing. This chapter has provided an overview of the fundamental aspects of report writing in age estimation cases from a forensic odontology perspective. It also outlines standard sample formats used in India, such as the Annexure-II format by the Sports Authority of India (SAI), which can serve as a reference for structuring age estimation reports. Adhering to these guidelines ensures that the reports are scientifically grounded, ethically sound, and legally acceptable, ultimately contributing to the credibility and reliability of the findings in age estimation cases. Proper training, standardization, and attention to detail in report writing are critical for the success of forensic age assessments [15].

12.8 Learning Outcomes

- You should be able to understand the standard format of an age assessment report in a medicolegal case.
- You should be able to understand the fundamental guidelines that need to be followed while preparing the DAA report.

12.9 Self-Evaluation Questions

- What do you mean by dental age assessment report?
- What are the parts of the medicolegal age assessment report?
- The DAA report by a forensic odontologist should be addressed to whom?

12.10 Multiple Choice Questions

Q1. Which organization provides standardized guidelines for forensic odontology report writing?
(a) WHO
(b) IOFOS
(c) ABFO
(d) Both b and c
Ans: d

Q2. What type of information is essential to include in a dental age estimation report for minors?
(a) Details of the methodologies used
(b) Consent from a guardian
(c) Population-specific references
(d) All of the above
Ans: d

Q3. What is a recommended guideline for preparing a DAA report?
(a) Use casual language to simplify findings
(b) Include disclaimers regarding the report's findings and limitations
(c) Rely only on a single age estimation method
(d) Avoid mentioning the date of the investigation
Ans: b

Q4. What is the primary purpose of an age estimation report in medico-legal cases?
(a) To determine dental health status
(b) To establish chronological age for legal decisions
(c) To evaluate forensic odontology methods
(d) To create detailed case studies
Ans: b

Q5. What is the significance of including population-specific methodologies in DAA reports?
(a) To ensure global applicability of findings
(b) To align findings with the subject's demographic characteristics
(c) To reduce the need for radiographs
(d) To simplify report writing
Ans: b

12.11 Mind Map (Fig. 12.1)

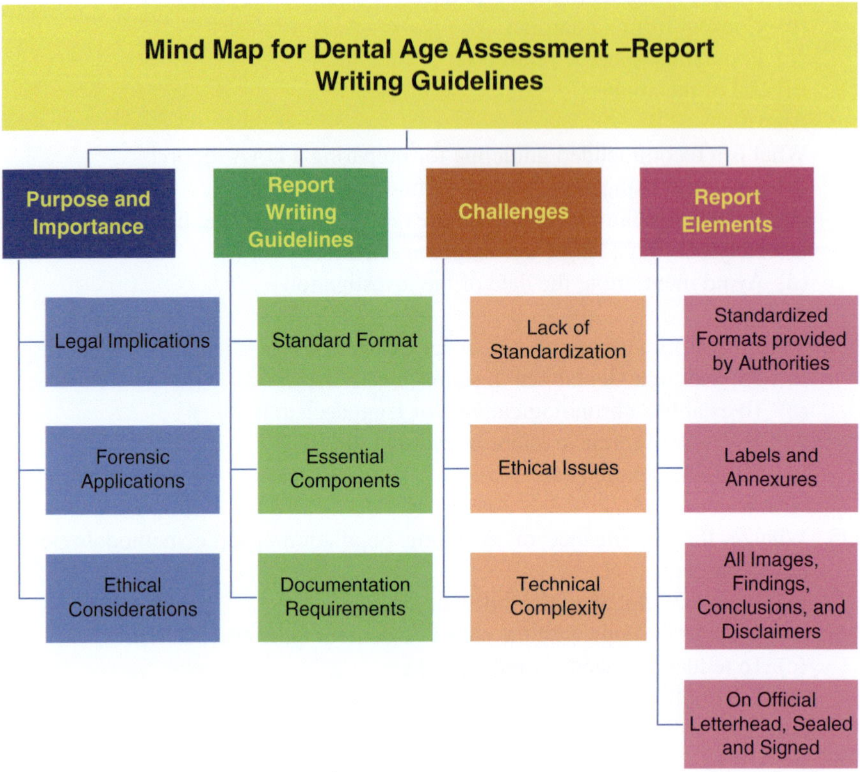

Fig. 12.1 A simplistic mind map to understand the report writing guidelines for dental age assessment

References

1. Al Qahtani S. Age estimation reports: where do we stand? J Forensic Sci Res. 2019;3:004–8.
2. Hackman L, Black SM. Age estimation in the living. In: Encyclopedia of forensic and legal medicine. Elsevier Inc; 2016. p. 34–40.
3. United Nations. Committee on the Rights of the Child (CRC) [online]. 2008. Available: http://www2.ohchr.org/english/bodies/crc/docs/AdvanceVersion/C.
4. Ritz-Timme S, Cattaneo C, Collins M, et al. Age estimation: the state of the art in relation to the specific demands of forensic practise. Int J Legal Med. 2000;113:129–36.
5. Franklin D, Flavel A, Noble J, Swift L, Karkhanis S. Forensic age estimation in living individuals: methodological considerations in the context of medico-legal practice. Res Rep Forensic Med Sci. 2015:53–66.
6. Rösing FW, Graw M, Marré B, Ritz-Timme S, Rothschild MA, Rötzscher K, et al. Recommendations for the forensic diagnosis of sex and age from skeletons. Homo. 2007;58(1):75–89.
7. https://www.law.cornell.edu/wex/daubert_standard. Accessed on 1 Dec 2023.

8. Lesciotto KM. The impact of Daubert on the admissibility of forensic anthropology expert testimony. J Forensic Sci. 2015;60(3):549–55.
9. Bajpai M, Pardhe N. Legal reporting in forensic odontology. J Forensic Anthropol. 2016;1:104. https://doi.org/10.4172/jfa.1000104.
10. Swganth. Age Estimation. The Scientific Working Group for Forensic Anthropology. 2013. Available from: http://www.swganth.org/products%2D%2Ddrafts.html.
11. European Asyllum Support Office (EASO). Practical guide on Age assessment. 2nd Ed; 2018. Accessed online: https://euaa.europa.eu/sites/default/files/easo-practical-guide-on-age-assessment-v3-2018.pdf.
12. Fradella HF, O'Neill L, Fogary A. The impact of Daubert on forensic science. Pepp L Rev. 2003;31(2):323–62.
13. ABFO Diplomate's Reference Manual, section IV, standards, and Guidelines. Available: https://abfo.org/resources/abfo-manual.
14. Liu F, Lei G, Jia XD, He SY, Dang YH. Worldwide trends of forensic dentistry: a 20-year bibliometric analysis in Pubmed. Rom J Leg Med. 2016;24(3):236–41.
15. Merdietio Boedi R, Mânica S, Franco A. Sixty years of research in dental age estimation: a bibliometric study. Egypt J Forensic Sci. 2023;13(1):41.

Dental Age Assessment Standards and Guidelines

13

Rizky Merdietio Boedi, Nikolaos Angelakopoulos, and Ademir Franco

13.1 Introduction

The process of dental age assessment entails the evaluation of dental development and maturation patterns, which serve as biological indicators for estimating an individual's chronological age. Normally, the chronological age (also referred to as documental age or even "real" age) expresses in the form of time the period that was lived from birth. The estimated (or biological) age reflects the effects of time on anatomic structures, such as the teeth. In an ideal scenario, the estimated age should match the chronological age. Depending on the circumstances, the age of a person is requested by the judicial authorities regarding the age thresholds of legal interest. The most common threshold is the age of legal majority, for instance, when an individual is formally recognized as an adult by law. Hence, the forensic experts must clarify and indicate whether the examined individual is below or above the age of majority (18 years in most countries). Conversely, some authorities might ask for the estimated age interval of a person to make legal decisions based on scientific forensic evidence. In these circumstances, the report should point out the lower and upper age limits estimated based on biological features, or even the probability of being below or above the ascertained legal age. The process of assessing the biological features, however, varies based on many factors.

R. Merdietio Boedi
Department of Dentistry, Universitas Diponegoro, Semarang, Indonesia
e-mail: rizkymerdietio@lecturer.undip.ac.id

N. Angelakopoulos
Department of Orthodontics and Dentofacial Orthopedics, University of Bern, Bern, Switzerland
e-mail: nikolaos.angelakopoulos@unibe.ch

A. Franco (✉)
Division of Forensic Dentistry, Faculdade São Leopoldo Mandic, Campinas, Brazil
e-mail: ademir.junior@slmandic.edu.br

© The Author(s), under exclusive license to Springer Nature Switzerland AG 2026

A. Chowdhry, P. Kapoor (eds.), *Dental Age Assessment*,
https://doi.org/10.1007/978-3-032-08788-1_13

One of the aspects is the availability of technological resources. Forensic practice might face challenges that can jeopardize experts' performances. An example is the use of radiological devices. It is understood nowadays that forensic imaging is a fundamental aspect of the forensic sciences that can support best practices. The visualization of human hard tissue and the way it changes over time is essential to achieve more realistic forensic assessments. Some countries, however, might not have the technology promptly available and may face difficulties in practice. What must be emphasized is that age assessments solely based on external (clinical) body inspection are becoming less common given the subjectivity of the process and the inherent errors that it may involve. Hence, the application for radiology has been advised.

Another aspect is the stage of life in which the individual is examined. Age assessment approaches change if the examined person is a child or an adult. In children, the age assessment process benefits from the multiple structures of the human body that are developing at the same time, while in adults there is a scarcity of developmental parameters leading to the need for alternative examinations of degenerative changes. Moreover, the age assessment strategies change if the examination is performed on the living or on the deceased, or according to the state of preservation of the dental remains on skeletal remains, for example, invasive and even destructive methods might be applied (methods that extract and destroy body parts during the analysis), while on the living, only noninvasive methods (such as the radiographic ones) are ethically allowed.

Human teeth are the most durable structures of the human body and can resist the effects of the environment to a large extent. Because of the persistence of the teeth in the oral cavity after death, they can be used for age assessment. Another advantage of human teeth is the fact that, normally, humans might have up to 32 teeth (not considering supernumerary). All these teeth develop throughout life up to the age of about 21.5 years—a moment in which only the third molars remain in development. Combined, all the available developing teeth can culminate in improving dental age assessment, providing each valuable contribution to the estimated age. Differently, in adults, the teeth are not developing anymore, except for the third molars in early adulthood. Hence, the error rate in this age group increases as the observation relies on post-formation changes that has multiple external factors affecting it (i.e., attrition, periodontal resorption, etc).

Therefore, to mitigate the observed increase in error rates and to strengthen both the methodological approach to forensic casework and the effectiveness of its presentation in expert reports, a series of recommendations was developed. When it comes to recommendations, it is worth mentioning that this chapter will use the terms *Standard* and *Guidelines* following the definition of the Standards and Guidelines for Dental Age Assessment of the American Board of Forensic

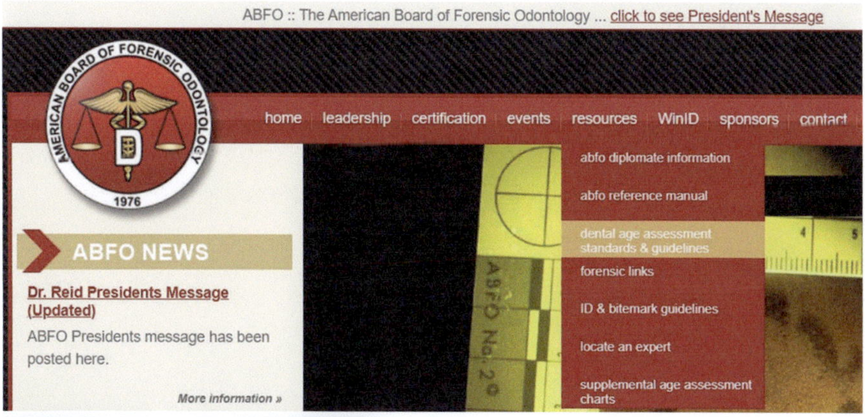

Fig. 13.1 Website (https://abfo.org) of the ABFO showing the location to find the Standards and Guidelines for Dental Age Assessment. Interface registered in January/2024. Download feasible through the QR code on the right

Odontology (ABFO). In this context, standards refer to protocol procedures that are mandatory and should be followed to enable the "minimum level of practice." Guidelines, on the other hand, are recommended procedures that help guide practice but are not mandatory.

In order to establish an architecture for the present chapter, two main documents were consulted, summarized, and presented for consultation of forensic odontology students, instructors, experts, and interested readers. These documents are (I) the ABFO's Standards and Guidelines for Dental Age Assessment (Fig. 13.1) and (II) the Recommendations for Quality Assurance in Dental Age Estimation of the International Organization for Forensic Odonto-Stomatology (IOFOS) (Fig. 13.2).

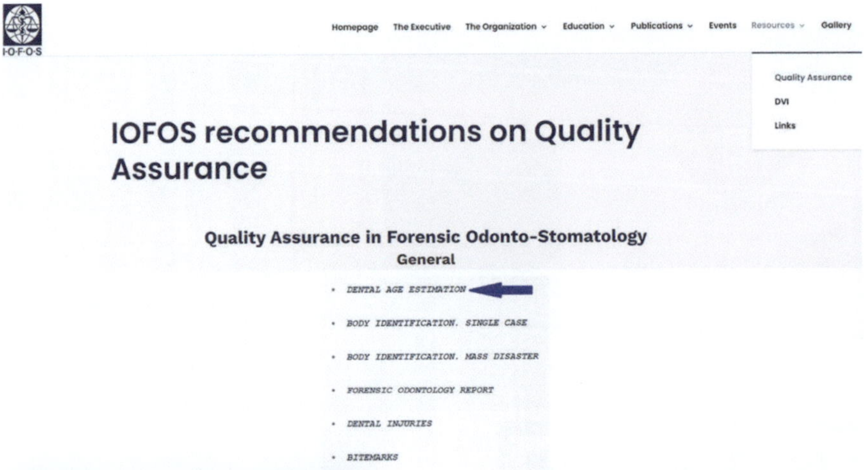

Fig. 13.2 Website (https://iofos.eu) of the IOFOS showing the pathway for the quality assurance resources and the latest version of the Recommendations for Quality Assurance in Dental Age Estimation. Interface registered in January/2024

13.2 American Board of Forensic Odontology

13.2.1 Standards and Guidelines for Dental Age Assessment

13.2.1.1 Background

The ABFO originated within the framework of the American Academy of Forensic Science (AAFS) in 1976, initiated by the proactive efforts of charter members, including Dr. E. Woolridge, R. Souviron, C. Mertz, and others. These pioneers underwent a rigorous process to meet the required criteria on education, experience, and forensic criteria, and become the first diplomates of the ABFO. Their leadership significantly shaped professional and public relations, laying a foundation for the ABFO itself. As the inaugural president, Dr. C. Mertz played a crucial role in defining the Board's early trajectory.

While certification and recertification remain central to the ABFO's mission, the Board has consistently recognized the need for education, research, and the promotion of public and professional relations regarding the importance of forensic odontology. The first guideline developed by the ABFO was the scientific analysis of bitemarks in 1984 through their workshop, marking their commitment to advance forensic odontology. These standards and guidelines then later collectively evolved and grew, leading to the current state of ABFO's guidelines including body identification, bitemark, and, of course, dental age assessment.

ABFO defines two primary terms in their dental age assessment primary document: guidelines and standards. Guidelines are characterized as suggestions, giving recommendations without mandatory enforcement. It offers a recommended course of action but lacks a mandatory or obligatory nature. On the other hand, standards are defined as a model to be followed, distinguished by a more stringent and restrictive nature when compared to guidelines. Standards set a compulsory, minimal level of practice, serving as a benchmark that must be adhered to within a specific context or field.

The ABFO Standards and Guidelines for Dental Age Assessment underwent a recent update, now referred to as "American Dental Association Technical Report No. 1077 for Human Age Assessment by Dental Analysis," surpassing the prior version from 2017. This current edition provides point-by-point definitions, guidelines, and standards, showcasing improvements over the previous document. The term "forensic dental age assessment" is explicitly defined as "the estimation of an individual's chronologic age through scientific evaluation of the dentition and maxillofacial structures." The primary objective of this assessment lies in its medicolegal applications, spanning from aiding the identification of missing or unidentified individuals by narrowing the search in the antemortem data pool to estimating the legal age or adhering to other age thresholds dictated by specific country laws. Several crucial aspects highlighted in this document will be summarized and further elaborated upon.

13.2.1.2 Specific Techniques

Various methods are available for assessing dental age; however, due to differences in populations, developmental patterns, and methodological approaches, there is no universally accepted standard for dental age estimation. Each method, found in scientific literature, is customized based on specific conditions, primarily the dental age intervals, the state of preservation of the dental remains and the individual's status (living or deceased). In essence, selecting the most suitable technique for a given case can lead to more accurate age estimation results. The goal is to emphasize the tailored nature of these methods, considering factors like age intervals, the degree of preservation and whether the individual is alive or deceased. The ABFO further facilitates the dental age assessment process by offering supplemental age assessment charts. This simplifies the need to search for specific techniques tailored to certain age intervals and an individual's status, providing a convenient and accessible resource for age estimation.

The ABFO establishes a distinct categorization of dental age intervals, classifying individuals into three main groups: infant/child, adolescent, and adult. This categorization plays a pivotal role in determining the appropriate methodology for assessing each respective interval. In the case of children, dental age intervals can be evaluated based on the stage of morphologic development of the primary or secondary dentition. For adolescents, the assessment is more limited, focusing primarily on the third molar as other teeth have completed their developmental stages. In the adult age interval, the methodology shifts towards utilizing post-formation changes that occur regressively after the cessation of morphologic dental development. This systematic approach, defined by the guideline, allows forensic odontologists to choose the appropriate analysis of dental age within each distinct interval.

In children's dental age intervals, a radiographic evaluation is recommended, whether for living or deceased individuals. This approach relies significantly on utilizing the morphological development of the permanent dentition. While clinical observation, such as monitoring gingival or alveolar emergence, is an alternative method, it tends to be less accurate due to a higher likelihood of bias in observing the timing of clinical emergence. Therefore, a radiographic image is preferred as it allows for a more comprehensive examination and reduces the potential for observational bias, contributing to more accurate results in assessing the progress of dental morphological development in children. Considering this, of the methodologies can be used in children's dental age intervals, such as: Moorrees et al. [17] staging, Demirjian et al. [6] staging, or Cameriere et al. [2] open apices measurement.

The adolescent age intervals also rely on observing morphological development and radiographic evaluation, specifically focusing on the third molars. ABFO acknowledges the high degree of morphological developmental variability in third molars. Nevertheless, this method is considerably more useful and accurate compared to the post-formation changes utilized in adult age intervals. In addition to prediction of chronological age, the third molar technique is heavily utilized in legal age estimation by reporting the probability of an individual being above or below a certain age threshold. The supplemental age assessment charts recommend the same methods as for children if the permanent dentition is still developing. However, when using only the third molar, ABFO recommends, Mincer et al. [16] formula which adapted the Demirjian staging system and recalculated it for a sample of white North American population.

The techniques recommended by ABFO differ in adult dental age assessment, with separate evaluation branches for the living and the deceased. This distinction arises due to the examination of post-formation changes, achievable through either clinical or radiographic observation. ABFO guidelines describe six post-formation changes based on research by Gustafson [9]: root translucency, secondary dentin deposition, periodontal attachment, cementum apposition, attrition, and root resorption. However, it is important to note that not all these variables are observable in radiographic observation examination. Radiographic observation is imperative in living subjects. In the deceased, factors such as sample preservation or ethical considerations aspects need to be considered, as invasive methods to observe these post-formation changes require extraction or tooth sectioning. The ABFO dental age assessment procedures chart outlines the use of Kvaal et al. [12] or Cameriere et al. [4] methods for radiographic age assessment in the living, and Maples [14], Lamendin et al. [13], or Bang and Ramm [1] for the deceased, involving extraction or sectioning methods. Additionally, aspartic acid racemization radiocarbon dating can be utilized for all age intervals, but due to the need for tooth destruction, it is exclusively applicable to the deceased.

13.2.1.3 Techniques and the Availability of Dental Evidence

While ABFO provides a selection of recommended techniques, it does not assert that these are the exclusive methods available for dental age assessment. The field sees a continuous influx of scientific papers proposing new techniques or validating existing ones for diverse populations, as discussed in the next section (13.2.1.4.). Consequently, selecting a technique demands a profound understanding of the scientific and statistical foundations behind each method.

Examiners must initially assess the approximate age interval, the availability of dental evidence and other resources, as the choice of techniques hinges on these factors. An examiner can determine estimate the approximate age interval of the subject by observing the development of permanent teeth, and subsequently the examiner can opt for an appropriate technique based on the available dental evidence.

Dental radiographs are mandatory for dental age assessment in children and adolescents. Examiners must ensure that this procedure aligns with ethical guidelines and federal or state regulations, given its nonmedical or dental referral status. Specific techniques may necessitate radiograph imaging, and the examiner must verify that the radiograph taken adheres to the specifications outlined in the respective techniques. For example, Cameriere et al. [2] open apices measurement study was originally conducted using panoramic radiograph. This means that the method should be applied to the same image modality in practice. If there is a should be scientifically revalidated apply the Cameriere et al. technique to another type of modality, the technique needs to be revalidated and go through a peer-reviewed process to be sound. In postmortem examinations for adults, the choice of technique for examining post-formation changes clinically relies heavily on dental evidence processing. For example, when a tooth can be extracted and sectioned, the method proposed by Maples et al. [14] may be applied. However, if sectioning is not feasible, the Lamendin et al. method constitutes a suitable alternative [13].

13.2.1.4 Reference Population and Validation Studies

The ABFO standards and guidelines underscore the importance of including sex information and utilizing population-specific reference data in dental age assessment. If a study specific to a population or sex is available, its technique, description, and formulation should be applied, rather than relying on the original study if conducted on a different population or lacking significant differences between sexes. There were multiple reports of sex differences that may affect the result of dental age assessment, especially on the chronologiy of tooth development stages. However, the significance of these differences varies and must be tested in individual studies. For instance, the original ABFO study on third molars by Mincer et al. [16] observed a significant sex dimorphism in maturation rate among white Americans but not among American blacks, possibly due to small sample sizes. Given the variation in maturation rates, the outcomes of dental age assessment, including model selection and error rates, may differ. Therefore, utilizing sex information, when available, is essential. However, if definitive sex identity is not possible, ABFO recommends selecting a method without sex as a variable or using the assessment for both sexes.

The term "population" is categorized under the description of "Identifiable Human Group," denoting a group of individuals based on ancestry or population specificity that reflects a similar genetic, geographic, and environmental background. This was due to the difference that may occur in dental development, post-formational changes, and other techniques. Utilizing a technique with a similar population reference could enhance the probability that the examined individual was represented by a population with comparable genetic and developmental characteristics,Thevissen et al. [28] noted significant differences in third molar development among nine country populations, but the actual differences in values were small and fluctuated across the age range. Recognizing this variability, ABFO recommends that if a study with a reference population like the individual being assessed is unavailable, the closest matching reference population study should be employed. In the absence of such a study, a thorough description of limitations, including potential errors introduced by using a different population in dental age assessment, must be reported.

13.2.1.5 Variables in the dental age estimation process

The application of dental age assessment techniques requires a profound understanding of statistics or, ideally, collaboration with a statistician. This is because the result of dental age assessment is not an exact pinpoint answer; rather, it stems from a correlation and prediction process through statistical modeling, introducing a margin of error. The correlation involves the observation of dental age-related data and the subsequent prediction of chronological age. As the progress of dental age-related changes is not always directly proportional to chronological age due to various factors (such as sex, population, genetics, and habits), a margin of error is introduced. This error is typically reported in scientific studies through metrics like standard deviation, mean squared error, or other methods, indicating the potential deviation in predictive results. The error result should be reported, and if possible, to explain why such an error occurs.

As mentioned earlier, the selection of dental age assessment techniques must be tailored to specific circumstances and evidence. However, ABFO recommends that examiners utilize multiple independent statistical methodologies. For instance when the legal age is estimated using the third molar, dental age assessment, the techniques and models developed by Gunst et al. [8] and Cameriere et al. [5] could be applied. It's important to note that this does not mean combining two dental age assessment results into one (e.g., if technique A results in an age range of 16–18 years old and technique B results in 17–19 years old, the result is not the intercept of the prediction, or 17–18 years old). Instead, practitioners should carefully apply their expert judgment to the most relevant statistical data while considering factors such as the individual's sex, population specificity, and known environmental influences to choose the method that better represents the examined individual.

Despite following respective scientific publications, the dental age assessment technique can be subjective given the examiner-depending procedures. This process introduces bias and can be influenced by human perceptions or systemic factors. ABFO mandates a blinding process in the age assessment procedure, ensuring that the examiner is unaware of the alleged chronological age. chronological age (if any) of the individual. This helps prevent the examiner from favoring a measurement or a dental age maturation stage that is closer to the chronological age. Additionally, to control the subjective interpretation of the observed dental age variables, ABFO encourages the use of an independent assessment of inter- and intra-variability for the examiner when handling a case, with a documented method of recording every examiner's result and resolution of differences.

13.3 International Organization for Forensic Odonto-Stomatology

13.3.1 Recommendations for Quality Assurance in Dental Age Estimation

13.3.1.1 Background

The IOFOS has a rich history that traces its origins to the need for collaboration and advancement in the field of forensic odontology. IOFOS was founded in Paris back in 1973, initially under the name of the International Society of Forensic Odonto-Stomatology (ISFOS). The inception of ISFOS can be attributed to the growing recognition of the vital role that forensic odonto-stomatology plays in legal and investigative processes. As a discipline dealing with dental evidence and its application in legal matters, forensic odontology has seen a surge in importance, leading to the establishment of international organizations to foster collaboration and standardization. Key individuals in the early steps of this new Organization were Professor Gösta Gustafson from Malmö (Sweden) and Soren Keiser Nielsen from Denmark. They both played a pivotal role in the establishment and expansion of the organization as they both served as presidents. The current IOFOS name dates from 1981 when initiatives were taken to establish a more organized and structured organization. Over the last five decades, IOFOS has flourished and evolved into a robust international organization, embodying the shared objectives pursued by its previous presidents. These objectives include facilitating connections among (legal) forensic odontology societies worldwide, fostering goodwill, promoting advancements and research in forensic odontology, and consistently publishing newsletters. Throughout the years, the IOFOS has forged collaborations and partnerships with other organizations such as FDI, WHO, Interpol, and the ICRC, illustrating the growth and influence of IOFOS. IOFOS has initiated the publishing of the scientific Journal of Forensic Odonto-Stomatology (JFOS).

When it comes to dental age assessments, the IOFOS initially published recommendations in 2008, reviewing them in 2018 to ensure they reflect current best practices. The guidelines provide a comprehensive framework for quality assurance, emphasizing that procedures should only be employed if they adhere to local legal and ethical standards.

The recommendations prioritize clear communication and management of expectations from the expert. Specifically, the expert is tasked with explicitly advising the instructing authority regarding the limitations of age assessment and clarifying what can realistically be achieved. This ensures that the assigning parties understand the boundaries of the scientific evidence before an investigation begins. Furthermore, comprehensive background information such as the individual medical history, socioeconomic status, and nutritional background needs to be present, as these factors might influence the final assessment.

Regarding the technical aspects, the IOFOS places an emphasis on scientific rigor. It is critical that the methods selected are not only applicable to the individual but are also scientifically verified. Experts must check the utilized methodology reference sample composition, statistical soundness, and reproducibility. Additionally, methods should be applied exactly as they were originally described in peer-reviewed literature, avoiding ad-hoc modifications with appropriate citations.

Finally, the guidelines enforce strict quality control measures to mitigate subjectivity and bias. A standard clinical and radiographic examination that adhere with ALARA (As Low as Reasonably Achievable) principle and checked for optimal quality. Most importantly, every age assessment should be conducted by two independent experts who much reach consensus in case of disagreement.

13.4 Study Group on Forensic Age Diagnostics of the German Association of Forensic Medicine (AGFAD)

13.4.1 Criteria for Age Estimation in Living Individuals

Due to cross-border migration within the European Union, several European countries have observed an increase in the presence of foreigners lacking valid identification documents. This trend has prompted a growing demand for forensic age estimation of individuals in question. To address this, the "10th Lübeck Talk of

German Forensic Doctor" was convened, providing a platform for a comprehensive analysis of the current state of forensic age diagnostics. During this congress, a proposal was put forth to establish a study group comprising forensic doctors, dentists, radiologists, and anthropologists. The primary aim of this initiative was to develop guidelines that facilitate expert opinions, aiming to standardize varied approaches and ensure the quality of such opinions. The interdisciplinary "Study Group on Forensic Age Diagnostics" was officially founded on March 10, 2000, in Berlin. The inaugural meeting concluded with the acknowledgment that age diagnostics of both living individuals and deceased bodies, including skeletons, fall within the purview of the study group's responsibilities. Ideally, the conduct of forensic age estimations among these countries should adhere to the recommendations set forth by AGFAD, which was last updated in 2008.

These recommendations advocate for a comprehensive approach involving three pillar examinations: an anamnesis and physical examination (to exclude developmental disorders or illnesses which could influence the sexual and the bone development), a dental examination (X-ray examination of the dentition, dental status), and an evaluation of the skeletal development by examining an X-ray of the left hand/wrist (relying on Greulich and Pyle's atlas) [7] and, in case of complete maturation of the hand/wrist skeleton, a computed tomography (CT) scan of the sternoclavicular joints (with a recommended slice thickness $\leq$1 mm). Each pillar examination needs to be performed and analyzed by a specialist with training and experience in forensic age estimations.

A comprehensive summary should be written then with an interpretation of all the results and conclusions. Forensic centers worldwide, members of the AGFAD study group, undergo annually the proficiency tests organized by the AGFAD to ensure the optimal and continuous quality of their reports.

13.4.2 Examination Methods

The three-pillar examinations proposed by AGFAD include the following:

- Conducting a physical examination to determine anthropometric measures (body height and weight, constitutional type), inspect signs of sexual maturation, and identify any age-relevant developmental disorders.
- Performing X-ray examination of the left hand.
- Carrying out a dental examination to assess the dental status and performing an X-ray examination of the dentition.
- If skeletal development of the hand is complete, an additional examination of the clavicles should be conducted, preferably through conventional X-ray examination and/or CT-scan [11, 26].

Using these methods collectively enhances diagnostic accuracy and improves the identification of age-relevant developmental disorders.

The justification for X-ray examinations should be verified in accordance with the regulations applicable in the respective country. Consideration of additional radiological features for determining individual maturation should only occur if the relevant radiographs and scans are already available [24].

13.4.3 Reference Studies

The same study group presented some important observations on what is considered a reference study. According to them, a reference study employs a specific methodology to evaluate data within a random sample, involving the conversion of an ontogenetic process into a chronological scale. For forensic age estimation, such studies must meet certain criteria, including an adequate sample size, verified age of subjects, even age distribution, separate analysis for both genders, information on the examination's timing, precise definition of examined features, detailed method descriptions, and data on the reference population's genetic/geographic origin, socioeconomic status, and health. Additionally, information on sample size, mean value, and range of scatter for each examined feature is essential. They suggested the following reference studies: Greulich and Pyle [7], Gunst et al. [8], Kahl and Schwarze [10], Mincer et al. [16], Olze et al. [18–20], Ruhstaller [22], Schmeling et al. [25], Tanner et al. [27], and Thiemann et al. [29].

13.4.4 Examination

Regarding the examination procedure, AGFAD suggests that prior to engaging in an expert evaluation for an individual case, it is imperative to ascertain whether the posed questions can be addressed with a sufficiently high degree of reliability through the application of rigorous scientific methods. The examinations to be conducted must be justified by a court order.

Individuals slated for examination should be duly informed about the nature and purpose of the assessment. Additionally, the court issuing the order must be apprised that the involvement of an interpreter may be necessary.

Each facet of the examination should be carried out by a specialist experienced in the formulation of expert reports and actively engaged in regular proficiency tests to ensure quality assurance.

In instances where ionizing radiation is utilized, adherence to national regulations is mandatory. From a scientific perspective, the minimization principle should be rigorously applied, necessitating the execution of each examination with the utmost consideration for minimizing radiation exposure and abstaining from any unnecessary exposure.

The coordinating expert is tasked with providing a comprehensive assessment based on the various components of the evaluation conducted by the respective specialists.

13.4.5 Reporting

AGFAD Study Group has also published the principles of good reporting. The primary forensic objective of an expert report is to provide the most probable age of the examined individual and/or the likelihood that the reported age accurately reflects the individual's true age or surpasses the pertinent legal age limit.

The expert report is required to specify the methods and reference studies upon which the age estimation is founded. For each analyzed feature, the report must specify both the most probable age and the range of variability within the reference population, as outlined by Rösing [21]. It is important to acknowledge that empirical observer error may contribute to an increased range of tolerance.

The report should delve into age-related variations arising from factors such as differing genetic/geographic origins, distinct socioeconomic status, potentially varying rates of acceleration, and individual developmental disorders. A comprehensive discussion of these factors, along with their impact on the estimated age, is essential. If feasible, a quantitative assessment of such effects should be provided, drawing on research by Cameriere et al. [3], Meijerman et al. [15], Olze et al. [19], and Schmeling et al. [23].

The individual's most likely age is estimated based on all partial diagnoses, coupled with a critical examination of the individual case. While summarizing age estimations derived from the employed methods generally leads to a reduction in the range of variability, the extent of this reduction has been approximated thus far.

Depending on the nature of the request, it might be necessary to verbally evaluate the legally relevant age limits and/or articulate the probability of the age specified in the court order.

13.4.6 Quality Assurance

Quality assurance plays a major role plays a major role in forensic dental age assessment and reporting, and for this reason, the AGFAD study group committee arranges annual proficiency tests as part of ongoing quality assurance efforts. Additionally, an expert has the option to seek an assessment of age estimation before the actual report is drafted. Their current recommendations undergo annual revision by the study group committee, taking into consideration new scientific and practical findings. Updates are made as necessary. The latest version of these recommendations is accessible on the study group's website at: http://rechtsmedizin.klinikum.uni-muenster.de/agfad/index.htm

References

1. Bang G, Ramm E. Determination of age in humans from root dentin transparency. Acta Odontol Scand. 1970;28(1):3–35. https://doi.org/10.3109/00016357009033130.
2. Cameriere R, Ferrante L, Cingolani M. Age estimation in children by measurement of open apices in teeth. Int J Legal Med. 2006;120(1):49–52. https://doi.org/10.1007/s00414-005-0047-9.

3. Cameriere R, De Angelis D, Ferrante L, Scarpino F, Cingolani M. Age estimation in children by measurement of open apices in teeth: a European formula. Int J Legal Med. 2007;121(6):449–53. https://doi.org/10.1007/s00414-007-0179-1.
4. Cameriere R, Ferrante L, Cingolani M. Variations in pulp/tooth area ratio as an indicator of age: a preliminary study. J Forensic Sci. 2004;49(2):317–9.
5. Cameriere R, Ferrante L, Liversidge HM, Prieto JL, Brkic H. Accuracy of age estimation in children using radiograph of developing teeth. Forensic Sci Int. 2008;176(2–3):173–7. https://doi.org/10.1016/j.forsciint.2007.09.001.
6. Demirjian A, Goldstein H, Tanner J. A new system of dental age assessment. Hum Biol. 1973;45(2):211–27.
7. Greulich W, Pyle S. Radiographic atlas of skeletal development of the hand and wrist. Stanford: Stanford University Press; 1959.
8. Gunst K, Mesotten K, Carbonez A, Willems G. Third molar root development in relation to chronological age: a large sample sized retrospective study. Forensic Sci Int. 2003;136(1–3):52–7. https://doi.org/10.1016/S0379-0738(03)00263-9.
9. Gustafson G. Age determinations on teeth. J Am Dent Assoc. 1950;41(1):45–54. https://doi.org/10.14219/jada.archive.1950.0132.
10. Kahl B, Schwarze CW. Aktualisierung der Dentitions- tabelle von I. Schour und M. Massler von 1941. Fortschritte der Kieferorthopadie. 1988;49:432–43.
11. Kreitner KF, Schweden FJ, Riepert T, Nafe B, Thelen M. Bone age determination based on the study of the medial extremity of the clavicle. Eur Radiol. 1998;8(7):1116–22.
12. Kvaal SI, Kolltveit KM, Thomsen IO, Solheim T. Age estimation of adults from dental radiographs. Forensic Sci Int. 1995;74(3):175–85. https://doi.org/10.1016/0379-0738(95)01760-g.
13. Lamendin H, Baccino E, Humbert J, Tavernier J, Nossintchouk R, Zerilli A. A simple technique for age estimation in adult corpses: the two criteria dental method. J Forensic Sci. 1992;37(5):1373–9.
14. Maples W. An improved technique using dental histology for estimation of adult age. J Forensic Sci. 1978;23(4):764–70.
15. Meijerman L, Maat GJ, Schulz R, Schmeling A. Variables affecting the probability of complete fusion of the medial clavicular epiphysis. Int J Legal Med. 2007;121(6):463–8. https://doi.org/10.1007/s00414-007-0189-z. PMID: 17909834; PMCID: PMC2039830.
16. Mincer HH, Harris EF, Berryman HE. The A.B.F.O. study of third molar development and its use as an estimator of chronological age. J Forensic Sci. 1993;38(2):379–90.
17. Moorrees C, Fanning EA, Hunt EE. Age variation of formation stages for ten permanent teeth. J Dent Res. 1963;42(6):1490–502. https://doi.org/10.1177/00220345630420062701.
18. Olze A, Schmeling A, Rieger K, Kalb G, Geserick G. Untersuchungen zum zeitlichen Verlauf der Weisheitszahnmineralisation bei einer deutschen population. Rechtsmed. 2003;13:5–10.
19. Olze A, Taniguchi M, Schmeling A, Zhu B-L, Yamada Y, Maeda H, Geserick G. Studies on the chronology of third molar mineralization in a Japanese population. Legal Med. 2004;6:73–9.
20. Olze A, van Niekerk P, Schmidt S, Wernecke K-D, Rösing FW, Geserick G, Schmeling A. Studies on the progress of third molar mineralization in a Black African population. Homo. 2006;57:209–17.
21. Rösing F. Forensische Altersdiagnose: Statistik, Arbeitsregeln und Darstellung. In: Oehmichen M, Geserick G, editors. Osteologische Identifikation (Research in Legal Medicine/Rechtsmedizinische Forschungsergebnisse). Lübeck: Schmidt-Römhild; 2000.
22. Ruhstaller P. Zahnärztliche Altersdiagnostik durch röntgenologische Evaluation der Entwicklungsstadien des unteren Weisheitszahnes: Auswertung von 1260 Orthopantomogrammen von Jugendlichen und jungen Erwachsenen. Med Diss, Zürich. 2006.
23. Schmeling a, Reisinger W, Geserick G, Olze A. Age estimation of unaccompanied minors. Part I. General considerations. Forensic Sci Int. 2006;159(1):61–4. https://doi.org/10.1016/j.forsciint.2006.02.017.
24. Schmeling A, Reisinger W, Geserick G, Olze A. The current state of forensic age estimation of live subjects for the purpose of criminal prosecution. Forensic Sci Med Pathol. 2005;1(4):239–46. https://doi.org/10.1385/FSMP:1:4:239.

25. Schmeling A, Schulz R, Reisinger W, Mühler M, Wernecke KD, Geserick G. Studies on the time frame for ossification of the medial clavicular epiphyseal cartilage in conventional radiography. Int J Legal Med. 2004;118(1):5–8. https://doi.org/10.1007/s00414-003-0404-5.
26. Schulz R, Mühler M, Reisinger W, Schmidt S, Schmeling A. Radiographic staging of ossification of the medial clavicular epiphysis. Int J Legal Med. 2008;122(1):55–8. https://doi.org/10.1007/s00414-007-0210-6.
27. Tanner JM, Healy MJR, Goldstein H, Cameron N. Assessment of skeletal maturity and prediction of adult height (TW3 method). London: Saunders; 2001.
28. Thevissen PW, Fieuws S, Willems G. Human third molars development: comparison of 9 country specific populations. Forensic Sci Int. 2010;201(1–3):102–5. https://doi.org/10.1016/j.forsciint.2010.04.054.
29. Thiemann H-H, Nitz I, Schmeling A. Röntgenatlas der normalen Hand im Kindesalter. Stuttgart/New York: Thieme; 2006.

Dental Age Assessment in Archaeological Remains

14

Hrvoje Brkić

Abbreviations

^{14}C Carbon 14

Concepts and Definitions

- *Archaeological sample*:
  Excavating, collecting, and researching archaeological samples at a specific site or set of artifacts.
- *Palatal suture*:
  The median palatal suture is at the midline of the hard palate, while the transverse palatal suture is at the interface between the maxilla and palate.
- *Tooth wear*:
  Tooth wear refers to loss of tooth substance by means other than dental caries. This is a normal physiological process occurring throughout life, but with increasing lifespan of individuals and increasing retention of teeth for life. Tooth wear varies substantially between people and groups, with extreme attrition and enamel fractures common in archaeological samples.
- *Root translucency*:
  Root translucency develops as the dentinal tubules within a tooth root begin to mineralize from the root apex toward the crown.
- *Incremental lines*:

H. Brkić (✉)
Department of Dental Anthropology, School of Dental Medicine University of Zagreb, Zagreb, Croatia
e-mail: brkic@sfzg.hr

© The Author(s), under exclusive license to Springer Nature Switzerland AG 2026

A. Chowdhry, P. Kapoor (eds.), *Dental Age Assessment*,
https://doi.org/10.1007/978-3-032-08788-1_14

Lines seen in a tooth in section showing the periodic depositions of dentin, enamel, and cementum occurring during the tooth's growth.

- *Carbon-14*:
  Radiocarbon or carbon-14 dating is a method for determining the age of an object containing organic material by using the properties of radiocarbon, a radioactive isotope of carbon.

14.1 Introduction

Dental age assessment is currently carried out in the following areas: clinical dental work, forensic analyses of living persons and cadavers, and archaeological analyses of found human remains.

In this chapter, we will focus on dental age assessment in archaeological remains using the results of numerous studies and scientifically based methods. Bioarchaeology is the scientific discipline that deals with the identification and interpretation of biological remains, most often bones and teeth, from archaeological sites. It is an interdisciplinary science that closely cooperates with a number of other sciences from the biomedical, social, and natural sciences [1].

Since the science of bioarchaeology is very broad, it can be said that the center of interest of bioarchaeological research is an integral part of various disciplines. Their common goal is to learn about the life, health, illness, and treatment of ancient populations, all in the context of clarifying evolutionary processes.

In bioarchaeological analyses, there are usually four indicators: age, sex, height, and race. Estimating the age of human remains was one of the most difficult challenges in ancient biology, because chronological age shows different biological ages in different people. Since teeth are more stable and permanent than other tissues, they are more commonly used for the evaluation of human remains [2].

The sample included in bioarchaeological and paleo-dental research comprises the remains of the viscerocranium and teeth. After a person's death, unless the appropriate body preservation techniques were applied, soft tissue decays, unlike calcified tissues, bones, and teeth which can remain preserved in their original form for centuries. The reasons for this are firmly mineralized tissues such as the enamel, dentin, and dental cementum, of which the tooth is composed. The proportion of calcium hydroxyapatite in them is so high (65–98%) that it gives exceptional hardness, strength, and durability. Teeth in an unchanged form, which corresponds to the moment of death, can remain preserved for thousands of years. As such, they are a rich source of information and data about an individual's life, such as age, sex, race, lifestyle, eating habits, professional activities, illnesses, etc., and can be analyzed using almost identical techniques that are applied to living people. If the alveolar bone or the entire skull is preserved along with the teeth, the data obtained can be even more detailed and complete [3].

The analysis of skeletal remains assess the biological or bone age of an individual. Biological aging refers to the accumulation of generative and degenerative processes, the consequent change in the size, condition, and functionality of tissues and the aging of the human body's physiological, chemical, sensory, and psychological functions. On the other hand, chronological age represents only the sum of an individual's years since birth, and the assessment of chronological age from bone age is based on measures of growth and development for younger individuals and on indicators of biological age for adults. Chronological and bone age overlap to a certain extent, and chronological age in archaeological samples is determined by bone age. Dental remains show a high rate of preservation in an archaeological context and can be used as indicators of age, which could complement traditional skeleton-based demography [4].

Age, sex, and race are the three basic demographic and anthropological characteristics of each individual. Techniques for assessment the age at the time of death differ depending on whether they are determined in childhood when the growth and development of the teeth is not yet complete or are applied in adulthood after the growth and development of the teeth is complete. In the phase of tooth growth and development, age assessment is based on knowledge of the biological changes that characterize the growth and development of teeth. Chronology of these changes depends on numerous factors such as genetic factors, body constitution, endocrine status, diet, and race; hence, age can only be assess approximately. Methods for determining dental age in children and adolescents are identical to those used in forensic analyses of recent humans. These are Cameriere, Havvikko, Demirijan, Moores, and others [5–8].

The assessment of dental age of adult archaeological remains is also very similar to that of recent humans in forensic analyses, especially when observing internal tissues such as accumulation of secondary dentin, translucency of apical dentin, and amount of precipitated cementum. The wear of enamel and dentin in the area of the dental crown differs due to different lifestyles and eating habits from the ancient period until today [9].

The samples that are the subject of paleo odontological research, primarily teeth, jaws, and skulls, are parts of archaeological skeletal collections from various archaeological sites and archaeological bone collections. The first and most visible change in dental crowns is wear of the dental crown or abrasion. Tooth abrasion, apart from being a reliable indicator of an individual's age at the time of death, can also be an indicator of his eating habits or the studied group. Namely, the frequent consumption of hard and solid food increases the abrasion of the teeth, hence they wear down more. The angle of abrasion is also one of the possible sources of data on the lifestyle habits of an individual. Thus, the flat type of abrasion is typical of populations who were engaged in hunting and fruit gathering, and the oblique type is typical of populations who were engaged in agriculture.

Estimation of dental age can point to the difference in the age of death from ancient and prehistoric societies. Understanding the living conditions that people faced throughout history is possible through the reconstruction and analysis of the remaining human remains. All changes in growth and development as well as possible diseases during lifetime can be read from bones and from teeth [10].

The appearance of age markers on the bones and teeth is different depending on the living conditions of each person. Most methods of assessment the age of adults that are related to changes in body appearance are based on the analysis of macroscopic characteristics of various osseous and dental structures. These methods do not give precise results, which is why dental age is estimated rather than determined [10].

Methods of estimating age at death are always expanding and improving, but it seems that methods based on changes in teeth due to aging are more accurate than other methods based on bone findings. Thus, teeth are much more useful than bones due to their great resistance to physical and chemical factors. While most bones are destroyed due to various environmental factors, most teeth remain healthy. Microscopic and biochemical methods, apart from being very complicated and expensive, destroy dental tissue, thus preventing the use of tooth morphology for further studies.

Classification of age groups is often used in the classification of human tooth remains

- Fetal (before birth)
- Infants (0–3 years old)
- Childhood (3–12 years old)
- Adolescent (12–20 years old)
- Adults (over 25 years old)

Assessment of the age of children and adolescents seems to be under strong genetic control. In an archaeological context, dental evolution is the most widely used method for estimating the age of juvenile remains. Traces of aging can be examined in three different ways in the processes of development of the dental system: calcification of enamel, dentin, and dental cement; teeth growing and eruption from the jawbone; and complete closure of the root apex.

14.2 Methods for Estimating Dental Age in Archaeological Samples

Age assessment is a very complex analysis because bones and teeth from archaeological sites are often very poorly preserved. Therefore, it is important to handle the samples carefully to prevent further damage.

Age estimates based on dental and bone remains are fairly accurate for adolescents or young adults. On the other hand, the remains belonging to elderly individuals pose great challenges. When dealing with ancient populations, it is difficult to be sure that significant age changes occurred at the same time and showed the same group variability as in modern populations. Therefore, it is best to combine several methods to increase the confidence level and percentage of success in age assessment.

Methods for assessing dental age applicable in adults can be divided into morphological and radiological techniques. Although there are many methods available, it is recommended to use only methods based on nondestructive analysis of the sample in bioarchaeological research. Therefore, the age estimation methods most often used by anthropologists and bioarchaeologists are macroscopic [11].

The four most common nondestructive age assessment methods: analysis of palatal suture closure, occlusal tooth wear, tooth root translucency, and pulp/tooth surface ratio [12].

14.2.1 Closure of the Palatal Suture

The pattern of cranial suture closure has been studied by many researchers for nearly a century as a marker of age. Unfortunately, its reliability is still debated as it does not give an exact age. This is due to the large intrasutural variability seen along its length. It is rare to see completely fused cranial sutures in the second decade of life or apparently non-fused sutures in the elderly. Meindl and Lovejoy mentioned that critical forensic questions involve the degree and nature of synostosis occurring in later years rather than the regularity of closure in early adulthood [11].

Obliteration of the palatal suture is defined as any part of the suture that is no longer visible. If obliteration of the suture is complete, it is considered that the person was over 40 years old at the time of death. If the suture was open or partially open, the person was considered to be less than 40 years of age at the time of death, Fig. 14.1.

14.2.2 Tooth Wear

With the emergence of the first permanent tooth in the oral cavity, namely the lower central incisors and the first permanent molars, the biting surface begins to wear down.

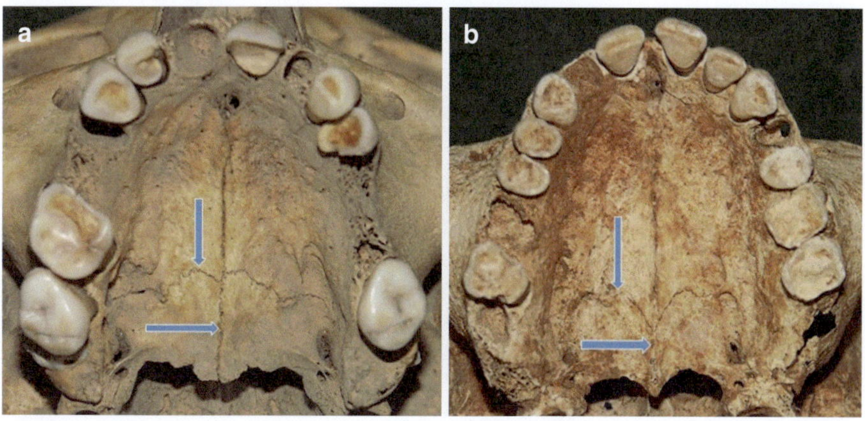

Fig. 14.1 Palatal suture on two skeletal remains: (**a**) sample younger than 40 years at the time of death and (**b**) sample older than 40 years at the time of death

Each subsequent tooth that erupts into the oral cavity will have a smaller pattern of tooth wear. In addition, wear will be affected by the strength of chewing, the type of diet, the thickness of dental structures, etc.

If the amount of wear in a population is almost the same, it can be concluded that the prevalence of wear in that population is a function of increasing age and, therefore, can be used to estimate the age of individuals. This method has also been tested in modern populations, and the relationship between age and tooth wear is well established. We should be aware of cases of very serious wear that can occur due to pathologies or the use of teeth as tools. The first step in age assessment using the tooth wear method is to use samples that show the stages of tooth growth and wear from the age sequence. For the first time, in 1963, Miles published a wear scale based on the process of tooth development. When the second permanent molar erupts at the age of 11.5, the first molar has been exposed to wear for about 6 years, Fig. 14.2, [13, 14].

In 1985, Lovejoy, by examining bones from prehistoric populations and preparing large collections with age sequence and tooth wear, concluded that tooth wear is an important and reliable measure of age at death in humans. Lovejoy et al. concluded that tooth wear is the single best measure of age at death in a skeleton. They found that the tooth wear with age rating scale has high accuracy and consistency, free from bias [15, 16].

Most researchers and authors tend to conclude that tooth wear is visible only after 20 years of life. While the previous methods are qualitative, today, a more

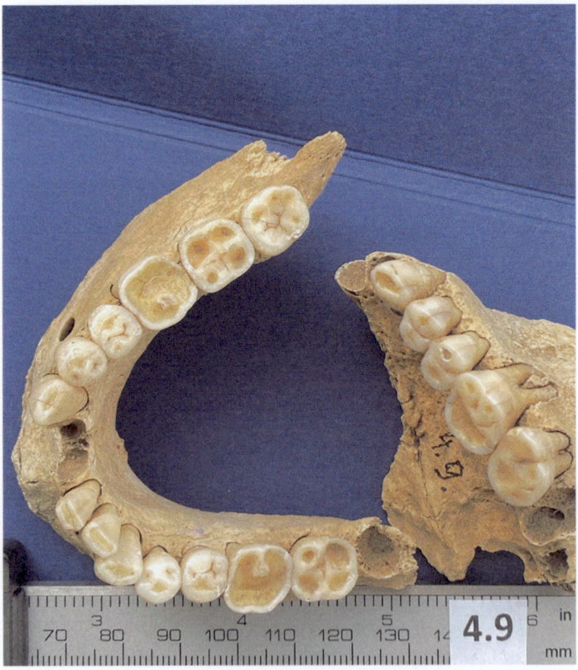

Fig. 14.2 Different degrees of tooth wear on the occlusal surfaces of teeth from the third century BC

modern quantitative method of digitized measurement for tooth wear surfaces using different software programs has been developed. VistaMetrix 1.38 software is a program that allows quantitative measurement on digital images of samples in a ratio of 1:1 to obtain metric data, Fig. 14.3, [17].

14.2.3 Root Translucency

During the lifetime, the dentinal tubules narrow, thus causing a translucent appearance in the dentin. The emergence of translucency begins in the third decade of life and has nothing to do with dental health or sex. Studies conducted on healthy and endodontically treated teeth showed the same level of apical dentin translucency. In forensic medicine, an increase in the size of sclerotic dentin in the apical root area of human teeth is used as a method to assess age. Measurement of translucency length in millimeters can be done with proper accuracy. In 1970, Bang and Ramm devised a method by which the length of translucent dentin at the end of the root was examined in two ways: incisors and complete teeth in human remains. Their formula, which was tested on modern human remains of known age and archaeological remains of unknown age, has proved to be applicable [18].

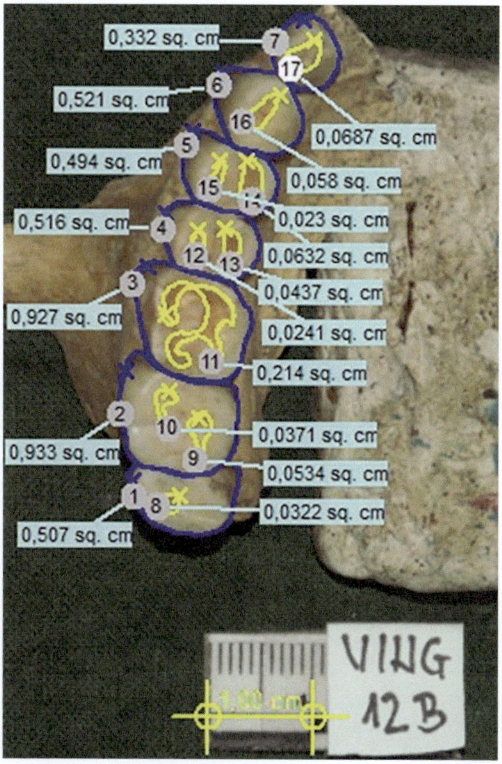

Fig. 14.3 Quantitative calculation of tooth wear with the software VistaMetrix 1.38

The roots of the permanent teeth are placed towards the light source, and the translucency of the apical dentin is observed. It is a consequence of the sclerosing of the dentine tubules that occurs during aging. Sclerosed dentin gives a transparent dentin color that is visible to the naked eye. Dentin translucency involvement is measured with a digital caliper. According to the results of numerous researchers in the field of paleostomatology and dental anthropology, this method is applicable to the teeth of recent humans and to samples of teeth from ancient times, Fig. 14.4.

14.2.4 Pulp/Tooth Surface Ratio

Deposition of secondary dentin occurs by continuous deposition of predentin produced by odontoblasts at the periphery of the dental pulp. Secondary dentin is a tissue that is naturally and physiologically slowly formed by the cells that form dentin. It is built linearly with very narrow tubes that are called dentin tubules. The formation of secondary dentin begins after the completion of the root. There is a slight difference between primary and secondary dentin that can sometimes be seen under a microscope. Continued formation of secondary dentin appears to be a biological response to aging. Therefore, since the wear of the dental crown increases with age, the surface of the pulp of the tooth core gradually decreases due to the

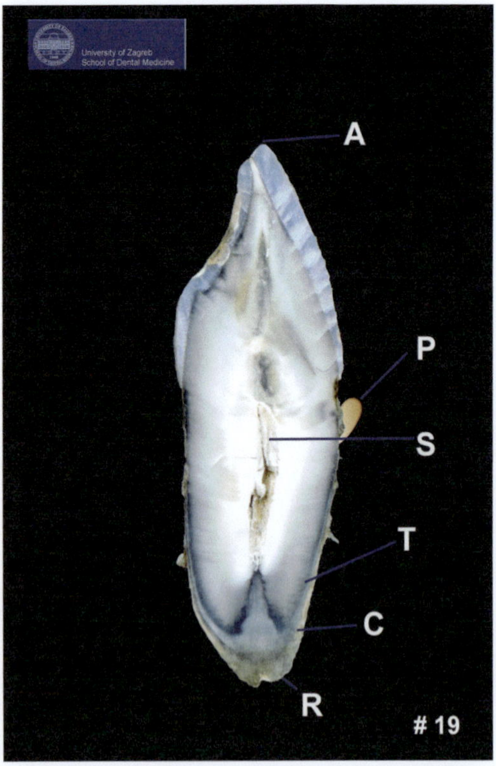

Fig. 14.4 Longitudinal section of human teeth showing (A) attrition, (P) level of periodontal ligament, (S) secondary dentin, (T) translucency, (C) cementum deposition, and (R) root resorption

continuation of the secondary deposition of dentin. Measuring the process of this reduction can be used as an indicator in age estimation. Today, there are several fast, simple, reliable, and nondestructive methods that use X-rays and radiographs, such as the Kvaal method, the Ikeda method, and the method according to Cameriere. According to Cameriere, radiographic images of upper canines are used to determine age using the pulp/tooth surface ratio. Cameriere et al. tested the reliability of pulp/tooth ratio age assessment in upper canines in historical samples of known age and found that the pulp/tooth ratio method is not only a useful technique for estimating the chronological age of living individuals, but is also a reliable age assessment tool at the time of death in skeletal remains [19–21].

14.2.5 Incremental Lines of Hard Dental Tissues

Mineralization of hard dental tissues occurs during the growth and development of enamel, dentin, and dental cementum. Calcium hydroxyapatite is the basic and most common inorganic substance that is incorporated into collagen networks that precede the final formation of the aforementioned tissues. The process of depositing minerals is not constant but takes place at intervals of several days or months. Each break in mineralization leaves a thin line in the tissue that is visible under a light microscope as a dark line and is called an increment line or growth line. They are named after the authors who first observed and investigated them. Apart from forming the basis of the histological structure of dental tissues, they have no other function, but can be used in forensic and archaeological research to estimate dental age. These methods are invasive and require the preparation of teeth in thin histological sections that are observed under a light microscope, and the distance between increment lines is measured [22].

Incremental lines in enamel are called Retzius lines according to the Swedish anatomist Retzius. The first Retzius line appears at birth and is given a special name, the neonatal line. It reflects the disturbed functioning of the ameloblast, which is a consequence of the change from the intrauterine to the extrauterine environment. Prenatal enamel is devoid of Retzius lines. Only primary teeth and first permanent molars possess prenatal enamel and will have a neonatal line. Retzius lines represent weekly changes in enamel mineralization. They are laid obliquely from the amelodentinal junction to the surface of the enamel, where they create a series of furrows called perikymata. The average human incisor contains about 150 brown stripes, and the distance between the stripes represents a growth of about 7 days. Retzius lines are used to determine the age of death in archaeological samples and their modern human contemporaries. Incremental lines in dentin are called von Ebner lines. Fine lines run almost perpendicular to the dentinal tubules from top to bottom on a thin section. Von Ebner lines represent the cyclic activity of odontoblasts during dentin formation. These incremental lines illustrate the diurnal pattern of dentin deposition which advances about 6 μm per day in the crown and about 3.5 μm per day in the root. These lines appear in regular increments. These lines can be also seen on demineralized tin sections [22, 23].

Incremental lines in cement have been named in a number of ways, often leading to confusion and misinterpretation. However, they are already known in the medical literature as "Lines of Salter," a term that would be more appropriate to adopt later in the study of dental cementum. Incremental lines of Salter indicate the so-called resting lines, darker in color, which alternate with lighter bands of tissue when seen under a transmitted light microscope. Their flow is irregular even though they are parallel to each other. They are most visible in the cellular cement that is created after the tooth root is formed, that is, during the lifetime. However, the debate on the nature and mechanism of their deposition still continues, Fig. 14.5.

14.2.6 Carbon-14

Carbon-14 (^{14}C) is the longest-lived radioactive isotope of carbon, the decay of which makes it possible to accurately determine the age of archaeological artifacts. An American physicist, Willard F. Libby, proposed the ^{14}C dating technique. For this development, he was awarded the Nobel Prize in Chemistry in 1960. It has proven to be a versatile technique for dating archaeological samples from 500 to 50,000 years old.

^{14}C, which is present in atmospheric carbon dioxide molecules, enters the biological carbon cycle. Green plants absorb it from the air, and then it is transferred to animals through the food chain. ^{14}C slowly decays in a living organism, and the lost amount is continuously renewed as long as the organism takes in air or food. However, when an organism dies, it stops absorbing ^{14}C; hence, the amount of the isotope in its tissues is constantly decreasing. ^{14}C has a half-life of 5730 ± 50 years. Since ^{14}C decays at this constant rate, an estimate of when an organism died can be made by measuring the amount of ^{14}C left behind [10, 24].

Once produced in childhood or adolescence, there is no change in enamel during the lifetime, and the concentration of ^{14}C in enamel reflects the level in food sources at the time of enamel formation. Since human teeth form at different, well-documented ages during childhood, the concentration of ^{14}C in tooth enamel can be used to determine the approximate date of birth. The absence of bomb-pulse carbon from the enamel indicates a date of birth no later than the early 1940s.

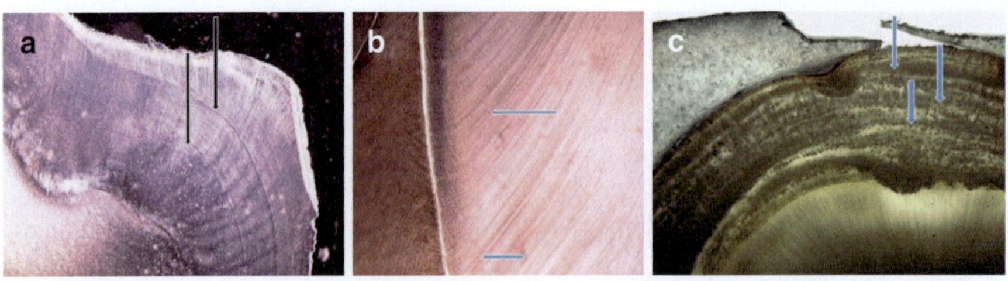

Fig. 14.5 Incremental lines in hard dental tissues: (**a**) Retzius lines in enamel, (**b**) von Ebner lines in dentine, and (**c**) Salter's lines in cementum

Enamel isolated from human teeth is processed into graphite, and ^{14}C levels are measured by accelerator mass spectrometry. Since there is no replacement of the enamel after it is formed, the ^{14}C levels in the enamel represent the ^{14}C levels in the atmosphere at the time of its formation.

In addition to the application of ^{14}C on archaeological remains to determine the time when they died, other stable isotopes are also used in archaeological analyses that prove the type of diet and possible migration [10, 24].

14.3 Examples from the Literature

Numerous studies performed by scientists in the field of bioarchaeology and anthropology around the world try to analyze and describe the bone and dental samples found. In this, the old continents lead the way, where numerous migrations, wars, and the collapse of civilizations took place.

Europe and Africa are such locations with a rich history where ancient civilizations existed before and after Christ. The Mediterranean area is very interesting because seas and rivers have always been the best locations for life, but also for occupations and conquests of territory. Throughout this rich history, numerous civilizations disappeared, leaving behind numerous biological and archaeological materials for analysis [25].

One of the most impressive examples is the discovery of the tomb of the youngest Egyptian pharaoh in 1922, which was initially very intriguing during the excavations and research. Besides, it was scientifically and archaeologically very provable. When the sarcophagus was opened, a mummy was found which, according to external anthropological parameters, pointed to Tutankhamun. Further analyses proved this, and based on the development of the roots of the third molars, his age at the time of death was estimated. Although the manner of Tutankhamun's death has not yet been proven, the analysis of radiological scans of his teeth has confirmed his age at the time of his death (1323 BC). He was between the ages of 18 and 19. Despite the importance of the boy king in contemporary history, his reign was short and relatively unimportant in the history of ancient Egypt. He became an important figure only after his death with the discovery of his tomb and mummy, both of which were remarkably well preserved and provided valuable insights into the history of ancient Egypt [26, 27].

The ancient Greek civilization and the Roman Empire were studied precisely on the basis of their biological, anthropological, and archaeological evidence, which is of interest to everyone today. Teeth played an important role in these analyses because they have survived to this day and are used for numerous micro and macroscopic analyses to confirm the time of their life, the type of food they consumed, socioeconomic status, whether they migrated or lived in one location, age, and sex at the time of death. The aforementioned facts can be proven by the methods described previously, as well as by the development of new interdisciplinary analyses [26, 28].

Research conducted on archaeological remains through the Croatian project "Analysis of teeth in forensic and archaeological research"—IP-2020-02-9423, mostly teeth and objects found in the tombs of the necropolis of Kopila on the island of Korčula in the Adriatic Sea, Croatia, not only confirms previous knowledge, but also leads to some new knowledge. According to the findings, the teeth and jaws from the tombs were made separately for children and separately for adults. Based on the assessment of the dental age of primary and permanent teeth, the age of deceased males and females was estimated using some standard methods described in previous chapters. Apical dentin translucency and tooth crown wear were used for dental age estimation in adults [29].

Furthermore, a new root variant was observed in Kopila, which is a buccal groove on the roots of the lower first and second premolars. This feature is unique, and it is not described in the Arizona State University Dental Anthropology System; hence, it is possible that this trait was typical of the ancient inhabitants of Korčula [29, 30].

Based on the analysis of ^{14}C from the teeth and skeletal remains of the Illyrian population from the Kopila necropolis on the island of Korčula in Croatia, the researchers determined that the anthropological remains date from the fourth to the first century BC. The results show that the island was inhabited by people engaged in agriculture and animal husbandry. Stable isotope analysis confirmed that they did not consume marine resources, at least not regularly or on a large scale. It was found that the dental status of the community was good, with a very low incidence of dental caries. This indicates that the community enjoyed good health and socioeconomic status, which improved over a long period of time under the influence of Hellenistic culture. The Illyrian population was the indigenous population of the island, and the inhabitants originally belonged to the West Eurasian geographical population group* [29].

14.4 Learning Outcomes

- You should be able to understand the importance of dental age in archaeological remains.
- You should be able to comprehend the different changes in the tooth like tooth wear, root translucency, pulp/tooth surface ratio, and incremental lines in hard dental tissues are studied to further correlate their applications in research analyses.

14.5 Self-Evaluation Questions

- Why are teeth favorable for age estimation in archaeological samples?
- Why are teeth more suitable than bone analysis in assessing age?
- What else can we evaluate with the help of teeth?
- Are destructive or nondestructive methods better for the analysis of teeth from archaeological remains?

14.6 Multiple Choice Questions

Q1. How can a tooth help us in the analysis of archaeological samples?

(a) Dental Age
(b) Sex
(c) Races
(d) All of the Above

Ans: d

Q2. Does tooth wear analysis require a destructive tooth procedure?

(a) Yes
(b) No
(c) I'm not sure
(d) None of the above

Ans: b

Q3. In which part of the tooth do we observe translucency?

(a) Tooth wear
(b) Tooth crown
(c) Tooth root
(d) None of the above

Ans: c

Q4. On which tooth is it possible to see the neonatal line?

(a) Permanent first molar
(b) Deciduous first molar
(c) Deciduous second molar
(d) All of the above

Ans: d

Q5. Is it possible to analyze the type of food from the teeth before death?

(a) No
(b) Maybe
(c) Yes
(d) None of the above

Ans: c

References

1. Šlaus M. Bioarheologija: demografija, zdravlje, traume i prehrana starohrvatskih populacija. Zagreb: Školska knjiga; 2006.
2. Vodanović M, Dumančić J, Galić I, et al. Age estimation in archaeological skeletal remains: evaluation of four non-destructive age calculation methods. J Forensic Odontostomatol. 2011;29(2):14–21.

3. Brkić H, Dumančić J, Vodanović M. Biology and morphology of human teeth. Jastrebarsko: Naklada Slap; 2021.
4. Iscan MY, Loth SR. Osteological manifestations of age in the adult. In: Reconstruction of Life from the Skeleton. New York: Liss; 1989. p. 23–40.
5. Cameriere R, Ferrante L, Belcastro MG, Bonfiglioli B, Rastelli E, Cingolani M. Age estimation by pulp/tooth ratio in canines by peri-apical X-rays. J Forensic Sci. 2007;52(1):166–70. https://doi.org/10.1111/j.1556-4029.2006.00336.x.
6. Haavikko K. The formation and the alveolar and clinical eruption of the permanent teeth. An orthopantomographic study. Suom Hammaslaak Toim. 1970;66:103–70.
7. Demirjian A, Goldstein H, Tanner JM. A new system of dental age assessment. Hum Biol. 1973;45:211–27.
8. Moorees CFA, Fanning EA, Hunt EE. Age variation of formation stages for ten permanent teeth. J Dent Res. 1963;42(6):1450–502.
9. Gustafson G. Age determination of teeth. J Am Dent Assoc. 1950;41:45.
10. Brkić H, Leesig R, Alves da Silva RE, Pinchi V, Thevissen P. Forensic odonto-stomatology by IOFOS. Jastrebarsko: Naklada Slap; 2021.
11. Scott GR, Turner CG, Townsend GC, Martinón-Torres M. The anthropology of modern human teeth: dental morphology and its variation in recent and fossil Homo sapiens. Cambridge: Cambridge University Press; 2018.
12. Kvaal S, Solheim T. A non-destructive dental method for age estimation. J Forensic Odontostomatol. 1994;12(1):6–11.
13. Buikestra JE, Ubelaker DH. Standards for data collection from human skeletal remains. Arkansas Archaeol Surv. 1994;44:18.
14. Scott EC. Dental wear scoring technique. Am J Phys Anthropol. 1979;51:213–8.
15. Miles AEW. Dentition in estimation of age. J Dent Res. 42:255–63.
16. Lovejoy CO. Dental wear in the libben population: its functional pattern and role in the determination of adult skeletal age at death. Am J Phys Anthropol. 1985;68:47–56.
17. Družijanić A, Vodanović M, Šlaus M, Čapkun V, Brkić H. Correlation of chronological age with tooth wear in archaeological populations. Coll Antropol. 2019;43:191–200.
18. Bang G, Ramm E. Determination of age in humans from root dentin transparency. Acta Odontol Scand. 1970;28(1):3–5.
19. Kvaal SI, Kolltveit KM, Thomsen IO, Solheim T. Age estimation of adults from dental radiographs. Forensic Sci Int. 1995;74(3):175–85.
20. Ikeda N, Umetsu K, Kashimura S, Suzuki T, Oumi M. Estimation of age from teeth with their soft X-ray findings. Jpn J Legal Med. 1985;39(3):244–50.
21. Cameriere R, Brogi G, Ferrante L, Mirtella D, Vultaggio C, Cingolani M, et al. Reliability in age determination by pulp/tooth ratio in upper canines in skeletal remains. J Forensic Sci. 2006;51(4):861–4.
22. McFarlane G, Guatelli-Steinberg D, Loch C, White S, Bayle P, Floyd B, Pitfield R, Mahoney P. An inconstant biorhythm: the changing pace of Retzius periodicity in human permanent teeth. Am J Phys Anthropol. 2021;175(1):172–86.
23. Birimiša M, Dumančić J, Vodanović M, Anić Milošević S, Marić M, Brkić H. Forensic determination of dental age by cementum thickness of human teeth. J Forensic Odontostomatol. 2021;39(3):41–8. Published online 2021 Dec 1.
24. Uberlaker DH, Parra RC. Radiocarbon analysis of dental enamel and bone to evaluate date of birth and death: perspective from the southern hemisphere. Forensic Sci Int. 2011;208(13):103–7.
25. Sedig JW, Olade I, Patterson N, Harney É, Reich D. Combining ancient DNA and radiocarbon dating data to increase chronological accuracy. J Archaeol Sci. 2021;133:105452.
26. Belcastro G, Rastelli E, Mariotti V, Consiglio C, Facchini F, Bonfiglioli B. Continuity od discontinuinity of the life-style in Central Italy during the Roman imperial age- early middle ages transition: diet, health and behavior. Am J Phys Anthropol. 2007;132(3):381–94.
27. Pausch NC, Naether F, Krey KF. Tutankhamun's dentition: the pharaoh and his teeth. Braz Dent J. 2015;26(6):701–4.

28. Vodanovic M, Brkic H, Slaus M, Demo Z. The frequency and distribution of caries in the mediaeval population of Bijelo Brdo in Croatia (10th–11th century). Arch Oral Biol. 2005;50(7):669–80. https://doi.org/10.1016/j.archoralbio.2004.11.014.
29. Marić M, Radić D, Dumančić J, Vodanović M, Birimiša M, Radovčić D, Brkić H. Teeth macroabrasion for determination of dental age and diet in the Illyrian population from the Kopila necropolis on the Island of Korčula, Croatia. Homo. 2022;73(1):49–60.
30. Vila-Blanco N, Varas-Quintana P, Tomás I, Carreira MJ. A systematic overview of dental methods for age assessment in living individuals: from traditional to artificial intelligence-based approaches. Int J Legal Med. 2023;137(4):1117–46.

15 Age Estimation in Criminal Investigations and Human Rights Frame

Emilio Nuzzolese, Hemlata Pandey Gala, Scheila Mânica, and Maurizio Cardanobile

Abbreviations

ANCI	Italian National Association of Italian Municipalities)
UFM	Unaccompanied Foreign Minors (UFM)
ECHR	European Court of Human Rights
DPCM	Italian Presidential Decree of the Council of Ministers
CRC	Convention on the Rights of the Child
EASO	European Asylum Support Office
ASGI	Association for Legal Studies on Immigration

15.1 Age Assessment and the Law

The assessment of an individual's age is of fundamental importance primarily in the legal field, especially in the context of criminal law, as it dictates the treatment an individual will undergo during the judicial process and the execution of the sentence.

Age significantly impacts both accountability and the procedure to be followed, which vary across Countries. The age of criminal responsibility varies widely across the world, reflecting different cultural, legal, and social perspectives on when a

E. Nuzzolese (✉)
University of Turin, Turin, Italy

Juvenile Court of Bari, Bari, Italy
e-mail: emilio.nuzzolese@unito.it

H. Pandey Gala · S. Mânica
University of Dundee, Dundee, UK

M. Cardanobile
Juvenile Court of Bari, Bari, Italy

© The Author(s), under exclusive license to Springer Nature Switzerland AG 2026

A. Chowdhry, P. Kapoor (eds.), *Dental Age Assessment*,
https://doi.org/10.1007/978-3-032-08788-1_15

young person can be held accountable for their actions. In many countries, the minimum age of criminal responsibility is set between 12 and 14 years, such as in Canada and Germany, where children below this threshold are considered too young to fully understand the implications of their behavior. In contrast, countries like Scotland have raised the age to 12, while others, like Japan and some Scandinavian nations, set it at 15. In some parts of the United States, however, children as young as 6 can face legal proceedings, though this is controversial and often revisited by lawmakers. Generally, there is a global trend toward raising the minimum age to align with developmental psychology insights, recognizing that children need age-appropriate approaches within the justice system [1].

In Italy, according to Article 85 of the Criminal Code, individuals under the age of 14 are not considered legally accountable, meaning they cannot undergo criminal proceedings or be punished for an offence. This principle reflects the legislator's intention to protect younger individuals, deemed incapable of fully understanding the consequences of their actions, or at least not yet possessing the necessary maturity to be held criminally responsible. In Germany, for various legal issues such as criminal, family, social, and immigration law, the age range is between 14 and 21 years [2]. In Portugal, the Portuguese penal code promotes the protection of juvenile individuals between the ages of 12 and 14 years, the legal ages. For the application of criminal law, the practice of an act committed by a minor under the age of 16 that would otherwise constitute a crime is not considered imputable [3]. In Brazil, criminal liability starts at 18 years of age, as determined by Article 228 of the Federal Constitution since 1988 [4].

The capacity to understand involves comprehending one's actions; in other words, it pertains to the ability to orient oneself externally and perceive reality truthfully. In essence, it involves the ability to distinguish between what can be done and what cannot be done by acknowledging and accepting the consequences [5]. Therefore, age assessment is also crucial in determining whether the procedure should follow the rules of ordinary or juvenile justice. The latter, governed by Italian Presidential Decree 448/1988, is based on an approach aimed not only at punishment but at the rehabilitation and reintegration of minors into society, recognizing the sensitivity and vulnerability of those who have not yet reached the age of majority.

The juvenile justice system adopts measures focused on the recovery of the minor (also in compliance with Article 27 of the Italian Constitution) as alternatives to detention, aiming to limit the negative impact that a judicial process could have on a young person's future.

In situations where an individual's age cannot be definitively established through documents or traditional identification methods, Article 8 of Presidential Decree 448/1988 is invoked, allowing for a noninvasive examination to estimate the subject's biological age. This is particularly relevant in cases of unaccompanied minors or migrants lacking identification documents.

Different countries employ varied approaches to juvenile justice and age determination, especially for undocumented minors. In the UK, age assessment involves a series of interviews and examinations conducted by social workers to evaluate physical appearance, behavior, and maturity [6]. Medical examinations are used only as a last resort. In France, the process includes judicial oversight, where age assessment may involve dental and wrist X-rays [7]. Germany prioritizes noninvasive assessments but may also use medical evaluations in situations involving unaccompanied minors, ensuring minimal psychological and physical impact on the minor [8].

In the United States, juvenile justice practices prioritize rehabilitation over punishment, similar to Italy. Age assessments often involve interviews and physical examinations, especially in cases of undocumented minors, though states may vary in their procedures. The U.S. Department of Health and Human Services sometimes oversees age assessments for migrant youth, often employing noninvasive methods but occasionally using medical imaging as a last resort [9]. In Australia, age determination practices for juveniles—especially for undocumented asylum seekers or those involved in legal matters—often include a range of assessments. While dental, wrist, or clavicle X-rays are sometimes used, their reliability is widely debated. X-ray age assessments, particularly wrist X-rays, have been used in the past but are now approached with caution due to potential inaccuracies. Australian authorities have increasingly adopted noninvasive techniques, focusing on interviews and document verification, and emphasizing ethical standards to ensure assessments respect minors' rights and health concerns [10].

The examination may include tests such as bone radiography, assessment of dental development, and other assessments comparing the physical development of the individual with medical age standards.

However, if the examination results are not precise or conclusive enough, the principle of *favor minoris* prevails, imposing an absolute presumption of the minority. This legal principle is based on the idea that, in case of doubt, the individual as a minor is preferable, applying the guarantees and protections provided for minors accordingly. This choice is driven by the need to protect young people from potential errors that could jeopardize their future, ensuring they are not subjected to a punitive regime unsuitable for their condition. This presumption is particularly significant in areas such as criminal law, immigration law, and other legal matters where the age of an individual plays a key role in determining their rights, responsibilities, or protection.

Age assessment is not merely a technical step but a central element in ensuring that the individual receives the most appropriate treatment based on their psychophysical maturity, in line with the principles of justice and protection envisaged by the legal system. Age estimation is vital for assessing the risk of reoffending. Research suggests that minors are more likely to be rehabilitated than adults, particularly when their offences are nonviolent [11]. If an individual is wrongly classified as an adult due to age estimation errors, they may be subjected to harsher penalties and deprived of rehabilitation opportunities to reduce recidivism. If a person is identified as a minor, they may be directed toward intervention programs designed for young offenders, which focus on education, psychological counselling, and skill development, aiming to prevent future crimes.

Age affects courtroom procedures, such as the right to a fair trial and the type of court in which an individual is tried. Minors are often entitled to more legal protections, such as closed hearings or the appointment of a guardian ad litem, who ensures that the minor's interests are represented [12]. Age estimation is crucial in determining whether these protections are afforded. In some jurisdictions, the ability to stand trial or the competence to understand legal proceedings is age-dependent. Children may not be considered competent to stand trial due to their cognitive and emotional development, and age estimation can be used to determine whether the individual is fit to face legal proceedings.

The issue of age assessment becomes even more critical in cases of unaccompanied foreign minors, given that they are recipients of many safeguards, especially at the international level. Often, these individuals arrive in the destination country without suitable documents to verify their age (due to loss, confiscation by traffickers, nonexistence, or following different calendars) and may not always be able to present them later.

Yet, age identification is crucial as it is a prerequisite for applying the protection and assistance measures prescribed by current regulations, such as the right to be welcomed into a minor's facility, to have a guardian, and not to be expelled or detained in an Identification and Expulsion Center.

For this reason, various regulations have been gradually introduced to overcome procedural shortcomings in Italy. A significant step in this direction was taken with Article 5 of Law 47/2017, which introduced a unified procedure for identifying unaccompanied foreign minors. This procedure begins when the minor arrives in Italy and involves immediate assistance and placement in initial reception facilities for up to 30 days. During this period, a meeting is guaranteed not only to determine their identity but also to understand their personal and family experiences and the reasons for their journey. This meeting, conducted by specialized personnel and assisted by a cultural mediator, plays a crucial role in verifying the declared age.

Age estimation has far-reaching implications in the criminal justice system, influencing everything from the legal process and sentencing to ethical considerations and human rights protections. It plays a fundamental role in ensuring that minors are treated appropriately and that justice is served fairly.

15.2 Definition of Unaccompanied Foreign Migrants

The legal frameworks governing the protection of unaccompanied foreign minors (UFM) differ across countries, but many international conventions set standards for their treatment. The European Union has established various directives and regulations to protect unaccompanied minors, notably the EU Directive 2013/33/EU, which lays down standards for the reception of applicants for international protection. It mandates special treatment and care for minors, ensuring they are treated with dignity and respect and that their best interests are a primary consideration in decisions made about them [13]. The Dublin Regulation (EU) No 604/2013 establishes the criteria for determining the country responsible for an asylum application.

However, there are exceptions for minors to ensure they are not returned to a country where they would face harm [14].

The United States treats unaccompanied minors (under 18 years old) as a special category within immigration law. The Trafficking Victims Protection Reauthorization Act mandates that UFMs from non-contiguous countries (such as Central American countries) are placed into the care of the Office of Refugee Resettlement and are provided with legal protections [15]. Unaccompanied minors seeking asylum are typically not subject to expedited removal processes but instead must go through immigration court procedures, where their age and vulnerability are considered.

In the United Kingdom, under the Children Act 1989 (England and Wales), the welfare of all children is paramount, including unaccompanied minors. Local authorities are required to assess the needs of UFM and provide appropriate care and accommodation. The Immigration Act (2016) includes provisions for the protection and care of unaccompanied minors within the asylum system. It also mandates the appointment of an independent guardian to represent their best interests.

The legislation concerning Unaccompanied Foreign Migrants (UFM) has undergone significant evolution since the 1990s. Although the migration flows of these minors began in the 1960s, it was only after the fall of the Berlin Wall that a considerable increase in arrivals was recorded. During the last decade of the twentieth century, there was an intensification of boat landings from Albania and land entries of minors from the former Soviet bloc.

By the end of July 2013, according to data provided by the Ministry of Labor and Social Policies, the unaccompanied non-asylum-seeking minors reported in Italy were 7402.[1] In 2021, because of the crisis in Afghanistan, the number of unaccompanied foreign minors (UFMs) seeking asylum in a European Union member state exceeded 23,250 individuals. This represents an increase of over 72% compared to 2020.[2] The growing phenomenon led to the enactment of regulations on the subject, also considering the fact that the identification of minors is not immediate.

Before delving into the topic, it is necessary to first provide a legal definition of UFMs. This dates to 1999 when in Italy, following the ratification of the Convention on the Rights of the Child in New York (1989), the Committee for Foreign Minors was established within the Ministry of Labor and Social Policies by the Presidential Decree of the Council of Ministers (DPCM) 535/1999. This committee was tasked with ensuring that unaccompanied minors received the rights they were entitled to while in the country, all in line with the principles of the Convention itself. The committee was also responsible for promoting initiatives for the reception and monitoring of minors.

[1] Italian Ministry of Labor, Immigration General Direction, Division IV, National report on unaccompanied foreign minors, accessed http://www.lavoro.gov.it/md/AreaSociale/Immigrazione/minori_stranieri/Documents/Report%20MSNA%2031-07-2013.pdf . This report included 1452 untraced minors.

[2] EUROSTAT, Asylum applicants considered to be unaccompanied minors by citizenship, age and sex—annual data (rounded), July 2022, accessed https://appsso.eurostat.ec.europa.eu/nui/show.do?dataset=migr_asyunaa

However, since 2012, due to a reorganization stemming from public expenditure containment measures adopted by the Monti government, the committee's responsibilities were transferred to the Directorate General of Immigration and Integration Policies.

DPCM 535/1999 introduced the first official definition of UFM, describing it as a minor who is not an Italian citizen or a citizen of other EU states, present in Italy without assistance or legal representation from parents or responsible adults.

This definition disagreed with those adopted at the international and European levels [16], to the extent that the European Union urged member states to harmonize definitions and data collection methodologies to facilitate comparisons among different national realities.

In 2008, to improve the reception system and make it more uniform, the Ministry of Labor and the National Association of Italian Municipalities (ANCI) developed the National Program for the Protection of UFMs.

One of the 2008 summary reports highlighted how the lack of harmonization of definitions and sources hindered the understanding of the phenomenon at the European level, resulting in difficulties in collecting uniform data.

In 2015, Legislative Decree 142 updated the definition of unaccompanied minors, overcoming the distinction between unaccompanied minors and asylum seekers. According to this norm, an unaccompanied minor is defined as a foreign citizen under eighteen years of age present in the national territory without assistance or legal representation. However, some categories of minors, such as unaccompanied minor community members, remained excluded from this definition, as evidenced by migration flows from Romania.

The legislation on UFMs underwent further changes with Law 47/2017, known as the Zampa Law, which eliminated differences in treatment between migrant minors, including political asylum seekers in the category of UFMs, thus ensuring equal legal protection. The law defines an unaccompanied foreign minor as a minor who is not an Italian citizen or a citizen of the European Union present in Italy without assistance or legal representation and states that such minors enjoy the same rights of protection as Italian or European minors.

The Committee for Unaccompanied Foreign Minors has identified four main categories of unaccompanied foreign minors: those seeking to reunite with emigrated parents, victims of trafficking or exploitation, minors illegally entering Italy, and those seeking international or humanitarian protection. It is important to emphasize that the concept of "minor" is not a biological fact but a legal criterion, set at 18 years old, both in Italy and at the European level. The definition of "foreigner" refers exclusively to citizens of non-EU countries.

Finally, the concept of "unaccompanied" refers to minors in a state of abandonment, that is, without assistance and protection from a responsible adult. Italian legislation equates unaccompanied Italian and foreign minors, but there has been debate regarding minors living with relatives up to the third degree who are not formally appointed as guardians. In such cases, the Committee for Unaccompanied Foreign Minors clarified that minors entrusted to relatives up to the third degree with a formal decision are considered accompanied.

15.3 Victims of Human Trafficking

Trafficking in human beings (THB) is a modern form of slavery, and after the drug dealing and weapon industry, human trafficking is the third largest criminal activity in the world. Over 40 million people worldwide are victims of human trafficking [17], and UNICEF estimates that more than 1.2 million children are trafficked annually. Migrants, refugees, and internally displaced people are particularly at risk of being trafficked. Many traffickers exploit minors by providing them with false identities or documentation to misrepresent their age. In addition, many trafficked minors arrive without any identification, making it difficult to establish their age. This lack of documentation can lead to misclassification, resulting in minors being treated as adults and subjected to harsher legal consequences.

This situation often complicates the identification process, making it imperative for authorities to utilize reliable assessment methods that prioritize the best interests of the child. Children, especially immigrant and refugee children, are at risk of victimization and may experience considerable physical and mental health consequences [18]. This includes exploitation of a child for prostitution, sexual exploitation in travel and tourism, the mail-order bride trade and early forced marriage, the production of child sexual exploitation material (pornography), live online sexual abuse, and forced participation in sexual venues [19]. Reliable estimates of the incidence and prevalence of child trafficking are unavailable, but it can be essential during an investigation to assess the age of the victims to identify the most appropriate interventions and subsequent resource provision for victimized and high-risk youth.

Minors who are victims of human trafficking require medical attention and protection to prevent secondary victimization [20, 21]. Addressing human trafficking requires a multifaceted approach that includes effective age assessment. By ensuring that age determinations are conducted accurately and sensitively, authorities can better protect vulnerable minors from exploitation and provide them with the support they need to heal and reintegrate into society. Legal systems, policymakers, and practitioners must work together to create frameworks that prioritize the rights and well-being of children, ultimately contributing to the prevention of trafficking and the protection of survivors.

15.4 National and International Regulations

To fully understand the topic, it is necessary to examine the regulations at both the international and national levels. The regulations we will address partly concern minors (such as the United Nations Convention on the Rights of the Child of 1989, the Civil Code, and Law 184/1983 on custody and adoption), partly those related to immigration (Legislative Decree 286/1998—Consolidated Immigration Act), and partly those specific to unaccompanied minors (DPCM 535/1999) [22].

The child's right to receive special assistance was first established in the Universal Declaration of Human Rights in 1948. Since then, the United Nations has developed further international treaties, such as the Human Rights Covenants,[3] and specific documents for the protection of minors, like the Declaration of the Rights of the Child in 1959. Subsequently, there was a need to give these rights a binding legal character. For this reason, in 1979, during the International Year of the Child, the UN Human Rights Commission began working on the Convention on the Rights of the Child (CRC), which was adopted in 1989 and came into force in 1990.

Thanks to the ratification of the CRC by 192 countries[4] (excluding only the United States and Somalia), a framework of minimum guarantees for the protection of children's rights was established. The CRC is now considered the most comprehensive international instrument regarding the rights of minors. Each article of the Convention reflects a compromise reached during negotiations, given the wide range of participating countries. The Convention is important not only because it recognizes civil, political, economic, social, and cultural rights for minors, but also because it acknowledges them as holders of rights, not merely as recipients of protection.

From the Convention emerge the fundamental rights of minors that, as emphasized by General Comment No. 6 of the UN Committee on the Rights of the Child, must be guaranteed by all adhering states in age verification procedures, including (1) the principle of the best interests of the child,[5] which must prevail in all decisions concerning them (Art. 3); (2) the right to non-discrimination,[6] which guarantees the same rights to all minors, regardless of their origin (Art. 2); (3) protection from violence, abuse, exploitation, and trafficking (Arts. 19, 20, 35, and 38); (4) the right

[3] The International Covenant on Economic, Social and Cultural Rights (New York, December 16, 1966, entered into force March 23, 1976), the International Covenant on Civil and Political Rights (New York, December 16, 1966, entered into force March 23, 1976), and the Optional Protocol relating to the latter Covenant (New York, December 16, 1966, entered into force March 23, 1976).

[4] Italy ratified the CRC with Law No. 176 of May 27, 1991.

[5] The principle in question must represent the primary reason for initiating an age assessment procedure, and this should be considered before examining the age itself. This principle, enshrined in Article 3 of the Convention on the Rights of the Child, requires that the best interests of the child be the primary consideration in all decisions affecting them. General Comment No. 14 clarifies that this principle is both a substantive right and an interpretive rule, applicable at all decision-making stages concerning the child. At the European level, this principle is reiterated in the Charter of Fundamental Rights of the European Union (Article 24) and in the Treaty on European Union (Article 3.3). Moreover, any margin of error in the assessment procedure must be applied in favor of the child. A significant case examined by the UN Committee on the Rights of the Child in 2018 involved an unaccompanied asylum seeker from Côte d'Ivoire (case N.B.F. v. Spain, No. 11/2017). In that case, the Committee emphasized that the principle of the best interests of the child implies that age assessment should not be based solely on medical criteria but also on psychological maturity, ensuring the individual benefits from the doubt and is treated as a minor in cases of uncertainty.

[6] The principle of nondiscrimination requires that the person undergoing the age assessment procedure be treated as a minor, without distinction based on nationality, ethnicity, social origin, or other status (such as that of a migrant), in accordance with Article 2 of the Convention on the Rights of the Child. However, difficulties in determining the age of individuals from specific contexts can lead to discriminatory situations.

to information about their rights and duties (Art. 13); (5) The right to participate,[7] express their opinions, and be heard in proceedings concerning them (Art. 12); (6) the right to physical, mental, and social development and to adequate living conditions (Arts. 6,[8] 24, 27, 28, 29, and 31); and (7) The right to preserve their cultural identity (Art. 8).

States that are signatories to the CRC commit to aligning their domestic legislation with the principles of the Convention and to adopting all necessary measures to ensure respect for these rights. However, despite community efforts to harmonize norms and policies regarding unaccompanied minors, discrepancies and suboptimal practices still exist in various European contexts, as shown by the cases of Italy and the UK post-Brexit. For this reason, states must periodically report to the Committee on the Rights of the Child on the status of implementation of the Convention.

Among other significant international regulatory sources, the 1961 Hague Convention on the Protection of Minors, the 1980 Luxembourg Convention on the Recognition of Custody Decisions, and the 1997 European Council Resolution on unaccompanied minors from third countries should be mentioned.

Turning to national legislation, it is important to highlight that Italian laws governing the situation of unaccompanied minors derive from the interaction between child protection legislation and immigration law, two traditionally separate areas, with the former focused on protection and the latter adopting a more restrictive approach. Over time, these areas have developed differently, creating confusion and varying practices in different Italian municipalities. Indeed, it was only in the late 1990s that legislation began to address the condition of unaccompanied minors. Before Law 40/1998 and Legislative Decree 286/1998, there was no specific regulation for foreign minors, and the approach was primarily inspired by the 1989 New York Convention, with interventions aimed at placing unaccompanied minors under the jurisdiction of the Juvenile Court rather than the police authorities.

The only provisions at the central and local levels were contained in administrative circulars that, while not formal sources of law, gained significant importance over time, generating an "infra-administrative law" that led to heterogeneous practices. Between 1994 and 1998, some ministerial circulars established that unaccompanied minors could access the labor market and were not subject to expulsion once

[7] This right is fundamental to ensuring the effective participation of the minor in the age assessment procedure. An unaccompanied minor should undergo this evaluation only after obtaining the informed consent of the minor and their guardian. According to a 2018 report from the European Union Agency for Fundamental Rights, most EU member states require the consent of the minor and/or the guardian before initiating the procedure. In some countries, explicit consent from both is necessary.

[8] The right to development and the dignity of the human person, as established in Article 6 of the Convention on the Rights of the Child, implies that age determination should occur in the least invasive manner possible, as provided by Directive 32/2013 (Article 25.5), and that priority should be given to official documents and psychosocial assessments before resorting to physical examinations. Invasive medical exams, such as physical or radiographic tests, can indeed violate the prohibition of inhuman or degrading treatment, according to an extensive interpretation of Article 3 of the European Convention on Human Rights.

they reached adulthood, thus favoring integration. The juvenile jurisdiction, on the other hand, had the sole task of identifying the most appropriate protective solutions for the minor.

The Turco-Napolitano Law of 1998, included in the Consolidated Immigration Act, established the principle of the non-expulsion of foreign minors, with exceptions for reasons of national security or public order. Moreover, the principle of the "best interests of the child" was introduced as a guiding criterion in all decisions concerning them.

Despite these advancements, some issues persisted, such as the difficulty for unaccompanied minors to obtain a residence permit upon reaching adulthood. Only "fostered" minors could obtain permits for study or work, while those under guardianship were excluded, creating a disparity in treatment. Subsequent legislative interventions, such as Legislative Decree 133/1999, further modified the situation, introducing the possibility of repatriating unaccompanied minors through administrative decisions, thus limiting judicial guarantees.

In 2002, the *Bossi-Fini* Law worsened the situation, reducing the options for unaccompanied minors to remain in Italy after reaching adulthood and making it more difficult to renew residence permits. This law, combined with ministerial circulars, increased the precariousness of foreign minors, despite the intervention of the Constitutional Court, which in 2003 sought to correct some of the disparities in treatment.

The regulatory framework was further improved with the approval of Law 47/2017, known as the Zampa Law, which introduced important innovations for the protection of unaccompanied minors. Among the main changes is the absolute prohibition of pushbacks at the border and the expulsion of minors, except for reasons of national security, and only if repatriation does not pose risks to the minor. The law also strengthened the reception system and integrated existing regulations, ensuring more comprehensive protection of the rights of unaccompanied minors, in line with the Italian Constitution and the Convention on the Rights of the Child. Furthermore, the *Zampa* Law of 2017 standardized the process of age identification and assessment and promoted the adoption of a multidisciplinary approach.

Despite this, the implementation of this legislation has faced challenges due to the lack of implementing decrees and standardization of operational practices throughout the country. Consequently, there are still territorial disparities in the procedures followed, with cases where medical assessments remain the only criterion adopted.

The Multidisciplinary Protocol of 2020, approved by the State-Regions Conference, represents another step towards greater national coherence. It provides for a three-phase procedure aimed at ensuring that each step is conducted in respect of the best interests of the child.[9] This document incorporates many of the precautions already present in previous protocols, such as social interviews and

[9] Unified Conference, "Multidisciplinary Protocol for Determining the Age of Unaccompanied Foreign Minors," 2020.

psychological assessments, but also introduces measures to reduce the invasiveness of procedures.[10]

Despite progress, the implementation of regulations remains fragmented and heterogeneous. However, there is a growing convergence between local practices and the national regulatory framework, which raises hopes for increasingly effective protection for unaccompanied minors.

15.5 Age Assessment

EU member states generally follow guidelines set out by the European Asylum Support Office (EASO), the UNHCR, and the Council of Europe for age assessments, which emphasize a child's right to protection and the principle of the "best interests of the child." The EU Reception Conditions Directive mandates that unaccompanied minors must be treated as such unless proven otherwise.

Determining age is one of the most complex and debated aspects in identifying an unaccompanied foreign minor (UFM), especially when there is uncertainty about whether the individual is a minor or an adult. When unaccompanied minors arrive in Italy, it is both necessary and legally required to provide them with immediate assistance and protection.

For this purpose, they are provided with accommodation in appropriate facilities for the strictly necessary period (not exceeding 30 days) and undergo identification, which also includes age verification. According to Article 19 of the Zampa Law, which amended Legislative Decree 142/2015, a conversation with the minor must be guaranteed during their stay in the first reception facility. The objective is to delve into their personal and family history, collecting information useful for their protection. The aim is to clarify the minor's personal situation, the reasons for their departure from the country of origin, the circumstances of the journey, and their future expectations. Among the useful documents for age assessment are passports, identity cards, birth certificates, school certificates, clinical documents, and other attestations issued by competent foreign authorities, which can be presented by the minor or collected through a variety of sources (databases, family, schools, hospitals, refugee camps).

The conversation, conducted by qualified personnel from the facility, with the support, if possible, of entities or organizations specialized in child protection [23, 24], is necessary to proceed with the identification of the minor, and in case of doubts about the declared age, the public security authorities must verify the existence of civil documents, possibly involving diplomatic-consular authorities. According to the UNHCR guidelines on assessing international protection claims in relation to minors (UNHCR, Guidelines on International Protection No. 8), age assessment should also consider psychological maturity, and in exceptional cases, the same

[10]The proposed composition for this team includes a pediatrician with auxological expertise, a developmental psychologist or child neuropsychiatrist, a cultural mediator, and a social worker, all properly trained and periodically updated; see Unified Conference, "Multidisciplinary Protocol."

guidelines may apply to individuals over 18, demonstrating that chronological age is not the only determining factor in assessing the person's vulnerability.

However, these authorities cannot intervene if it could expose the minor to dangers, for example, if they have requested international protection or have refused the intervention of consular authorities. At this stage, to facilitate communication, the presence of a cultural mediator is necessary. If doubts about the age persist after the checks, the Public Prosecutor's Office at the Juvenile Court may order socio-health examinations to determine it. The minor or their guardian must be informed of the need for these exams, the possible results, and the consequences of refusal.

At this stage, the presence of a cultural mediator is required to facilitate communication, taking into account the minor's maturity and literacy level.

Article 19 specifies that age verification must take place in a suitable environment, with a multidisciplinary approach by qualified professionals. The methods must be as noninvasive as possible, respecting the presumed age, gender, and physical and mental integrity of the person, while avoiding any harm or infringement of dignity.

Since there is no scientific method that can determine age with absolute certainty, the techniques used only provide an estimate with a margin of error of about ±2 years, based on standards not always suitable for the populations of the evaluated minors.

The procedure foresees, as mentioned, a social interview, an auxological pediatric visit, and a psychological or neuropsychiatric evaluation. The social interviews aim to reconstruct the personal and family history, the journey, and the social context of origin, with the goal of cross-referencing the information collected, possibly also through contact with family members.

Article 5 of DPCM 234/16 establishes that health examinations must follow a progressive invasiveness criterion: if certain elements of minority emerge from one phase, further assessments are not carried out.

An assessment that determines adulthood based on a single examination, such as a wrist X-ray, is not valid, while to establish a minority, a single examination with a certain outcome may be sufficient. Considering the adults, the age assessment is more challenging; therefore, a few methods should be used in combination to increase the accuracy of age estimates [25].

The examination results must be communicated to the foreigner in a language comprehensible and appropriate to their age, maturity, and level of literacy. The guardian and the judicial authority that ordered the assessment must also be informed, and the margin of error of the examinations must be reported in the report.

There is also the possibility to challenge the decision on the assigned age, with the judge required to rule within ten days. Until then, any administrative and criminal proceedings related to identification as an adult are suspended. In case of persistent doubt about the age after the examinations, the law provides for the presumption of minority. The *Zampa* Law thus introduces the presumption of minority until there is evidence to the contrary.

It is necessary to clarify that the personnel conducting the interviews are not always trained in interviewing techniques and listening to minors, and should be familiar with the sociocultural context of the minor's origin. However, this critical aspect can be overcome through adequate training of the staff and the dissemination of specific guidelines or support tools, such as interview templates or checklists. Among these, the evaluation of physical development is highlighted: in Italy as in Europe, the most common approach is medical, particularly using wrist X-rays. The methods used also include visual examination, which includes a medical history and the evaluation of anthropometric indicators or pubertal development; measurement of skeletal maturity through auxological parameters, especially through wrist and hand X-rays, and to a lesser extent of the clavicle; analysis of dental development; and examination of epiphyseal fusion degree using non-radiological methods. The dental analysis is performed mainly by observing the development of wisdom teeth (or third molars) [26, 27] using radiographs. Mention should be made that limitations are present: third molars are highly variable, commonly extracted, and may be congenitally absent, and many studies claim that the development is population-specific [28].

The assessment of wrist and hand X-rays through the development of carpal bones and ossification of growth cartilages, which close at different ages depending on the subject's development [29], is analyzed; the examination of the clavicle, which represents one of the last bones to complete ossification in an individual [30] and the analysis includes the assessment of the medial clavicular epiphysis [31].

Despite the wide variety of methods, there is no consensus on the most reliable one or the most suitable professionals to conduct these assessments. However, the literature agrees that there are no scientific methods capable of precisely determining a person's chronological age, especially in adolescence. A medical examination only provides an estimate of chronological age, with a margin of error that can vary by about two years more or less than the estimated age. Since skeletal and dental growth occurs more rapidly in children and slows down as they approach 18 years, this margin of error is smaller in younger individuals but can increase by up to five years as adulthood approaches.

Additionally, there are issues related to the invasiveness of some methods, especially considering that these practices are not for diagnostic or therapeutic purposes. Pubertal development assessment could be traumatic for minors who have experienced sexual abuse. The use of ionizing radiation for nondiagnostic or therapeutic purposes is controversial due to potential health risks, with different implications depending on the exposed body part.

Lastly, it is important to highlight that medical assessments are not always carried out by adequately specialized personnel or individuals aware of the sociocultural context of unaccompanied minors' origin. Moreover, the reports often do not indicate or describe the scientific method used or the margin of error.

On July 9, 2020, the Unified Conference sanctioned an agreement between the Government, the Regions, and Local Authorities regarding the "Multidisciplinary Protocol for Determining the Age of Unaccompanied Foreign Minors." This agreement, under Article 9, paragraph 2, letter c) of Legislative Decree August 28, 1997, no. 281, aligns with the provisions of the Prime Minister's Decree of November 10, 2016, no. 234, and Law April 7, 2017, no. 47. The main objective is to define a uniform and appropriate procedure in the socio-health field for determining the age of unaccompanied foreign minors, to be applied uniformly at the national level. The Protocol, of a sequential and incremental nature, adopts a multidisciplinary approach that, in compliance with the best interests of the minor and upon request of the competent Judicial Authority, is applied in cases where there are well-founded doubts about the declared age, and this cannot be verified through identification documents or other procedures provided for by Article 5 of Law no. 47/2017.

The outlined procedure involves the intervention of a multidisciplinary team and is structured, as mentioned earlier, into three successive phases with increasing invasiveness: a social interview, a psychological or neuropsychiatric evaluation, and an auxological pediatric visit with possible health assessments, conducted in a manner as respectful as possible of the presumed age, gender, and psychophysical integrity of the minor. These examinations must be carried out in suitable environments, at the minor's accommodation facilities or in public healthcare facilities of the National Health Service (NHS), identified by the Regions and Autonomous Provinces based on specific competencies and territorial organizations.

If certain elements confirming minority emerge during any of the phases, further assessments are not carried out. However, if doubts persist even after the socio-health assessment, the law provides that the minority is presumed for all purposes. This protocol aims, therefore, to ensure an age determination process respectful of the rights of the minors, safeguarding their integrity and promoting harmonization of practices at the national level.

15.6 Italian and International Jurisprudence

The evolution of the procedure for determining the age of so-called unaccompanied foreign minors (UFM) has found reflection and, in some cases, support in both national and international jurisprudence. One of the main topics of debate concerns the multidisciplinary nature of the assessment. However, over time, the position of Italian jurisprudence on age assessment has changed. For example, the use of radiological examinations to establish age was addressed in a ruling by the Court of Cassation, which referenced ruling no. 18336 of 2003, reaffirming the reliability of results related to skeletal development. Nonetheless, the introduction of regulations favoring a more multidisciplinary and holistic approach has influenced jurisprudence, leading to greater scrutiny regarding the exclusive use of auxological examinations. An example of this shift is the ruling of the Turin Court in January 2014,[11]

[11] "But [...] it must be emphasized here that the reading of the opinion [of the Superior Health Council] (and especially the related attachments) clarifies one point: the mere radiographic examination is not capable of accurately estimating a person's chronological age in individual cases (except with a margin of error, which is also variable). The existence of a legitimate orientation that considers the assessment of the results of radiographic examinations that evaluate bone age to be satisfactory—for the purposes of determining chronological age—imposes a particular motivational carefulness" in Tribunal of Turin, Criminal Sect. III, January 27, 2014, R.G. No. 6288/13, rapporteur Natale.

which dealt with the case of an alleged minor without documents, who was declared an adult based on radiological examinations, despite consistent statements from the individual. The ruling highlighted the inaccuracies of radiological examinations, particularly concerning the individual's ethnicity, and stressed the importance of multidisciplinary assessment. In light of the uncertainties identified, the court acquitted the defendant, concluding that the results of the radiological examination were not sufficiently reliable.

Similar concerns were expressed by the Justice of the Peace in Genoa in a ruling from 2014,[12] which accepted an appeal against an expulsion decree based on a radiological assessment, giving greater weight to the documents presented by the defendant.

At the European level, the issue of exclusive reliance on radiological examinations has been raised in appeals to the European Court of Human Rights, as seen in the cases of Darboe and Camara v. Italy[13] and Bacary v. Italy.[14] In these cases, the applicants contested that their age was determined solely through X-rays, without applying the prescribed multidisciplinary procedures. Recently, the Court of Cassation emphasized the necessity of genuinely multidisciplinary procedures for age assessment, insisting on the importance of reporting the margin of error in radiological examinations and prioritizing civil documents. These developments indicate a gradual alignment between national jurisprudence and supranational jurisprudence, as well as between the rulings of ordinary courts and those of the Court of Cassation, moving towards a convergence of legislation, judicial interpretation, and practical application.

However, in a recent statement on March 15, 2024, the Committee of Ministers of the Council of Europe expressed concerns regarding Italy's implementation of the European Court of Human Rights (ECHR) ruling in the aforementioned case of Darboe and Camara v. Italy, where Italy was condemned for placing an unaccompanied foreign minor in an adult reception center for over 4 months without adequate healthcare and identifying them as an adult solely based on a radiological examination of the wrist. Furthermore, the minor was not granted the opportunity to appeal. In 2023, the Italian government requested the closure of the supervision procedure, claiming to have adopted sufficient measures to correct these violations. However, the Association for Legal Studies on Immigration (ASGI) emphasized, in two communications, that systemic violations of the European Convention on Human Rights continue to exist, particularly in the age assessment procedures for unaccompanied foreign minors. These issues have been further exacerbated by the enactment of Decree-Law 133/2023, converted into Law 176/2023.

The Committee of Ministers observed with concern that the legislation introduced in October 2023 significantly reduced the guarantees related to age assessment, which are central to the ECHR ruling, highlighting the need for further

[12] Justice of the Peace of Genoa, October 14, 2014, order No. 6579, rapporteur Gualandi, XXX (attorney Ballerini) v. Ministry of the Interior.

[13] ECHR, Darboe et Camara v. Italy, No. 5797/17, February 14, 2017.

[14] ECHR, Bacary v. Italy, No. 36986/17, July 5, 2017.

measures to ensure that unaccompanied foreign minors practically benefit from the presumption of minority and the protections provided by the 2017 regulations, even in an emergency.

Moreover, it was noted that the reception system in Italy remains inadequate, as many minors are placed in adult facilities with conditions that do not serve their best interests. In particular, the Committee criticized the 2023 legislation, which allows the placement of unaccompanied minors over 16 years old in adult facilities for periods of up to 150 days. The Committee reiterated the obligation of Italian authorities to prevent further violations, in accordance with the ruling in Darboe and Camara, and requested that information on any measures taken to address the identified issues be provided by September 2024.

This framework highlights a critical situation in the reception and age assessment procedures in Italy, necessitating urgent interventions to ensure the respect of the rights of unaccompanied foreign minors, following international regulations and Italy's commitments in the field of human rights.

Thus, age assessment is closely linked to human rights issues, including the registration of birth dates, strongly connected to the legal recognition of a person and access to fundamental rights, which all states are obliged to recognize, respect, and guarantee.

Furthermore, this act represents the legal basis for many of the fundamental rights of minors, [32] which, in the absence of such registration, could be compromised, putting at risk not only the safety and life of the minor but also their prospects, since they would be unable to exercise their right to vote, register for marriage, or obtain documents that certify their legal identity.

Among the fundamental rights of minors that could be compromised if there is no complete birth registration are the rights to legal identity, name, and citizenship, which are key elements for demonstrating a person's existence before the state, even outside their country of origin.

Therefore, the legal existence of an individual starts from the registration of the date of birth, granting them the right to exercise a series of civil, political, economic, and social rights. At the international level, this right is fully recognized in the Universal Declaration of Human Rights (UDHR) and the Convention on the Rights of the Child (CRC).

Despite these guarantees, birth registration remains one of the main challenges to overcome in various countries, especially those that are particularly poor and isolated. According to UNICEF data, millions of children worldwide are not registered at birth, particularly in sub-Saharan Africa and some areas of Asia and Latin America.

To address and overcome this issue, efforts should be made to improve registration systems, making them accessible to everyone, as well as to raise awareness among populations about the importance of registering their children, ensuring them a better and safer future.

15.7 Human Rights Considerations

Age assessment procedures are critical tools used in various sectors ranging from immigration services to criminal justice and welfare systems. Determining age accurately is pivotal because it affects the individual's legal rights and the type of support and protection they are entitled to receive. However, the methods and implications of age assessments raise substantial human rights concerns that need to be rigorously examined and addressed. Age is more than just a number, because it is a crucial determinant in access to rights and services, especially for minors. In legal contexts, age can determine whether one is treated as a juvenile or an adult, and this significantly affects the severity of legal consequences.

Ethical considerations highlight the importance of using multidisciplinary approaches, combining various methods to improve reliability and accuracy [33]. This ensures that decisions impacting an individual's rights are grounded in robust evidence. Collaboration among forensic odontologists, radiologists, anthropologists, and legal professionals, supported by population-specific data, is essential to safeguard the rights of vulnerable individuals while minimizing the risk of misclassification.

Dental age estimation methods are a valuable tool, and in combination with various techniques and technologies, such as biometric analysis and machine learning algorithms, the age estimation process will be able to ensure that margins of error do not compromise the dignity, safety, or well-being of those assessed, as demanded by the respect for human rights [34, 35]. The accuracy of dental age estimation methods varies depending on the specific technique, the age of the individual, and the population being studied, but human rights considerations play a crucial role in shaping how these methods are applied, particularly in cases involving minors. Techniques like Nolla and the London Atlas are among the most accurate for younger individuals, with margins of error of approximately 1.2–1.3 years, while methods such as Demirjian's are less precise, with deviations of about 2 years. However, accuracy declines significantly after 16 years of age as dental development completes, making it challenging to determine age beyond 18 years, with a 1-year margin of error falling below 50% reliability. This limitation is especially critical in contexts where legal or social thresholds, such as the age of majority, are being assessed. The variability in dental development due to ethnicity, sex, and individual differences necessitates caution to avoid discrimination or errors that could adversely affect the individual's rights. For instance, errors in age estimation could result in minors being placed in adult detention facilities or denied access to child-specific protections, violating their rights under international human rights law.

Ethical guidelines emphasize giving the benefit of the doubt to minors if age uncertainty exists, ensuring they are not unjustly categorized as adults, which might expose them to inappropriate legal or social treatment. For this reason, a human rights-oriented age estimation method is the critical step to ensure that children benefit from specific measures to protect their rights, avoiding delays and incomplete procedures. The guidelines advocate for the use of the least invasive methods first, such as interviews and psychological evaluations, before resorting to any medical or dental examination. Of course, age assessments should only be conducted when in the best interest of the child and never when a the individual is evidenlty a minor.

One last aspect of the age estimation process is informed consent, providing clear information about the procedures, their purpose, and potential legal consequences. Individuals have the right to refuse, and the presumption of the minority principle should always be applied. The informed consent must also include the information about the right to appeal in case they do not agree with the outcome of the age assessment.

Finally, it must always be considered that an age assessment, especially for children and adolescents, should only be conducted when it aligns with their best interests.

Respecting human rights in the age assessment of living individuals is not merely about choosing a multidisciplinary method, but also about implementing a procedure which respects the dignity, integrity, and privacy of the individual, considering the impact of these assessments on the lives and futures of those undergoing them. As international awareness of these issues grows it should involve the joint effort of policymakers, practitioners, and advocates to ensure that age assessments are conducted ethically, respecting the human rights of all individuals.

References

1. Child Rights International Network. Ages of majority – why do they matter? CRIN; 2023. [Internet]. Available from https://archive.crin.org/en/home/ages.html.
2. Schmeling A, Dettmeyer RM, Rudolf E, Vieth V, Geserick. Forensic age estimation: methods, certainty, and the law methods, certainty, and the law. Dtsch Arztebl Int. 2016;113:44–50. https://doi.org/10.3238/arztebl.2016.0044.
3. Augusto D, Pereira CP, Rodrigues A, Cameriere R, Salvado F, Santos R. Dental age assessment by I_{2M} and I_{3M}: Portuguese legal age thresholds of 12 and 14 year olds. Acta Stomatol Croat. 2021;55(1):45–55. https://doi.org/10.15644/asc55/1/6.
4. Kuhnen B, Fernandes CM d S, de Barros F, Andrade JM, Scarso Filho J, Gonçalves M, Serra M d C. Age estimation by analysis of dental mineralization and its forensic contribution. Res Soc Dev. 2021;10(11):e598101119481. https://doi.org/10.33448/rsd-v10i11.19481.
5. Garofoli R. Compendio di diritto penale. Parte generale e speciale. Rome: Nel Diritto editor; 2022. (in italian).
6. De Sanctis V, Soliman AT, Soliman NA, Elalaily R, Di Maio S, Bedair EM, Kassem I, Millimaggi G. Pros and cons for the medical age assessments in unaccompanied minors: a mini-review. Acta Biomed. 2016;87(2):121–31.
7. Musso S. The truth of the body as controversial evidence: an investigation into age assessments of migrant minors in France. In: Waiting and the temporalities of irregular migration. Routledge; 2020. p. 151–69.
8. Siefer T. Accommodation and inclusion of unaccompanied minors: an example from Berlin. In: Newcomer integration in Europe: best practices and innovations since 2015. Foundation for European Progressive Studies Rue; 2018. [Internet]. Available from: https://feps-europe.eu/wp-content/uploads/downloads/publications/integtration_web.pdf.
9. Office of Juvenile Justice and Delinquency Prevention. Chapter 4: Youth and the Juvenile Justice System – 2022 National Report. Washington, DC: U.S. Department of Justice; 2022.

[Internet]. Available from: https://ojjdp.ojp.gov/sites/g/files/xyckuh176/files/media/document/ncjj-chapter4.pdf.
10. Australian Human Rights Commission. Home. Australian Human Rights Commission. [Internet]. Available from: https://humanrights.gov.au/.
11. Kurlychek MC, Johnson BD. The juvenile penalty: a comparison of juvenile and young adult sentencing outcomes in criminal court. Criminology. 2004;42(2):485–515.
12. Novaković F. Guardians of justice: balancing rights and protection in the examination of minors and juvenile testimony in criminal proceedings. Zbornik Radova Centra Za Edukaciju Sudija I Tužilaca Rs. 2024;15(15):286–309.
13. Peek M, Tsourdi L. Asylum Reception Conditions Directive 2013/33/EU. In: Hailbronner K, Thym D, editors. EU Immigration and Asylum Law 2016. Verlag CH, Beck oHG, Nomos Verlagsgesellschaft mbH & Co KG. p. 1382–478.
14. Desimpelaere K. The dublin regulation: past, present, future. Master thesis, University of Kent. 2015. [Internet]. Available at: https://libstore.ugent.be/fulltxt/RUG01/002/213/386/RUG01-002213386_2015_0001_AC.pdf.
15. Harrington B. Legalization framework under the immigration and nationality act (INA). Congressional Research Service; 2019. [Internet]. Available at: https://crsreports.congress.gov/product/pdf/R/R45993.
16. De Marchi L. A piccoli passi. Minori non accompagnati e cittadinanza attiva. Formigine: Infinito Edizioni; 2017.
17. International Labour Organization (ILO) Forced labour, modern slavery and human trafficking. http://www.ilo.org/global/topics/forced-labour/lang%2D%2Den/index.htm (2017).
18. Nazer D, Greenbaum J. Human trafficking of children. Pediatr Ann. 2020;49(5):e209–14. https://doi.org/10.3928/19382359-20200417-01.
19. Institute of Medicine and National Research Council, Confronting commercial sexual exploitation and sex trafficking of minors in the United States.Washington, DC, The National Academies Press, 2013.
20. Moore JL, Kaplan DM, Barron CE. Sex trafficking of minors. Pediatr Clin N Am. 2017;64(2):413–21. https://doi.org/10.1016/j.pcl.2016.11.013.
21. Rafferty Y. Challenges to the rapid identification of children who have been trafficked for commercial sexual exploitation. Child Abuse Negl. 2016 Feb;52:158–68. https://doi.org/10.1016/j.chiabu.2015.11.015.
22. Petti. The lesser evil: the protection of foreign minors as exclusion. Verona: Ombre Corte; 2004.
23. UNICEF. Age assessment practices: a literature review & annotated bibliography. 2011. [Internet]. Available at: http://www.unicef.org/protection/Age_Assessment_Practices_2010.pdf.
24. Aynsley-Green A. The assessment of age in undocumented migrants, march 2011; SCEP, Position Paper on Age Assessment in the Context of Separated Children in Europe. 2012. [Internet]. Available at: http://www.scepnetwork.org/images/16/163.pdf.
25. Schmeling A, Geserick G, Reisinger W, Olze A. Age estimation. Forensic Sci Int. 2007;165(2–3) https://doi.org/10.1016/j.forsciint.2006.05.016.
26. Cameriere R, Ferrante L, De Angelis D, Scarpino F, Galli F. The comparison between measurement of open apices of third molars and Demirjian stages to test chronological age of over 18 year olds in living subjects. Int J Legal Med. 2008;122(6):493–7. https://doi.org/10.1007/s00414-008-0279-6.
27. Aynsley-Green A, Cole TJ, Crawley H, Lessof N, Boag LR, Wallace RM. Medical, statistical, ethical and human rights considerations in the assessment of age in children and young people subject to immigration control. Br Med Bull. 2012;102:17–42. https://doi.org/10.1093/bmb/lds014.
28. Berkvens ME, Fairgrieve SI, Keenan S. A comparison of techniques in age estimation using the third molar. J Can Soc Forensic Sci. 2017;50(2):74–83. https://doi.org/10.1080/00085030.2017.1281632. Teodoro MT, Forte V, Mazzone V, Cascio O. Accertamento dell'età biologica in immigrato clandestino. Ital J Legal Med. 2014;3:1 (in italian).

29. Focardi M, Pinchi V, De Luca F, Norelli GA. Age estimation for forensic purposes in Italy: ethical issues. Int J Legal Med. 2014;128(3):515–22. https://doi.org/10.1007/s00414-014-0986-0.
30. Kreitner KF, Schweden F, Riepert T, Nafe B, Thelen M. Bone age determination based on the study of the medial extremity of the clavicle. Eur Radiol. 1998;8:1116–22. https://doi.org/10.1007/s003300050518.
31. Bonaiuti C. Right to birth registration: the first step towards the protection of minors. In MARS paper, 1, 2021.
32. Dow U. Birth registration: the 'first' right in United Nations Children's Fund. New York: The progress of Nations; 1998.
33. Nuzzolese E, Di Vella G. Forensic dental investigations and age assessment of asylum seekers. Int Dent J. 2008;58(3):122–6. https://doi.org/10.1111/j.1875-595x.2008.tb00186.x.
34. Galante N, Cotroneo R, Furci D, Lodetti G, Casali MB. Applications of artificial intelligence in forensic sciences: Current potential benefits, limitations and perspectives. Int J Legal Med. 2023;137(2):445–58. https://doi.org/10.1007/s00414-022-02928-5.
35. Franco A, Murray J, Heng D, et al. Binary decisions of artificial intelligence to classify third molar development around the legal age thresholds of 14, 16 and 18 years. Sci Rep. 2024;14:4668. https://doi.org/10.1038/s41598-024-55497-5.

Artificial Intelligence in Age Estimation 16

Mohd Yusmiaidil Putera Mohd Yusof
and Norhasmira Mohammad

16.1 Introduction

The increasing number of undocumented or irregular migrants has raised concerns, particularly in third-world countries. The biological profile, which provides vital bone demographic information such as age, is a critical piece of evidence for authorities when determining refugee status and sentencing criminals. In cases involving deceased bodies, this information allows for the narrowing down of missing persons' lists and positive or definitive identification of unidentified human remains.

Traditionally, age estimation relies on conventional radiographic examinations and human competence. Demirjian's technique, amongst others, is frequently used to establish an individual's age, where it involves manually rating all seven permanent mandibular teeth using panoramic dental imaging and a designated atlas. However, this method becomes significantly lagging during large-scale incidents, leading to increased workloads and extended working hours. This leads to delayed identification and thus imposes pressure on the authority and the next-of-kin. Moreover, the conventional method may introduce subjective interpretation bias, especially between young and experienced forensic odontologists.

To address these limitations, researchers have explored the use of artificial intelligence (AI) technology to estimate an individual's sex and age based on radiographic images. AI is seldom addressed as automation. By definition, AI is the

M. Y. P. Mohd Yusof (✉)
Faculty of Dentistry and Research Institute of Forensic Medicine (RI-ForM), Universiti Teknologi MARA, Sungai Buloh Campus, Sungai Buloh, Malaysia
e-mail: yusmiaidil@uitm.edu.my

N. Mohammad
Faculty of Cognitive Sciences & Human Development, Universtiti Malaysia Sarawak, Kota Samarahan, Malaysia

© The Author(s), under exclusive license to Springer Nature Switzerland AG 2026

A. Chowdhry, P. Kapoor (eds.), *Dental Age Assessment*,
https://doi.org/10.1007/978-3-032-08788-1_16

ability of a digital computer or computer-controlled robot to perform tasks commonly associated with intelligent beings. The term is frequently applied to the project of developing systems endowed with the intellectual processes characteristic of humans, such as the ability to reason, discover meaning, generalize, or learn from past experience.

Automation on the other hand, especially in health care, means using software that makes care and services better. In addition, for the sake of efficiency, this technology makes use of modern techniques and tools. It helps us monitor the safety, security, and health status of our family members. The automation system may benefit both healthcare services and patients. For example, in healthcare services, the automation system improved the operational and administrative areas [8]. The impact of automation includes faster data retrieval, improved ordering, and quicker billing.

Furthermore, early disease identification, greater precision and speed in medical diagnostics, superior and long-lasting technology, and potentially reduced errors are some of the primary benefits of health care automation for patients [3]. The sophisticated healthcare system has the potential to improve efficiency and uniformity significantly. This indicates that an automation system built and adapted from the traditional way performs well. Besides, automation may aid in the improvement of reproducibility especially in the automated age estimation system [30]. Through the learning process, the ideal dataset for training can reach a complete agreement between inter-rater observers. Technically, a larger dataset for training can boost an automated system's performance significantly.

Age estimation in children and adolescents often depends on morphological methods, such as radiological examination of skeletal and dental development. However, the pelvic bone is one of the best indicators of adult age, and cranial sutures are also good predictors of death age. As the standard way of estimating age usually refers to the "gold standard," this shortcoming has become one of the possible research areas for automating the method.

One of the earliest studies on the automated dental age estimation method was based on a computer vision application, which uses the image segmentation approach to segment the region of interest (ROI) to estimate dental age in adults. The development of automated line-by-line scanning of tooth-cementum annulations (TCA) software to assess an individual's age was presented where this approach was evaluated on an unknown individual's age and compared to manual TCA counting-based age estimation. However, no comparison results were reported by the authors [7]. The advancement of computer vision and artificial neural network technology enables interdisciplinary scholars to improve reproducibility in a wide range of dental applications, particularly the operator-dependent procedure.

16.2 Application

The AI, machine learning (ML), and deep learning (DL) have become the most talked-about technologies in today's business sector, as corporations use these advancements to create intelligent devices and apps. It could be used as a second opinion for clinicians in the health industry, assisting them with clinical diagnosis and treatment.

AI is used informally when a machine mimics "cognitive" functions that humans associate with other human minds, such as "learning" and "problem-solving." Machine learning, on the other hand, was defined by Munoz [25] as the branch of computer science that can learn without being explicitly programmed. Machine learning is the study and creation of algorithms that can learn from data and make predictions based on that data. Meanwhile, deep learning is a branch of machine learning that emphasizes algorithms that are inspired by the structure of the human brain. This system can handle massive amounts of structured and unstructured data.

Convolutional neural networks (CNN) are the prime example of DL. The architecture of CNN typically consists of convolutional, pooling, and fully connected layers. Figure 16.1 shows an example of the general architecture of CNN, which consists of two layers of both convolution and pooling. Studying successful applications is an excellent way to create effective CNN architectures. The LeNet-5 is often described as the first successful and important application of CNNs before the ImageNet Large Scale Visual Recognition Challenge or ILSVRC. The intense study and application of CNNs from 2012 to 2016 for the ILSVRC witnessed four different winning architectural innovations: AlexNet, VGG, Inception, and ResNet.

LeNet-5 [19] was probably the first CNN that was widely known and worked well. It was created to address the issue of handwritten character recognition. The system was tested on the MNIST standard dataset, attaining a classification accuracy of 99.2% (or a 0.8% error rate). The network was then defined as the key component of a larger system known as graph transformer networks. According to this paper, the CNN architecture has seven layers and inputs grayscale images with the shape 32 × 32, which corresponds to the size of images in the MNIST dataset.

On the other hand, AlexNet [18] could be credited with bringing back interest in neural networks and paving the way for deep learning to become the best way to do many computer vision tasks. The model was first made for the ILSVRC-2010 competition, in which people had to put pictures of things into thousands of different groups. The architecture of this model consists of five convolutional layers in the feature extraction section, in which the authors fixed the input images to a size of

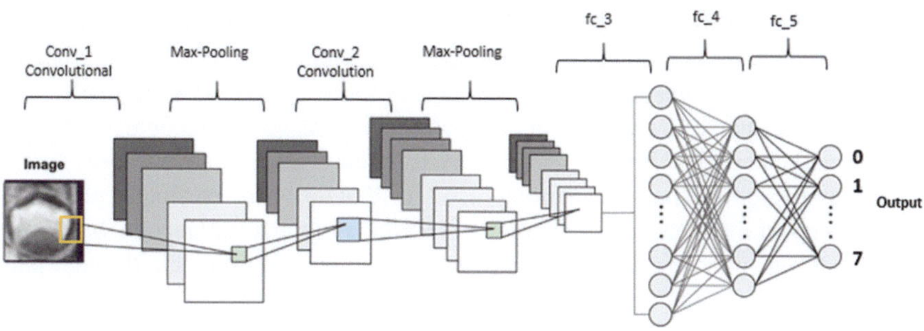

Fig. 16.1 Example of CNN architecture

224 × 224 with three colour channels. In contrast, the classifier section has three fully connected layers.

Another excellent intervention was published in 2014 called "Very Deep Convolutional Networks for Large-Scale Image Recognition," which aimed to standardize architecture design for deep CNN while also developing significantly deeper and better performing models [33]. VGG is the abbreviation for the Visual Geometry Group at Oxford, which is where they developed their architecture. For the ILSVRC-2014 competition, the VGG model was created. The employment of a large number of small filters is the first significant change that has established a genuine standard. Filters of sizes 3 × 3 and 1 × 1 with a stride of one, as opposed to the huge-sized filters in LeNet-5 and the smaller but still very large filters with a stride of four in AlexNet. The VGG models' design decisions have been the essential foundation and have become the starting point for simple and straightforward CNNs. In addition, the network architecture of the VGG model uses multiple convolutional layers stacked together before a max-pooling layer is used.

Instead of a simple and straightforward CNN, Szegedy et al. [35] show that a deeper parallel convolutional layer is a big step forward in how convolutional layers are used. It was suggested to use the inception architecture, and a model called GoogLeNet did very well in the ILSVRC-2014 competition. This model has a block of parallel convolutional layers with varying-sized filters such as 1 × 1, 3 × 3, 5 × 5, and 3 × 3 max-pooling layers, in which the outputs are then combined. This model was considered an intense and profound one as it has 22 layers.

Another significant advancement of the CNN model was the Residual Network (ResNet) [14] which has 152 layers. The model's development is based on the idea of residual blocks that use shortcut connections. A residual block is a pattern made up of two convolutional layers with ReLU activation. The output of the block is added to the input of the block. Basically, this model is inspired by the VGG model network. The idea is that the authors take exactly what is being proposed in the VGG network. However, no pooling layers between blocks were designed, resulting in a plain network. To define residual blocks, the plain network is transformed into a residual network by adding shortcut connections. The shortcut connection's input is usually the same size as the residual block's output.

The CNN model was one of the frequent network architectures for DL used in the field of dentistry, especially for the application of human identification that focuses on age estimation [11]. The abovementioned models are based on the CNN model, which at the beginning of its production only had a few layers of complexity that got more complicated and sophisticated as more inventions were made. The CNN is particularly useful for finding patterns in images to recognize objects, classes, and categories. It will learn directly from data. Because dental x-rays are a great diagnostic tool that is commonly used for diagnosis and treatment planning, the majority of the data was in images, and CNN is more advantageous than other traditional machine learning models because it can learn all the data through patterns and provides high reproducibility.

16.3 Previous Research in Age Estimation

The automation process of age assessment demonstrated exact reproducibility, just like the traditional method. The incomparability between the two methods, conventional and automated, was usually due to their different types of features. For example, if continuous features such as area and volume of anatomical structures are considered and the ROI is detected automatically, human observer action cannot compare to the automated staging system [9]. Therefore, only the performance of age estimation methods can be compared.

In 2015, Ge et al. [12] proposed a semi-automated system based on the volumetric measurements of the pulp/tooth chamber of the first molar. An open-source 3D image semi-automatic segmenting and voxel-counting software, ITK-SNAP 2.4, is used to calculate the volume of the pulp chamber. Logarithmic regression was used to estimate age using the volume obtained from the calculation using the software. In addition, the authors did the same study, but volumetric measurement was done on the 13 tooth types. Based on their findings, the authors discovered that the upper second molar volume is the most correlated with age [13].

Meanwhile, Asif et al. [4] studied a correlation between chronological age and pulp/tooth volume ratio for Malaysian adults, where two volumetric analysis methods of maxillary central incisors were employed. Method 1 used volumetric measurement of the pulp cavity/tooth ratio, and Method 2 used volumetric analysis of the pulp chamber/crown ratio. The authors used mimic software to process the images acquired from CBCT scans. Based on their findings, both methods show a strong correlation between chronological age and pulp/tooth volume ratio. On the other hand, method 2 yielded a better coefficient of determination value ($R2 = 0.78$) than method 1 ($R2 = 0.64$). In addition, an automated system that involves no human intervention during the preprocessing phase in Method 2 shortens the process and exhibits higher interobserver reliability. The authors also proposed using the method 2 regression equation in age estimation. Based on the studies above [4, 12, 13, 34], all of them used continuous data, such as the volume of the pulp chamber, to perform the dental age estimation, but none of them did a study on the development of the dentition.

The most common method of dental age estimation, which is based on tooth development, is based on Demirjian's staging system [10] where this method uses digital panoramic dental imaging to estimate the chronological age of an individual based on the mineralization of seven left permanent lower teeth. This method is also suitable for determining dental maturity states in individuals with known ages, rather than predicting an unknown age.

Several methods have been used in the past to segment dental radiographic images with good results. A semi-automatic approach which is based on a contour extraction method in order to overcome the limitation of fuzzy tooth contours caused by the low image quality has been proposed by Jain and Chen [16]. It involved three stages: image segmentation, pixel classification, and contour matching. Results showed that the proposed method can produce promising object segmentation using small sets of data. However, further improvement is needed as the algorithm had difficulties working on the blurry image, occluded objects, and irregular shapes of teeth that eventually led to the oversegmentation problem.

Another semi-automatic approach has been discussed by Banumathi et al. [5], which also involves three stages: morphological contour detection, Gaussian filtering, and an existing semi-automatic contour extraction method. Results affirmed that the proposed algorithm could achieve a precision rate of 0.7. However, the algorithm faced the same limitation as what has been proposed by Jain and Chen [16] when the blurry input image with the occluded object is used. Tuan et al. [37] proposed a new advanced approach in which the authors presented a new semi-supervised fuzzy clustering algorithm known as SSFC-FS based on Interactive Fuzzy Satisficing. The algorithm was tested on 56 dental radiographic images and was proven to produce better clustering results compared to other methods such as Fuzzy C-Means, Otsu, eSFCM, SSCMOO, FMMBIS, and another version of SSFC-FS with the local Lagrange method known as SSFC-SC.

A fully automated system for person identification using dental radiographic images requires a prior segmentation of the images into sections containing a single tooth. Dental shape extraction based on contour information is a common approach for feature extraction. Pushparaj et al. [29] used the integral intensity projection to segment the upper jaw, lower jaw, and individual teeth separately, followed by the shape extraction based on the fast connected component. The final stage includes the distance measurement using the Mahalanobis distance equation to measure the means of the matching distance. Results showed that the algorithm has produced better performance compared to their previous work, which is based on semi-automatic contour extraction [28]. An improvement of contour extraction has been made by Lin et al. [21], who used the point reliability measuring method and calculated the Hausdorff distance (HD) between the contours. Experimental results showed that this approach can achieve 100% accuracy for single tooth segmentation.

Another fully automated segmentation approach that is based on a thresholding method for dental age assessment has been proposed by Ahmad et al. [1]. The primary goal of this method is to optimise the threshold value, T, for use with the mean, median, and OTSU thresholding methods. Choosing the right value of T will produce a good segmentation result where the foreground and background image can be effectively separated. Meanwhile, a fundamental study on the region-based segmentation approach has been discussed by Razali et al. [31], where the comparison between the Canny and Sobel methods has been made in order to fulfil the requirements of the Demirjian method for assessing all of the tooth types in quadrants 2 and 3. Besides, the application of pixel-based image segmentation associated with the mathematical morphological operation for object extraction has been proposed by Amer and Aqel [2]. The result showed that the proposed method is able to produce the lowest mean absolute error (MAE) compared to other existing methods [26].

De Tobel et al. [9] proposed an automated technique for age estimation based on the mandibular third molar development using panoramic radiographs by employing pattern recognition and classification approaches to the target images. First, image contrast is being normalized for all data and ROIs which indicate the third molar was cropped using the Photoshop software. The performance of the CNN classifier was then evaluated in a five-fold cross-validation scenario, using different validation metrics to obtain the accuracy, Rank-N recognition rate, mean absolute difference, and linear kappa coefficient. As a result, the proposed method is able to stage lower third molar development according to staging by human observers. However, more data training is required as the pilot study was only tested on 20 images.

Muad et al. [24] have proposed a contour-based segmentation method to segment the second molar teeth. This has been accomplished by measuring the ratio of the mean and standard deviation of directional image derivatives over an entire closed contour boundary using the active contour algorithm. As a result, the authors obtained an overall segmentation accuracy of 95.3%.

Apart from that, the application of digital image processing on dental radiographs is broad and extensively used for dental disease detection, quantification of dental images, and detection of the dentition structure. Image classification techniques include image sensors, image pre-processing, object detection, object segmentation, feature extraction, and object classification. Yu [39] performed the teeth classification using the CNN classifier to classify all 28 permanent teeth by excluding the third molar. The training image was tested on two different CNN models, which are 4-layer and 16-layer. The result shows that the training time for the 4 layers of the CNN model was shorter, but the accuracy was lower than for the 16 layers of the CNN model.

The CNN algorithm was used by Prajapati et al. [27] to come up with a way to classify dental diseases. The dataset consists of 251 Radio Visiography (RVG) X-ray images that were trained using the CNN model to separate three different disease severity classes. The overall accuracy obtained is very promising. A similar study was also performed by Imangaliyev et al. [15] and Choi et al. [6], where the authors implemented the CNN to detect the dental plaque and carried out quantitative light-induced fluorescence (QLF) images and dental radiographs, respectively. Both results shown are encouraging. In addition, to evaluate the quality of the dental treatment, the CNN classifier is also applied by Yang et al. [38]. As a result, the F1 score of 0.749 is obtained, which is comparable to the performance of expert dentists and radiologists.

Recently, the deep learning convolutional neural network (DCNN) has been introduced to perform automated tooth segmentation, where these artificial intelligence methods have shown better performance compared to other mathematical approaches. De Tobel et al. [9] proposed a pilot study in which they modified the pre-trained model of the AlexNet network to stage lower third molar development on panoramic radiographs for age estimation. However, improvements have been made by Merdietio Boedi et al. [22], who use the DenseNet201 network for automated stage allocation. Based on the improvement, the authors made a new hypothesis that segmenting only the third molar could further improve the automated stage allocation performance. Another recent approach utilizing the region-based convolutional neural network, which required object segmentation before the classification, has been proposed by Lee et al. [20] and Kahaki et al. [17]. Image segmentation before classification might be needed for certain conditions, especially in dental age estimation, as literature states that the variation of the third molar might affect the accuracy of age estimation in different populations Tafrount et al. [36]. As such, for the automated approach, the classification accuracy may also be affected due to the morphology of the tooth and its surroundings. According to Merdietio Boedi et al. [22], the unwanted ROIs such as periodontal ligaments, bony structures, and the mandibular nerve canal influence the performance of automated stage allocation.

Also, the review article by Sharifonnasabi et al. [32] says that there will have to be a big change towards automated procedures. Image processing, feature extraction, image categorization, decision-making, and results are common processes in the reviewed studies. However, there is no good way to determine how old the dental age is because different studies use different methods to analyse and process images. As a result, recent AI technology, which provides a better end-to-end machine learning platform with a high-level API (application programming interface), enables AI practitioners to develop potential machine learning architectures, particularly based on the CNN model.

Transfer learning or modelling from scratch can be used to train the CNN or deep learning model. Seeing a lot of real-world problems, making much bigger datasets, and testing them with a model that has already been trained does not always lead to better results on the target tasks. The other alternative is to train a model from scratch, where the random weight initialization occurs in the early operations. The advent of deep learning platforms like Tensorflow makes it easier to build our own model based on real-world problems.

Mohammad et al. [23] developed their own deep CNN model from scratch using Tensorflow and Keras and compared the findings with the conventional method of estimating the individual's age. The performance of the proposed model is promising, as 97.74% and 78.13% of training and testing accuracy were obtained, respectively. In addition, moderate agreement (Kappa value = 0.58) between the human observer and the computer was identified. Nonetheless, a robust DCNN model was achieved, as there is no sign of the model's over- or under-fitting upon the learning process.

16.4 Conclusion and Future Research

In neural networks, the architecture is all that matters. A good performance of the neural network in making a prediction will significantly improve the classification accuracy and the inter-observer agreement. Deep learning approaches have been a major success due to their ability to learn task-specific feature representations automatically. It is one of the most often utilized models in data science applications today. It is also shown to be a successful model in various fields, including pictures, text, and voice and music. As the application of deep learning grows, applying it rapidly and being scalable becomes more important. Essentially, training the CNN model can be accomplished through transfer learning or modelling from scratch, and in certain real-world problems, the performance of the CNN model built from scratch outperformed that of transfer learning or vice versa.

Instead of focusing on the primary tool, which in the majority of the reviewed literature is the orthopantomogram obtained from the dental X-ray machine, other advanced imaging modalities such as cone-beam CT and MRI can be useful. Also, most of the proposed automated systems for figuring out a person's age use Demirjian's method, which looks at the eight stages of tooth growth. Demirjian's method is undeniably exceptional. This gold standard has been verified with numerous population-specific reference datasets. Also, this method is still relevant in the research area and is being employed and used as a benchmark for the newly proposed method of dental age estimation. Another recently established atlas on dental age estimation, which estimates the dental age based on tooth development and eruption and is known as the London atlas, provides a promising outcome. Thus, considering extending the deep CNN method with the London Atlas in the future might open a new topic of research interest that may gain the attention of interdisciplinary researchers.

References

1. Ahmad NS, Zaki ZM, Ismail W. Region of adaptive threshold segmentation between mean, median and otsu threshold for dental age assessment. In: 2014 International conference on computer, communications, and control technology (I4CT). IEEE; 2014. p. 353–6.
2. Amer YY, Aqel MJ. An efficient segmentation algorithm for panoramic dental images. Procedia Comput Sci. 2015;65:718–25.
3. Asan O, Bayrak AE, Choudhury A. Artificial intelligence and human trust in healthcare: focus on clinicians. J Med Internet Res. 2020;22:e15154.
4. Asif MK, Nambiar P, Mani SA, Ibrahim NB, Khan IM, Sukumaran P. Dental age estimation employing CBCT scans enhanced with mimics software: comparison of two different approaches using pulp/tooth volumetric analysis. J Forensic Leg Med. 2018;54:53–61.
5. Banumathi A, Vijayakumari B, Geetha A, Shanmugavadivu N, Raju S. Performance analysis of various techniques applied in human identification using dental X-rays. J Med Syst. 2007;31:210–8.
6. Choi J, Eun H, Kim C. Boosting proximal dental caries detection via combination of variational methods and convolutional neural network. J Signal Process Syst. 2018;90:87–97.
7. Czermak A, Czermak A, Ernst H, Grupe G. A new method for the automated age-at-death evaluation by tooth-cementum annulation (TCA). Anthropol Anz. 2006;64:25–40.
8. Davenport T, Kalakota R. The potential for artificial intelligence in healthcare. Future Healthc J. 2019;6:94.
9. De Tobel J, Radesh P, Vandermeulen D, Thevissen PW. An automated technique to stage lower third molar development on panoramic radiographs for age estimation: a pilot study. J Forensic Odontostomatol. 2017;35:42.
10. Demirjian A, Goldstein H, Tanner JM. A new system of dental age assessment. Hum Biol. 1973;45:211–27.
11. Ding H, Wu J, Zhao W, Matinlinna JP, Burrow MF, Tsoi JK-H. Artificial intelligence in dentistry–a review. Front Dent Med. 2023;4:9.

12. Ge Z-P, Ma R-H, Li G, Zhang J-Z, Ma X-C. Age estimation based on pulp chamber volume of first molars from cone-beam computed tomography images. Forensic Sci Int. 2015;253:133. e1-133. e7.
13. Ge Z-P, Yang P, Li G, Zhang J-Z, Ma X-C. Age estimation based on pulp cavity/chamber volume of 13 types of tooth from cone beam computed tomography images. Int J Legal Med. 2016;130:1159–67.
14. He K, Zhang X, Ren S, Sun J. Deep residual learning for image recognition. Proc IEEE Conf Comput Vis Pattern Recognit. 2016:770–8.
15. Imangaliyev S, Van Der Veen MH, Volgenant C, Loos BG, Keijser BJ, Crielaard W, Levin E. Classification of quantitative light-induced fluorescence images using convolutional neural network. *arXiv preprint arXiv:1705.09193*. 2017
16. Jain AK, Chen H. Matching of dental X-ray images for human identification. Pattern Recogn. 2004;37:1519–32.
17. Kahaki SM, Nordin MJ, Ahmad NS, Arzoky M, Ismail W. Deep convolutional neural network designed for age assessment based on orthopantomography data. Neural Comput Appl. 2020;32:9357–68.
18. Krizhevsky A, Sutskever I, Hinton GE. Imagenet classification with deep convolutional neural networks. Commun ACM. 2017;60:84–90.
19. Lecun Y, Bottou L, Bengio Y, Haffner P. Gradient-based learning applied to document recognition. Proc IEEE. 1998;86:2278–324.
20. Lee J-H, Han S-S, Kim YH, Lee C, Kim I. Application of a fully deep convolutional neural network to the automation of tooth segmentation on panoramic radiographs. Oral Surg Oral Med Oral Pathol Oral Radiol. 2020;129:635–42.
21. Lin P-L, Lai Y-H, Huang P-W. Dental biometrics: human identification based on teeth and dental works in bitewing radiographs. Pattern Recogn. 2012;45:934–46.
22. Merdietio Boedi R, Banar N, De Tobel J, Bertels J, Vandermeulen D, Thevissen PW. Effect of lower third molar segmentations on automated tooth development staging using a convolutional neural network. J Forensic Sci. 2020;65:481–6.
23. Mohammad N, Muad AM, Ahmad R, Yusof MYPM. Accuracy of advanced deep learning with tensorflow and keras for classifying teeth developmental stages in digital panoramic imaging. BMC Med Imaging. 2022;22:66.
24. Muad AM, Bahaman NSM, Hussain A, Yusof MYPM. Tooth segmentation using dynamic programming-gradient inverse coefficient of variation. Bull Electr Eng Inf. 2019;8:253–60.
25. Munoz A. Machine learning and optimization. 2014. https://www.cims.nyu.edu/~munoz/files/ml_optimization.pdf. Accessed 2016-03-02. [WebCite Cache ID 6fiLfZvnG].
26. Patanachai N, Covavisaruch N, Sinthanayothin C. Wavelet transformation for dental X-ray radiographs segmentation technique. In: 2010 eighth international conference on ICT and knowledge engineering. IEEE; 2010. p. 103–6.
27. Prajapati SA, Nagaraj R, Mitra S. Classification of dental diseases using CNN and transfer learning. In: 2017 5th international symposium on computational and business intelligence (ISCBI). IEEE; 2017. p. 70–4.
28. Pushparaj V, Gurunathan U, Arumugam B. Human forensic identification with dental radiographs using similarity and distance metrics. In: 2012 Annual IEEE India conference (INDICON). IEEE; 2012. p. 329–34.
29. Pushparaj V, Gurunathan U, Arumugam B. An effective dental shape extraction algorithm using contour information and matching by mahalanobis distance. J Digit Imaging. 2013;26:259–68.
30. Putra RH, Doi C, Yoda N, Astuti ER, Sasaki K. Current applications and development of artificial intelligence for digital dental radiography. Dentomaxillofac Radiol. 2022;51:20210197.
31. Razali MRM, Ahmad NS, Hassan R, Zaki ZM, Ismail W. Sobel and canny edges segmentations for the dental age assessment. In: 2014 international conference on computer assisted system in health. IEEE; 2014. p. 62–6.
32. Sharifonnasabi F, Jhanjhi N, John J, Alaboudi A, Nambiar P. A review on automated bone age measurement based on dental OPG images. Int J Eng Res Technol. 2020;13:5408–22.

33. Simonyan K, Zisserman A. Very deep convolutional networks for large-scale image recognition. arXiv preprint arXiv:1409.1556. 2014.
34. Star H, Thevissen P, Jacobs R, Fieuws S, Solheim T, Willems G. Human dental age estimation by calculation of pulp–tooth volume ratios yielded on clinically acquired cone beam computed tomography images of monoradicular teeth. J Forensic Sci. 2011;56:S77–82.
35. Szegedy C, Liu W, Jia Y, Sermanet P, Reed S, Anguelov D, Erhan D, Vanhoucke V, Rabinovich A. Going deeper with convolutions. Proc IEEE Conf Comput Vis Pattern Recognit. 2015:1–9.
36. Tafrount C, Galić I, Franchi A, Fanton L, Cameriere R. Third molar maturity index for indicating the legal adult age in southeastern France. Forensic Sci Int. 2019;294:218. e1-218. e6.
37. Tuan TM, Ngan TT, Son LH. A novel semi-supervised fuzzy clustering method based on interactive fuzzy satisficing for dental X-ray image segmentation. Appl Intell. 2016;45:402–28.
38. Yang J, Xie Y, Liu L, Xia B, Cao Z, Guo C. Automated dental image analysis by deep learning on small dataset. In: 2018 IEEE 42nd annual computer software and applications conference (COMPSAC). IEEE; 2018. p. 492–7.
39. Yu YJ. Machine learning for dental image analysis. arXiv preprint arXiv:1611.09958. 2016.

On-Field Assessment and Recovery of Dental Remains in Complex Scenarios

17

Abraham Johnson and Jyotirmoy Roy

> I will live in thy heart,
> die in thy lap,
> and be buried in thy eyes
> –William Shakespeare

17.1 Introduction

The tooth is the hardest structure in the human body. The outermost anatomic and histologic layer of the tooth, known as enamel, is resilient to traumatic natural and man-made events. It is able to withstand high temperatures, high pressure, and fares well in acidic and basic environments. Also, a tooth is extremely individualistic, bearing characteristic qualities of the organism it belonged to. The morphology and morphometric parameters of a tooth are determined by the environmental, evolutionary, and dietary factors. The attrition pattern, presence or absence of any pathology such as dental caries, and subsequent dental intervention such as dental fillings, crowns, etc. are all unique to the person to whom the tooth belongs. These properties make the tooth an invaluable source of evidence for any investigation, may it be forensic or academic. In forensic contexts, teeth are used primarily for positive identification and are particularly strong indicators of age. Archaeologically, dental studies that incorporate teeth include, for example, dietary reconstruction, assessment of biological distance, stable isotope analysis, and pathology. They are also sound reservoirs for ancient DNA. There are instances when taphonomic events/factors are significant enough to damage teeth to such an extent that certain analyses

A. Johnson (✉)
School of Medico-Legal Studies, National Forensic Sciences University, Gandhinagar, Gujarat, India
e-mail: abraham.johnson@nfsu.ac.in

J. Roy
Department of Oral & Maxillofacial Pathology and Microbiology, Guru Nanak Institute of Dental Sciences and Research, Khardaha, West Bengal, India

© The Author(s), under exclusive license to Springer Nature Switzerland AG 2026

A. Chowdhry, P. Kapoor (eds.), *Dental Age Assessment*,
https://doi.org/10.1007/978-3-032-08788-1_17

are hampered or even obviated. Mechanical processes need not be severe to fracture teeth; traumas, such as those seen in forensic settings where high-speed projectiles or blunt objects impact the face, can lead to dental fractures. However, even when major events such as mass disasters occur, it is possible that teeth will be available for examination. Therefore, it is important to understand dental anatomy and the physical properties of teeth in order to properly recover and study them.

Forensic taphonomy has been defined simply as the study of what happens to a human body after death. Since most of what happens to the body (and evidence) happens at an outdoor setting, the result of alteration or modification by natural agents such as plants, animals, soils, environment, gravity, and many other factors must be considered. The recognition and documentation of these specific roles played by each of these natural agents is critical to understanding and explaining why evidence ends up where it ends up, or why it looks as it looks at present. This allows us to focus on unusual patterns of dispersal or removal of evidence and remains that can provide indications of human intervention (e.g., moving/removing remains to hide evidence). The other primary assessment is that of postmortem interval (PMI), and how long the body has been at the location. This chapter provides examples where extreme postmortem mechanical and thermal events affect the conditions of teeth in terms of structure and appearance.

17.1.1 Forensic Taphonomy

Taphonomy is the study of how an organism's decay and becomes fossilized or preserved in the paleontological record. Soon, it was realized that the principles of taphonomic changes studied in archeology can be utilized in forensic investigations, and the discipline of forensic archaeology arose in the 1980s, just after the debut of forensic anthropology in the 1970s. The most effective tool for evidence collection of the outdoor scene was clearly archaeology. This was evident simply by comparing the coincidental primary goals of both disciplines which are the reconstruction of the past based on evidence found in highly altered contexts. In the 1970s and 1980s, discussion of the role of archaeology in forensics focused on the recovery of clandestine graves. Since that time, common archaeological methods and practices began to be employed in forensic scenes, including searches, burials, surface scatters, and, eventually, fatal fire and mass disaster scenes. These methods and practices, modified to meet forensic standards, were incorporated into a new discipline appropriately named forensic taphonomy. They have constructed the best methods for determining issues such as whether a particular fracture occurred antemortem or could instead be better attributed to natural postmortem damage or decay; whether the remains had been originally deposited at that location or had been transported there after death by different physical and biological processes; or how fast these changes occurred. With the introduction and quick adoption of taphonomy into anthropology and archaeology in the 1970s and 1980s, taphonomic methods and inference came to incorporate past human behavior, including how to distinguish alterations caused by humans from similar ones caused by natural agents, whether a deposit could represent an intentional burial or natural interment post-deposition. These are almost exactly the same questions posed by forensic scientists regarding forensic significance or manner of death, considering exactly the same natural processes playing a role at outdoor crime scenes and addressed by many of the same types of materials.

Taphonomic processes reduce the portions of a biological profile that can be generated and in particular lead to a loss of individualistic characteristics of the skeleton and tooth. Teeth trauma (gunshot wound, high-speed impact, etc.) is even more susceptible to further postmortem damage, especially the perimortem fracture surfaces with their distinctive characteristics. Teeth and bone do not have to pass through a singular taphonomic trajectory and in practical experience almost never do. Weathering of teeth and bone has been studied for decades, and this gradual process of bleaching and cracking can be distinguished from broadly similar changes such as cremation/calcination as well as give some indication of the PMI. Loss of teeth and bone may be understood by comparisons with known survivability rates and natural processes that delete teeth and bone. Therefore, in many cases, teeth and bone record their postmortem history by the alterations caused to them, cut marks, surface cracking and bleaching, adhering fauna, mineralization, marks from plant roots, algae growth, adherent sediments, thermal alteration, overall patterns of recovery, the loss of cortical surface, and epiphyses in patterned areas, or with retained tooth markings. Hence, it is the task of the forensic odontologist to sort out these conflicting signals and place them in correct temporal order to reconstruct the postmortem history backward from the recovered remains to their original living source.

17.2 Perimortem Changes Versus Postmortem Changes

Another important forensic taphonomic analytical category is the differentiation between human and natural alteration of teeth. Again, human alteration (perimortem trauma) is of specific interest to forensic expert, given that the reconstruction of the events surrounding the death is one of the main reasons that their analytical skills are sought by law enforcement agencies. Acts of violence may leave traces upon bone, which may be obscured or destroyed later, and unrelated taphonomic processes, or other postmortem forces, may cause damage to bone, which can be mistaken for perimortem trauma. More precisely, taphonomic analysis often focuses upon the differentiation between perimortem trauma from pseudotrauma (postmortem damage to a bone that superficially or more deeply appears to be perimortem in origin). Naturally, the presence of such postmortem alteration, if misdiagnosed as perimortem trauma, can result in serious legal ramifications for that case. This type of analysis includes differentiation between sharp force trauma vs. postmortem markings (incidental scratches, carnivore tooth marks, etc.); blunt force trauma vs. postmortem sources of teeth or bone breakage (animal gnawing, weakening through decomposition and postmortem erosion, etc.); and thermal alteration to fresh teeth and bone vs. dry, already skeletonized remains. This type of analysis is also restricted by a relative dearth of studies involving exactly how long the perimortem interval extends especially regarding how long bones and teeth have to age after death before they no longer fracture in the same manner as in a living or recently deceased individual. Natural alteration, however, also may include details of death information of significance to law enforcement. Death by wild animal attack is an obvious example, and this predation upon a human may lead to both perimortem trauma from the initial fatal attack damaging bone and to subsequent postmortem alteration as feeding on the deceased person proceeds and remains are dispersed. Death from accidental falls from height or drowning also has a high natural component, in the sense that the primary agency of death was a part of the natural world and as such may have had the largest amount of influence over immediate (massive perimortem blunt force trauma) or later (water transport and feeding by marine species) taphonomic changes to those remains.

17.3 Effects of Burial Environment on Tooth Remains

The most pervasive long-term destructive force acting upon calcified structure is soil acidity. In depositional environments with near-neutral or slightly basic pH, teeth and bone preservation typically are excellent. This is particularly true for deposits in limestone caverns. Limestone caverns have yielded the bulk of hominin fossil history into the beginning of the Holocene. Other factors interacting with the effects of soil acidity include the amount of groundwater flow. In an acidic soil water solution, the hydroxyapatite crystals, Ca5(PO4)3(OH), are depleted of calcium (Ca2+) ions by their replacement with hydrogen (H+) ions (derived from hydronium ions, H3O+) as equilibrium is reached with the soil water. If the water flow rate is high in this acidic environment, the effect upon skeletal remains is the constant replenishment of hydronium ions in their immediate soil solution vicinity. Any acid-neutralization effect brought about by the calcified structures' mineral content itself is quickly negated. Similarly, the concentration of phosphate (PO43−) ions in the soil water solution reaches equilibrium with the hydroxyapatite, but these ions combine with iron (Fe) and aluminum (Al) in highly acidic solutions and precipitate out. Any increase in water flow rate may increase the dissolution of the mineral component of the bone (constituting about 70%), even in mildly acidic conditions. Crow [1] found experimentally that mineral apatite was highly susceptible to dissolution with decreasing pH. The gross morphological result of these (and other related) processes is acidic soil corrosion, which tends to appear on all exposed surfaces of a buried element, including interior spaces where these have become in direct contact with sediments/soil solution.

Other organisms besides plants utilize buried teeth and bone and associated soft tissue as a source of nutrients and thereby may leave behind surface damage. Primary among these is the Kingdom Fungi, which along with bacteria are the major decomposers in most ecosystems. Fungi may also leave behind macroscopic surface damage to bone, and this effect may occur in conjunction with the exudates of plant roots as noted earlier. These can invade the porous structure of bone and leave behind focal damage. They also may grow on the surface of teeth and bone in large masses, often initially feeding on the soft tissue still attached or the residual organic content. The overall effect is to leave behind a roughened, eaten-away surface that forms through acidic dissolution similar to acidic soil corrosion. Fungal damage, however, may leave behind much more localized patches of surface erosion, with irregular edges. Calcified structures tend to take on the color of the medium into which they are deposited, due to their porous, wicking structure and initially pale coloration. Specific types of staining caused by different mineral deposits, including iron and copper oxides, are frequently encountered on buried remains. It is, however, an important and ubiquitous taphonomic clue as to the previous burial of teeth and bone, for example, in dark topsoil, the teeth and bone surface becomes stained dark brown, whether in patches or more uniformly. It is likely that organic compounds, in particular the tannins, are primarily responsible for this color change. Carbon resulting from organic breakdown is also a likely source of bone and teeth darkening.

17.4 Fluvial and Marine Environmental Alterations to Teeth

Human remains routinely enter fluvial systems through natural (i.e., erosion of cemeteries and archaeological sites), accidental (i.e., drowning), suicidal, and criminal (i.e., body disposal or intentional drowning) events. Regardless of the mechanisms of entry into a river, accidental or intentional, it is beneficial for human material to be recovered and subjected to a forensic or anthropological analysis. If the remains are the product of criminal activity, the discovery of additional remains may be beneficial for the prosecution by increasing the potential for identification, cause, and manner of death determination. Abrasion can take many forms on a tooth surface including smoothing, rounding, polish (sometimes shiny), scratches, gouges, frosting, pitting, denting, chipping, grooves, and notches; rarely are long grooves and scratches produced. In addition to these individual marks, the surface will generally become thinner, eventually leading to small openings (windows) that enlarge with further abrasion. Similarly, in bones, the lacunae and vascular canals (any natural opening) will gradually enlarge. Articular surfaces of bone rapidly thin to expose underlying cancellous bone, and in juvenile vertebrates, the epiphyses will detach if not fused. Edges of teeth and bone can be fractured or chipped as well. Acid etching of bone surfaces usually occurs over nearly the entire bone surface and presents as a delocalized surface roughening. Small pits form, expand outward, and finally connect, making irregular and rough galleries in the bone surface. Often, acid etching is accompanied by discoloration, probably caused by the same acids that are etching the biological material. Determining when acid etching will occur is primarily a function of the ions present in the solution surrounding the teeth and bone and their concentration. Acid etching of the surfaces usually occurs over nearly the entire surface and presents as a delocalized surface roughening. Discoloration can occur from a variety of agents, most of which are poorly understood or unknown. The most common color change is to a light or medium brown which appears to be caused by partial or complete burial in a river bed or through submersion in discolored water. A light green staining often accompanies the growth of algae on bone surfaces, a modification that can be found on bones in nearly all rivers, and which can occur in less than a year. Black staining has been observed. Sediment impaction within cracks, hollow spaces, and foramina is common in recovered hard tissue remains from sandy or coarse-bed rivers. The size, composition, and variety of clasts will be a function of the river from which the remains came; however, impacted sediment on or in a tooth is a good indicator of some aqueous history, freshwater or marine. If sand or gravel grains are wedged in cracks or holes, it can suggest a fluvial origin, since there are few processes operating in a standing body of water (lake or pond) that can wedge sediment into openings.

Coastal areas are a frequent setting for forensic investigations, given the frequency of deaths at sea from homicide, suicide, and accidents, burials at sea, the use of the ocean for deliberate remains disposal after terrestrial homicide, and the potential for transport of remains from river systems into the ocean. Coastal margins present an impenetrable barrier to the further transport of bodies or isolated skeletal elements moved by currents or wave action, with tidal fluctuations allowing objects to be deposited above the water line. Coastal margins also attract large numbers of people into a setting where any remains (skeletonized or fleshed) washing ashore are usually deposited in an exposed area devoid of plant cover. The overall effect is the concentration of many casual observers into a narrow area where exposed remains are typically easier to spot than in other terrestrial settings. Marine environments, especially coastal margins, present perhaps the most energetic environment for sedimentary abrasion and rounding of bone and tooth.

17.5 Thermal Alteration to Teeth

Burned dental remains are frequently found after natural disasters, airplane crashes, or house fires, as a result of either direct contact with open flames or exposure to high temperatures. Especially in cases of prolonged fires with temperatures above 700 °C, dental analysis stands alone as other materials used as primary (fingerprints and DNA) or secondary (e.g., clothing) means of identification are often destroyed. Andersen et al. [2] classified six grades of fire injuries to teeth and jaws: (0) no injury, (1) injury to anterior teeth, (2) injury to anterior and posterior teeth (unilaterally), (3) injury to anterior and posterior teeth (bilaterally), (4) fragments of jaw bone including teeth and/or roots, and (5) no dental remains. In their review of 292 single fire cases, the authors stated that 25% of the cases led to severe damage of the dentition (grades 2–5). Bohnert et al. [3] listed the effects of fire on the skull more specifically, based on observations of cremations carried out at 670° to 810 °C. After 8–10 minutes, the facial soft tissue is charred, and only sparse soft tissue remains visible; after 20 minutes, prominent parts of the facial skull are destroyed. Similar observations were reported by other experimental crematoria-based studies. Posterior teeth tend to be better preserved than anterior teeth due to their size and the heat protection offered by the tongue, layers of skin, mucosa, muscle, and adipose tissue, and are therefore more likely to be used in the odontological identification process. During the cremation process in modern crematoria, for the first 10 to 24 minutes, the soft tissue protection keeps the temperature inside the oral cavity as low as 87 °C, depending on the nutritional state of the body, age, temperature, and time of exposure. Lain et al. [4] and Bush and Bush [5] reported that teeth shrink and are often removed from their anatomical position as an effect of extensive heat exposure. Posterior teeth with multiple roots tend to remain in the alveolar bone sockets, whilst single-rooted teeth are mostly found isolated.

The enamel remains attached to the dentine in teeth at about 400 °C but gets partially separated from the coronal dentine or fragmented at about 500 and 700 °C and fully separated and fragmented at about 800 °C. Besides the separation and fragmentation of the enamel, heat-induced cracks and fractures are observed at high temperatures (Fig. 17.1). Fractures, referring to cracks that extend over an entire cross-section, could be visualized using conventional radiographs and micro-CT imaging. Micro-CT sections of all teeth of the lower temperature groups ($\leq$ 600 °C) show multiple cracks in the apical dentine and cementum as well as single, larger longitudinal cracks. At higher temperatures (700 to 1000 °C), multiple larger longitudinal and numerous transversal fractures are visible in the dentine, originating from the root canals and pulp cavity. Due to the fragmentation and separation of enamel, the analysis primarily focuses on the root. The shrinkage can generally be described as uniform, and the overall tooth morphology is well preserved in premolars and molars. Minor heat-induced contraction of the distal (apical) portions of the roots is found in the 3-D models of teeth heated at and above 800 °C, but is not identifiable on the standard digital radiographs.

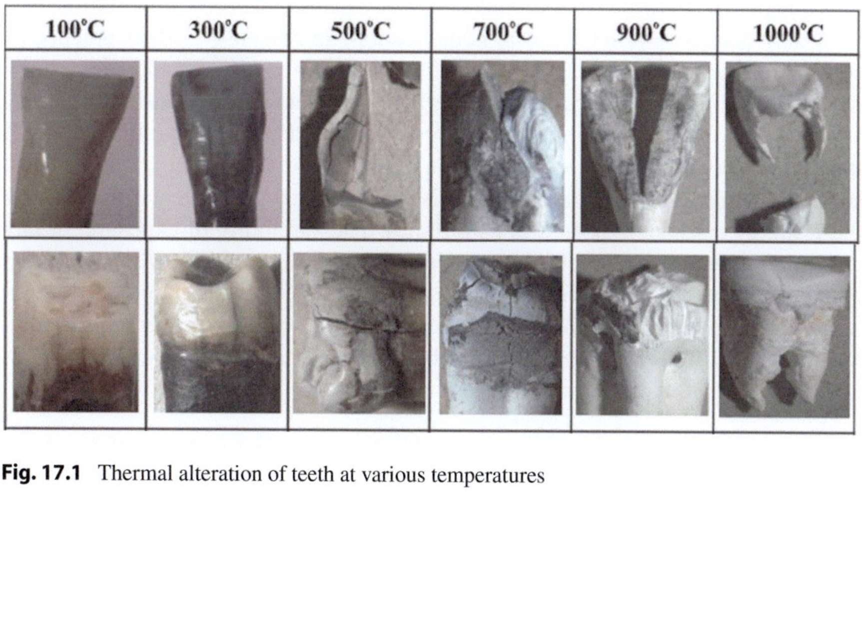

Fig. 17.1 Thermal alteration of teeth at various temperatures

17.6 Chemical Alterations to Teeth

There are several potential contexts in which human teeth may be exposed to corrosive chemicals: forensic cases involving the use of corrosive chemicals on a victim, the act of vomiting in bulimic individuals, industrial chemical hazards in the workplace, and methods in dentistry which regularly expose teeth to acidic chemicals for etching purposes. Dental fragments from the legendary Romanov case displayed convincing evidence that suggested exposure to a corrosive chemical. In this case, soil samples revealed high acidity and skeletal analysis noted corrosion and etching on the bones which supported claims that some sort of acidic property was poured over the remains. Examination of dental material revealed noticeable etching on the enamel surface of the teeth. Identification of the corrosive chemical was not made through analysis of the teeth, but rather through interview reports of the offenders and a receipt found for 400 pounds of sulfuric acid. Another forensic case documenting the use of a corrosive chemical concerns the killings and disposal of the victims of John George Haigh. Haigh utilized sulfuric acid to dispose of the bodies. The body of one victim was found after being submerged in a vat with 40 gallons of sulfuric acid for 4 days. Reports indicate that tooth fragments, along with bone fragments and various synthetic materials, were collected during the investigation. A description of the teeth fragments was not given, but it was hypothesized that if the body of the victim were to have remained in the vat for an entire month, no identifiable evidence of the victim would be found. A case examined by Ubelaker and Sperber found the use of another chemical tentatively identified as sodium hydroxide. Dental fragments were described as having a loss of sheen and polish from the enamel surface, corrosion, and a chalky white color. Despite this damage, the chemical did not significantly affect the restorative dental work of the victim, thus potentially allowing for identification. Individuals diagnosed with bulimia nervosa may display a variety of oral complications in response to their practice of self-induced vomiting. The labial (tongue) surface of the incisors and canines and the occlusal (biting) surface of the molars and premolars are frequently affected by stomach acid during vomiting. These morphological changes are a direct result of the gastric acid causing a demineralization of the enamel and thinning of the incisal edge of the maxillary incisors. Characteristic malformations on dental surfaces are the result of constant exposure to acid fumes. The variability of exposure, or any extrinsic factors such as dietary consumption, can account for the diverse effects that the tooth structure exhibits (Fig. 17.2). Reports state that the symptoms of long-term exposure to hydrochloric acid as producing erosion on dental surfaces. Similarly, exposure to sulfuric acid has been directly linked to enamel erosion in addition to a brownish stain covering the tooth surface.

ACIDS	4hrs	8hrs	16hrs	24hrs
Hydrochloric Acid Conc. HCl	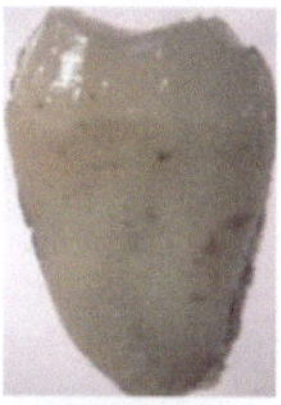	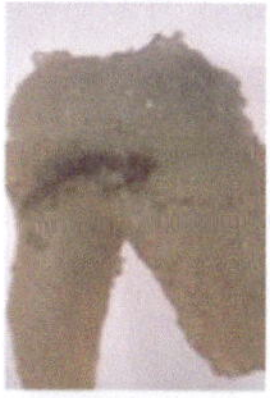	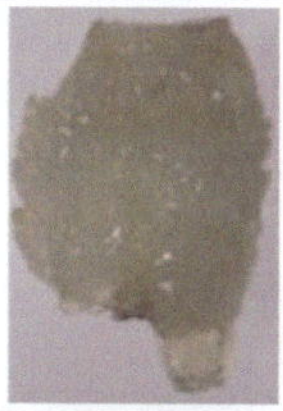	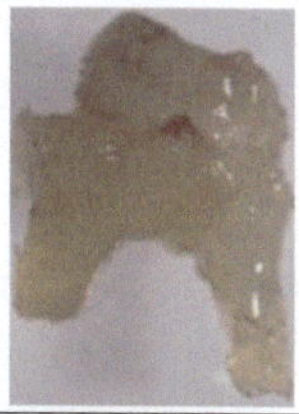
Nitric Acid Conc. HNO_3	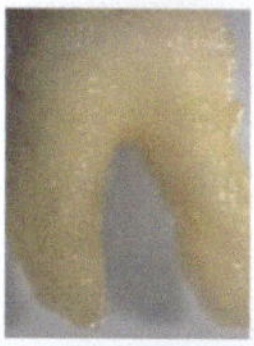	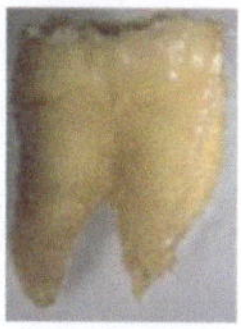	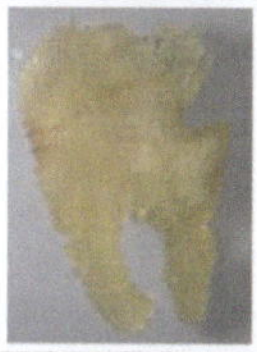	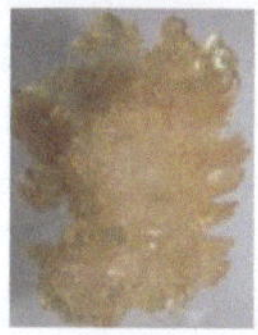
Suphuric Acid Conc. H_2SO_4	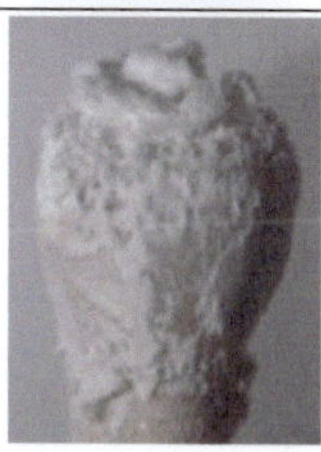	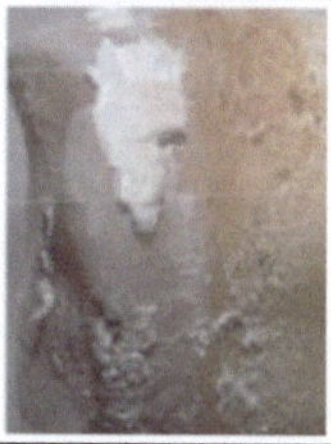	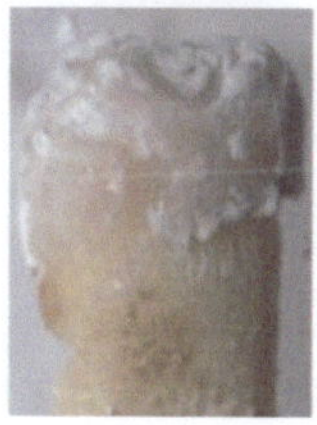	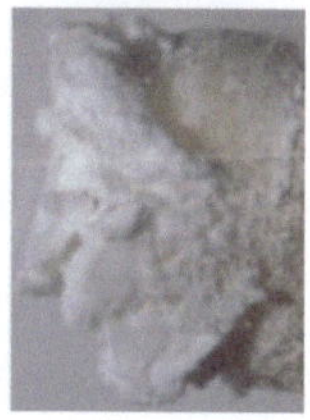

Fig. 17.2 Alteration of teeth by various acids/chemicals at different intervals

17.7 DNA Survivability

Molecular taphonomy is the study of those factors that influence molecular diagenesis and explores the impact of the various intrinsic and extrinsic forces influencing molecular integrity. Different molecules will degrade at different rates and are dependent upon the particular local environment, making a full understanding of the molecular diagenesis of DNA over long periods difficult due to the complexity and number of variables involved. While several variables have been identified as instrumental in the preservation or degradation of biological molecules, these variables do not work in isolation but rather within a complex web of interactions (discussed subsequently). In addition, as mentioned previously, DNA degradation is influenced by the rate and level of bone degradation, since the skeletal DNA binds to the hydroxyapatite. As the inorganic component of the bone degrades, the DNA is released from the hydroxyapatite and is no longer stabilized or protected. Multiple studies have demonstrated that depositional environment is a more important factor in DNA preservation than the absolute age of the DNA sample. A study by Perry et al. [6] attempted to use the degradation rate of DNA isolated from human ribs obtained at autopsy to estimate the PMI. They incubated the bones at either high or low humidity at room temperature and took samples for DNA analysis at selected time intervals. They found variation in the amount of degradation for samples that were collected at the same time interval, suggesting that DNA does not follow a specific degradation trajectory that can be used to predict time since death. They did find, however, that humidity had a more profound impact on DNA degradation, as the samples incubated at low humidity were much less degraded than those incubated at high humidity. Hagelberg et al. [7] investigated the relationship between gross bone preservation, histological preservation, and DNA recovery in human bone and found that their thirteenth-century bone samples had consistently produced better PCR amplification results than their seventeenth-century bone samples. They analyzed skeletal DNA isolated from human femora and found gross, microscopic, and molecular preservation to be better in the older skeletal remains. The authors suggested that this may be due to soil geochemistry or burial depth, supporting the observation that DNA preservation is not directly related to the time since death of the individual.

17.8 Handling of Forensic Samples

In order to preserve the integrity of the inquiry, a few steps must be taken prior to the gathering of evidence. The biological evidence is initially divided into a number of categories according to how mobile it is, and then its examination is given a priority according to criteria including how quickly the analysis must be finished and how quickly the evidence deteriorates over time. The rate at which the sample deteriorates is determined by a number of environmental and climatic conditions, including temperature, humidity, the presence of different external agents, and, at times, the presence of people at the crime scene. If the evidence is portable, it is packed and sent straight to the forensic science lab in its entirety. The segment holding the evidence is transmitted, or it is divided into other parts, and then sent to the laboratory for analysis if it is substantial in size or immovable. All biological samples, whether wet or dry, should be stored for transportation in breathable paper bags to prevent fungal growth with proper labelling and reference code number. Once the sample reaches the lab, it should be kept in a freezer to prevent any autolytic changes. A tooth being small may easily be missed in an outdoor or open crime scene; hence, grid-by-grid search methods should be employed where the actual location of each biological sample is noted and recorded in relation to a reference point. In specific conditions such as arson incidents or samples submerged in corrosive fluids, the tooth samples become extremely friable; in that case, moving the tooth sample to a forensic lab becomes challenging. Stabilization of the sample is required either with cyanoacrylate glue or by making a plaster cast mold around the tooth for maintaining the its integrity. Once stabilized, spot analyses such as metric and nonmetric analyses, radiographs, and high-quality images with an alternative light source (ALS) can be conducted. A forensic odontologist posted on field should

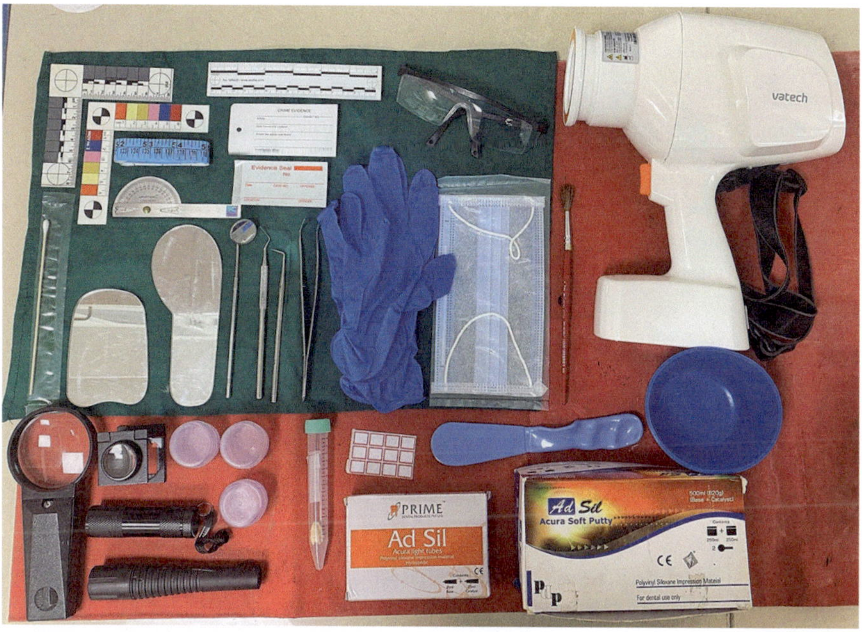

Fig. 17.3 Various armamentarium and instruments used for the examination of forensic dental evidence

have a well prepared kit bag (Fig. 17.3) which must contain gloves mask and disposable gowns for personal protection; a magnifying glass for easy identification of fragmented remains; multiple paper bags and labels for collection of sample; a camera and ALS for proper documentation of crime scene and circumstantial evidence; armamentarium to stabilize friable samples; various scales for metric analysis; reference guides for analysis of non-metric parameters; a portable X-ray and RVG sensor for radiographic documentation; and finally a personal notebook to record the step by step actions taken by the expert.

17.9 Multiple Choice Questions

Q1. Forensic taphonomy utilizes the –

(a) Principles of archeology
(b) Principles of paleontology
(c) Principles of forensic science
(d) Principle of all three doctrines
Ans: d

Q2. What is the major difference between burial in a fluvial and a marine environment –

(a) Polishing and rounding of the tooth
(b) Development of cracks and deposition of sand in them

(c) Superficial staining
(d) Loss of soft tissue attachment

Ans: b

Q3. What happens to a tooth exposed to temperatures of 400 °C or above –

(a) The enamel remains attached to the dentine
(b) The becomes brittle and sheds off
(c) Whole tooth is pulverized
(d) Only the crown is pulverized

Ans: a

Q4. What are the surface characteristics of fungal growth –

(a) Pitting and denting of the surface layer
(b) Loss of shine and polish of the surface layer
(c) Cracks on the surface layer
(d) Limited areas of etching of the surface layer

Ans: d

Q5. What should a Forensic odontologist do if encountered with friable tooth remains –

(a) Stabilize the sample with cyanoacrylate glue
(b) Start making photographic and radiographic documentation
(c) start performing metric and non-metric analysis
(d) Leave the sample as it is

Ans: a

References

1. Crow P. Mineral weathering in forest soils and its relevance to the preservation of the buried archaeological resource. Journal of Archaeological Science. 2008 Aug 1;35(8):2262–73.
2. Andersen L, Juhl M, Solheim T, Borrman H. Odontological identification of fire victims—potentialities and limitations. International journal of legal medicine, 1995;107:229–34.
3. Bohnert M. Morphological findings in burned bodies. Forensic pathology reviews, 2004;3–27.
4. Lain R, Taylor J, Croker S, Craig P, Graham J. Comparative dental anatomy in disaster victim identification: lessons from the 2009 Victorian Bushfires. Forensic science international, 2011;205(1-3):36–9.
5. Bush PJ, Bush MA. The next level in victim identification: materials properties as an aid in victim identification. In Forensic Dental Evidence. 2011:pp. 55–72. Academic Press.
6. Perry III WL, Bass WM, Riggsby WS, Sirotkin K. The autodegradation of deoxyribonucleic acid (DNA) in human rib bone and its relationship to the time interval since death. Journal of Forensic Sciences. 1988;33(1):144–53.
7. Hagelberg E, Gray IC, Jeffreys AJ. Identification of the skeletal remains of a murder victim by DNA analysis. Nature, 1991;352(6334):427–9.

Dental Age Assessment: An Indian Perspective

18

Hemlata Pandey Gala and Parul Khare Sinha

18.1 Introduction: Age Estimation in India

Forensic applications of age estimation in India involve assessing both living as well as deceased individuals. Age estimation is a common tool utilized in both civil and criminal investigations. The human age is a measure, typically stated in years, of the period lived since birth, so the indubitable registration of the date of birth is critical to estimate an individual's chronological age. Scientific techniques assess age as a measure of the biological, psychological, and social changes that occur during the course of a lifetime.

India faces several unique challenges that affect the practice and accuracy of dental age estimation. One of the primary challenges is the lack of reliable birth records in some regions. According to the United Nations Children's Fund (UNICEF), a significant percentage of children in India, around 28%, are not registered at birth, which creates difficulties in legal and administrative processes where age verification is essential [1]. In cases of child abuse, trafficking, and adoption, the absence of an official record heightens the risk of exploitation, making forensic age estimation an indispensable tool in ensuring justice.

H. Pandey Gala (✉)
Forensic Dentistry, Centre for Forensic and Legal Medicine and Dentistry, School of Dentistry, University of Dundee, Dundee, UK
e-mail: HPandeygala001@dundee.ac.uk

P. K. Sinha
Department of Oral & Maxillofacial Pathology & Oral Microbiology, School of Dental Sciences, Sharda University, Noida, UP, India
e-mail: Parul.khare@sharda.ac.in

© The Author(s), under exclusive license to Springer Nature Switzerland AG 2026

A. Chowdhry, P. Kapoor (eds.), *Dental Age Assessment*,
https://doi.org/10.1007/978-3-032-08788-1_18

Another challenge is the variation in medical infrastructure across urban and rural areas. While metropolitan cities like Delhi, Mumbai, and Bengaluru have relatively easy access to medical facilities, including tertiary hospitals and forensic experts, rural regions often lack such resources. This disparity in access to forensic expertise further complicates age estimation procedures, leading to inconsistent practices and potential misjudgments. To address this, there is a need for a nationwide effort to standardize age estimation practices and ensure that expert panels are accessible across all regions.

Additionally, the practice of age estimation in India is often influenced by societal and legal pressures. For instance, in juvenile justice cases, accused individuals may attempt to manipulate their age to be tried under juvenile laws, which carry more lenient sentences. Similarly, in cases of child marriage or illegal employment of minors, there may be attempts to falsify ages. These situations underscore the importance of accurate age estimation to uphold the integrity of the law. One solution to this challenge is the development of more accurate, reproducible, and legally recognized methods for age estimation that can withstand scrutiny in court settings.

18.1.1 Key Themes of Dental Age Estimation in India

One of the central themes is the critical role that dental age estimation plays in a variety of legal and forensic contexts in India. From cases of juvenile justice and child labour to human trafficking and child marriage, the ability to accurately assess age is vital to ensure the protection of individuals and uphold legal standards. Age estimation is especially significant in India due to issues such as unregistered births, child exploitation, and the growing prevalence of age-related fraud in sports. As explored, Indian law provides for different age thresholds that have direct implications for criminal responsibility, eligibility for marriage, child protection, and various social benefits, making accurate age estimation indispensable.

Another prominent theme is the challenge of age estimation methods. Dental age estimation has emerged as one of the most reliable techniques due to the robust correlation between tooth development and chronological age. Various methodologies such as the Demirjian, Kvaal, and Cameriere techniques are being used in the Indian population, along with population-specific formulas modified to better suit the Indian population. While these methods have proven effective, they often require calibration to account for ethnic, nutritional, and regional variations within India. This customization, while important, also poses challenges in terms of standardization across the country, making it difficult to create universally applicable formulas for age estimation.

Age estimation in India is often required to be done in cases of infanticide (Section 315, IPC), child adoption (Section 38, Juvenile Justice Act 2015 and Section 10, Hindu adoption and maintenance act, 1956), child marriage (Prohibition of Child Marriage Act, 2006), child labour (Child Labour Prohibition and Regulation) Amendment Act, 2016, domestic employment (Domestic Workers

Registration, Social Security and Welfare) Act, 2008, human trafficking (Section 370, 370 A IPC and Immoral Traffic Prevention Act 1986), and pension claims of the elderly (Maintenance and Welfare of Parents and Senior Citizens Act 2007). The Juvenile Justice (Care and Protection of Children) Act 2015 defines child abuse as any physical, sexual, emotional, or economic maltreatment of a child. This includes neglect, abandonment, exploitation, and any other form of harmful treatment [2, 3]. As shown in Table 18.1, age thresholds vary significantly by legal context with different statutes assigning distinct legal responsibilities and protections at various ages, depending on the applicable legislation [28].

The most common cases requiring age estimation are related to the Juvenile Justice Act, 2015, Child Labour Amendment Act, 2016, Prohibition of Child Marriage Act, 2006, Protection of Children from Sexual Offences (POCSO) Act, 2012, and Sports and Academic eligibility cases [29].

Table 18.2 outlines the common referral contexts for age estimation in India, highlighting the diverse medicolegal scenarios in which forensic odontologists may be called upon, including juvenile justice proceedings, child labour disputes, and age-related eligibility for sports participation.

Table 18.1 Key legal age thresholds across Indian statutes

Age	Significance in law	Relevant law
20 weeks I.U.	Opinion of only one doctor is required for termination of pregnancy up to 20 weeks of gestation and two providers for 20–24 weeks of gestation	Medical Termination of Pregnancy Amendment Act 2021 [4]
20–24 weeks IU	Opinion of two doctors is required for termination of pregnancy of 20–24 weeks of gestation	Medical Termination of Pregnancy Amendment Act 2021 [4]
24 weeks IU	Upper gestation limit for special categories of women including survivors of rape, victims of incest, and other vulnerable women (like differently abled women, minors) etc.	Medical Termination of Pregnancy Amendment Act 2021 [4]
1 year	Infanticides (crime against newborn child) (0 to 1 year)	Section 315, Indian Penal Code [5]
Up to 5 years	Free travel in Indian railways	IRCTC Press Release, 2022 [6]
5 years	(a) A minor who has not completed the age of 5 years shall ordinarily be in the custody of the mother.	Section 6 (a) of The Hindu Minority and Guardianship Act 1956 [7]
5–12 years	(a) To collect (half) fare in railways.	IRCTC Press Release, 2022 [8]
6–14 years	The right to free and compulsory education in a neighborhood school till the completion of elementary education	The Right of Children to Free and Compulsory Education Act, 2009 [9]

(continued)

Table 18.1 (continued)

Age	Significance in law	Relevant law
7 years	Criminal responsibility—nothing is an offence which is done by a child under 7 years of age	Section 82 of the Indian Penal Code 1860 [10]
7–12 years	Criminal responsibility—nothing is an offence which is done by a child above 7 years of age and under 12, who has not attained sufficient maturity of understanding to judge of the nature and consequences of his conduct on that occasion	Section 83 of the Indian Penal Code 1860 [10]
10 years	Whoever kidnaps or abducts any child under the age of 10 years with the intention of taking dishonestly any movable property from the person of such child, shall be punished with imprisonment of either description for a term which may extend to 7 years, and shall also be liable to fine	Section 369, the Indian Penal Code 1860 [11]
<12 years	The punishment for sexual assault on a child under the age of 12 years is imprisonment for a minimum of 20 years, which may extend to life imprisonment	Protection of Children from Sexual Offences Act (POCSO), 2019 [12]
12 years	(a) Criminal responsibility—exception section 84 and 85 of the Indian Penal Code 1860 (b) Whoever being the father or mother of a child under the age of 12 years, or having the care of such child, shall expose or leave such child in any place with the intention of wholly abandoning such child, shall be punished with imprisonment of either description for a term which may extend to 7 years, or with fine, or with both (c) Nothing which is done in good faith for the benefit of a person under 12 years of age, or of unsound mind, by or by consent, either express or implied, of the guardian or other person having lawful charge of that person, is an offence by reason of any harm which it may cause, or be intended by the doer to cause or be known by the doer to be likely to cause to that person. (d) < 12—oath not necessary—Indian Oaths Amendment Act 1939. (e) Considered an adult for drug therapy (f) To collect full fare in all modes of transport.	The Indian Penal Code, 1860 [13] Section 317, the Indian Penal Code [13] Section 89 of the Indian Penal Code 1860 [13]
12–18 years	For sexual assault on a child between the age of 12 and 18 years, the punishment is imprisonment for a minimum of 10 years, which may extend to life imprisonment.	Protection of Children from Sexual Offences Act (POCSO), 2019 [12]

(continued)

Table 18.1 (continued)

Age	Significance in law	Relevant law
14 years	Section 2 (i) "child" means a person who has not completed his 14th year of age or such age as may be specified in the Right of Children to Free and Compulsory Education Act, 2009, whichever is more Section 3 No child shall be employed or permitted to work in any occupation or process. (Except helping their family or family enterprise or working as an artist in the audio-visual entertainment industry provided that no exception affects the school education of the child) Section 2 (ii) "adolescent" means a person who has completed his 14th year of age but has not completed his 18th year Section 3 (A) No adolescent shall be employed or permitted to work in any of the hazardous occupations or processes	The Child and Adolescent Labour (Prohibition and Regulation) Act, 1986 [14] The Child Labour (Prohibition and Regulation) Amendment Act, 2016 [14] Child And Adolescent Labour (Prohibition and Regulation) Act, 1986 [14]
> 14 years (boys) > 16 years (girls)	Where a children's court is satisfied on inquiry that a child has committed an offence, then the children's court may (c) make an order directing the child to be sent to a special school, (i) in the case of a boy over 14 years of age or of a girl over 16 years of age, for a period of not less than 3 years	Section 21, The Children Act, 1960 [15]
Above 15, below 18 years	An adolescent employee in a factory	The Child Labour (Prohibition and Regulation) Amendment Act, 2016 [14]
< 16 years	Whoever commits penetrative sexual assault on a child below 16 years of age shall be punished with imprisonment for a term which shall not be less than 20 years, but which may extend to imprisonment for life, which shall mean imprisonment for the remainder of the natural life of that person, and shall also be liable to fine.	Protection of Children from Sexual Offences Amendment Act (POCSO), 2019 [12]
16 years (male) 18 years (female)	Kidnapping from lawful guardianship. —Whoever takes or entices any minor under 16 years of age if a male, or under 18 years of age if a female, or any person of unsound mind, out of the keeping of the lawful guardian of such minor or person of unsound mind, without the consent of such guardian, is said to kidnap such minor or person from lawful guardianship.	Section 361 of the Indian Penal Code [13]
< 18 years	Rape—with or without her consent, when she is under 18 years of age	Section 375, The Criminal Law (Amendment) Act, 2013 [16]

(continued)

Table 18.1 (continued)

Age	Significance in law	Relevant law
18 years	Majority: "child" means a person who has not completed 18 years of age Every person domiciled in India shall attain the age of majority on completing the age of 18 years and not before. (a) Consent for procedures involving risk of life—nothing which is not intended to cause death, or grievous hurt, and which is not known by the doer to be likely to cause death or grievous hurt, is an offence by reason of any harm which it may cause, or be intended by the doer to cause, to any person, above 18 years of age, who has given consent, whether express or implied, to suffer that harm; or by reason of any harm which it may be known by the doer to be likely to cause to any such person who has consented to take the risk of that harm. Every person is competent to contract who is of the age of majority according to the law to which he is subject and who is of sound mind and is not disqualified from contracting by any law to which he is subject. "child" means a person who, if a male, has not completed 21 years of age and, if a female, has not completed 18 years of age (legal age for marriage) No pregnancy of a woman, who has not attained the age of 18 years, or who, having attained the age of 18 years, is a lunatic, shall be terminated except with the consent in writing of her guardian. "adult" means a person who has completed their 18th year of age Whoever takes or entices any minor under 16 years of age if a male, or under 18 years of age if a female, or any person of unsound mind, out of the keeping of the lawful guardian of such minor or person of unsound mind, without the consent of such guardian, is said to kidnap such minor or person from lawful guardianship. Every citizen who is 18 years old on the qualifying date (January 1 of the year in case) unless disqualified, is eligible to be enrolled to cast votes for local bodies assembly and Parliament elections. No person under the age of 18 years shall drive a motor vehicle in any public place. Minimum age of entry to any type of employment or work, which is likely to compromise the health, safety, or morals of young persons shall not be less than 18 years.	The Juvenile Justice (Care and Protection of Children) Amendment Act, 2021 [17] The Indian Majority Act, 1875 [18] Section 87, Indian Penal Code 1860 [13] Indian Contract Act, 1872 [19] The Prohibition of Child Marriage Act, 2006 [20] Section 4 A, The Medical Termination of Pregnancy Act, 1971 [4] Indian Factories Act 1948 [21] Sections 361–366 of the Indian Penal Code 1860 [13] Citizenship Act 1955, Election Commission of India [22] Motor Vehicles Act, 1988 [23] International Labour Organization (UN), Convention No. 138, 1973 [24]

(continued)

Table 18.1 (continued)

Age	Significance in law	Relevant law
21 years	Majority of those under the guardianship of the Court of Wards "child" means a person who, if a male, has not completed 21 years of age, and if a female, has not completed 18 years of age (legal age for marriage) Importation of a girl (under the age of 21) from a foreign country with the intention or knowing it is likely to be that she will be forced or seduced to illicit intercourse with another person, is punishable under this Section with imprisonment for a period of up to 10 years and a fine.	The Guardians and Wards Act, 1890 [25] The Prohibition of Child Marriage Act, 2006 [20] *The Prohibition of Child Marriage (Amendment) Bill, 2021 seeks to raise the minimum age of marriage for women to 21 years (from the present 18 years) Section 366 B of the Indian Penal Code 1860 [13]
25 years	The minimum age for becoming a candidate for the Lok Sabha/Assembly election shall be 25 years.	Article 84 (b) in the Constitution of India 1949 [26]
30 years	The minimum age for becoming a candidate for the Rajya Sabha election shall be 30 years.	Article 84 (b) in the Constitution of India 1949 [26]
55–62 years	The general retirement age range of state government employees is 55 to 62 years.	Each state government is entitled to amend its respective Public Employment Act to regulate the age of superannuation of its employees [27].
60–65 years	Retirement age for all central government employees To obtain a concession in fares for senior citizens in the railways and Indian Airlines	Fifth Central Pay Commission report dated May 30, 1998 [27]

Source: Compiled by authors from multiple Indian legal documents (e.g., IPC, JJ Act, POCSO, MTP Amendment Act, etc.)

Compiled and adapted from Aggrawal [28]

*The *Prohibition of Child Marriage (Amendment) Bill, 2021* proposes to increase the minimum legal age of marriage for women from 18 to 21 years, thereby aligning it with the legal age prescribed for men. Introduced in the Lok Sabha on 21 December 2021, the Bill aims to establish uniformity in the legal framework governing marriage across all communities in India. Following its introduction, the Bill was referred to a Parliamentary Standing Committee for further examination and recommendations. As of the latest legislative update, the Bill remains under deliberation and has not yet been enacted into law

Table 18.2 Common referral scenarios for forensic age estimation in India

Case type	Relevant laws	Purpose	Process
Juvenile justice cases	The Juvenile Justice (Care and Protection of Children) Amendment Act, 2021 [17]	To determine if an accused or victim is a juvenile (under 18) at the time of the alleged offense, as juveniles are subject to separate legal processes and rehabilitative, rather than punitive, measures.	Medical examinations ordered by court, including dental and skeletal tests, are often used to establish age in the absence of valid age documentation.
Child labor and employment disputes	Child Labour (Prohibition and Regulation) Amendment Act, 2016 [14]; Minimum Wages Act, 1948 [30]	To verify if a minor is illegally employed in a hazardous occupation. The act prohibits the employment of children under 14 years in most jobs and regulates the employment of adolescents (14–18 years).	Employers or authorities may request age estimation if documentary evidence is unavailable to determine if someone falls under prohibited or restricted age groups for specific types of work.
Marriage disputes	Prohibition of Child Marriage Act, 2006 [20]; Hindu Marriage Act, 1955 [22]; Indian Christian Marriage Act, 1872 [31]	To confirm if individuals meet the minimum age requirement for marriage (18 for females and 21 for males). If a marriage is contested due to age, such as in cases of alleged child marriage, age estimation can substantiate claims.	Courts may order age verification tests to confirm the legality of the marriage, particularly if official documentation is lacking or contested.
Sexual offense cases	Protection of Children from Sexual Offences Amendment Act (POCSO), 2019 [12]; Indian Penal Code (IPC), Section 375 and Section 376 [13]	To ascertain if the victim of a sexual offense is a minor, as sexual relations with a minor (under 18) are considered statutory rape, regardless of consent.	Age determination is crucial for implementing stringent legal protections under POCSO and can influence sentencing. Courts may rely on medical age estimation to verify claims.
Missing and trafficked persons cases	Immoral Traffic (Prevention) Act, 1956 [32]; The Juvenile Justice (Care and Protection of Children) Amendment Act, 2021 [17]	To determine the age of rescued individuals in trafficking or missing person cases, as minors receive specialized legal protections.	Age estimation can help decide the appropriate legal recourse and rehabilitation measures, particularly when documentary evidence is unavailable.

(continued)

Table 18.2 (continued)

Case type	Relevant laws	Purpose	Process
Property and inheritance disputes	Indian Succession Act, 1925; Hindu Succession Act, 1956 [33]	In cases of inheritance, age determination can confirm if an heir was a minor at the time of the benefactor's death, impacting property distribution and guardianship decisions.	Courts may request age verification to uphold inheritance claims for minors, particularly if the minor's legitimacy is questioned or if age affects succession rights.
Employment injury and compensation cases	Employee's Compensation Act, 1923 [34]	To establish age for compensation purposes, as compensation amounts and eligibility for minors or younger individuals often differ.	Age estimation may be required if documentary proof is unavailable, and the age of the individual impacts the compensation due.
Immigration and refugee claims	Foreigners Act, 1946; Citizenship (Amendment) Act 2019 [35]	To determine the age of unaccompanied minors or young asylum seekers. Age verification is essential to ensure they receive age-appropriate protections and services.	Immigration authorities may rely on age estimation techniques to verify age claims in the absence of documentation.
Sports and academic eligibility cases	Guidelines by the Ministry of Youth Affairs and Sports; Education Department Regulations [36]	To prevent age fraud in sports competitions and academic settings. Some age-based categories in sports and education require verification to ensure fairness.	Institutions may request age estimation when discrepancies arise or when individuals lack valid proof of age.
Medical termination of pregnancy cases	Medical Termination of Pregnancy Amendment Act 2021 [4]; Protection of Children from Sexual Offences Act (POCSO), 2019 [12]	To establish the age of the individual seeking a termination, as it impacts the legal requirements for consent and reporting. For minors (under 18), consent must also be provided by a guardian. Additionally, if the pregnancy is a result of sexual activity involving a minor, it may necessitate mandatory reporting under POCSO.	When age documentation is unavailable or unclear, healthcare providers may request age estimation. Establishing age can help verify the legal requirements for consent and reporting, ensuring compliance with both the MTP and POCSO Acts.

Source: Compiled by authors based on relevant laws and forensic guidelines

18.2 National Code Against Age Fraud in Sports

To eliminate age fraud in sports and promote fair play, it was essential to establish a robust regulatory mechanism to take appropriate action against athletes found guilty of age fraud. The government therefore decided that all sports federations, associations, and governing bodies should implement measures to combat age fraud, as it constitutes cheating and undermines the fundamental spirit of sport [36].

In light of this, it is necessary to adopt a National Code against age fraud in sports, supported by a clear and well-defined mechanism to prevent, detect, and penalize such offenses. Figure 18.1 illustrates the age estimation reporting format recommended by the Ministry of Youth Affairs and Sports under the National Code Against Age Fraud in Sports [36], providing a standardized structure for presenting radiographic and clinical findings in age verification cases.

18.3 Procedure and Format for Age Estimation Reporting in India

The 18-year-olds are of specific importance, according to Indian law, as this age demarcates a child from an adult. Consequently, trial or sentencing of the accused in this age threshold is directed in the juvenile or adult justice system, respectively. Convicted young adults often claim to be a minor with the hope of being tried in a juvenile justice court for a lenient sentence.

According to a study which reviewed data published by the National Family Health Survey, 2015–2016, the birth registration level was lower than the national average (80.21%) in the 254 districts in India. In Uttar Pradesh, 12 out of 71 districts recorded lower than 50% birth registration. Also, some districts from Arunachal Pradesh, J&K, and Rajasthan recorded lower than 50% birth registration. It was found that a lower proportion of children were registered among children of birth order three and above (62.83%) and rural residents (76.62%). Children of mothers with no formal education, no media exposure, the poorest wealth quintile, belonging to OBC, and of Muslim religion have lower level of birth registration [37]. Age estimation forms a major portion of forensic odontology work done in India, as numerous investigations, both civil and criminal, require age assessment of an individual.

In India, non-therapeutic age estimation is routinely performed by medical officers, forensic medicine experts, civil surgeons, and autopsy surgeons, according to the availability of expertise and nearby government hospitals, medical colleges, health centres, etc.

In metropolitan cities with easy access to medical colleges or tertiary hospitals, the onus of forensic age estimation lies with the forensic medicine expert. Age estimation has been acknowledged as a multi-disciplinary process, and the forensic medicine expert or the Head of Department or the Dean of the institute presides over the expert panel for age estimation. Members of the panel would include experts from gynecology, pediatrics, psychiatry, radiology, and dentistry. Additional

ANNEXURE-II

(para 7.1.1 refers)

Age Estimation Format

Space for colour photograph attested by Gazetted officer

a **Informed consent**

b I .... S/D/O or Guardian of ....voluntarily give my consent for complete medical examination for the purpose of age estimation. I understand that this examination may involve physical examination including genital examination, dental examination and radiography. The purpose, procedure and use of such examination have been explained to me in the language which I understand.

Signature of the candidate/ guardian:

Signature of the accompanying person/witness:
(Note: Consent by guardian is essential in respect of athletes below 12 years)

c **Preamble**

1. Age category..
2. Sports Discipline...
3. Events to be participated ....
4. Case Serial No...
5. Name..
6. Age as stated (Any documentary evidence like birth certificate)
   ....
7. Sex...
8. Permanent Address..
   ....
   ....
9. Corresponding address..
   ....
   ....
10. Name of school/college/Institute..
11. Tel. No. & e-mail...
12. Father's name..
13. Mother's name...
14. Name of the person accompanying..
15. Date and Time of examination..
16. Place of examination...
17. Marks of identification (Scar/mole/deformity, etc.):
    1...
    2...
18. Thumb impression (right in female and left in male)
17. Signature

d **General Physical Examination**

1. Height (cm):
2. Weight (kg):
3. Chest girth at the level of nipples:
4. Abdominal girth at the level of naval:
5. For calculating Body development index (BDI):
   I. Biacromial breath(cm):
   II. Bulbospinal breath (cm):
   III. Forearm circumference(cm) in males:
   IV. Mid-thigh circumference(cm) in females:
6. Voice (Hoarseness of voice):

e **Dental Examination**

i. Dental Data: (S) 8 7 6 5 4 3 2 1 1 2 3 4 5 6 7 8 (S)
(Rt.)..(Lt.)
(S) 8 7 6 5 4 3 2 1 1 2 3 4 5 6 7 8 (S)

a. Temporary
b. Permanent
c. Space for third molar(S)
d. Partially erupted/completely erupted

ii. Dental X- ray : Oral pantogram (OPG)
iii. Dental X- ray findings :

f **Radiological Examination/MRI/CT Scan (as applicable)**

Note : A single film of hand and wrist is sufficient for age below 13 years. Wherever radiological examination is not indicated MRI/CT Scan may be done.

1. X-ray advised (as per requirements):
   i. Shoulder joint : A.P view
   ii. Elbow joint : A.P and lateral view
   iii. Hand with wrist : A.P view
   iv. Pelvis with hip joint : A.P view
2. Date of radiological examination:
3. Name of the radiographer :

Radiological findings:

S.no.	X-ray advised	Findings	Age inference

g **Age Certificate**

After performing general physical, dental and radiological examination, we are of the considered opinion that the biological age of the person is about... years which is consistent /not consistent with birth certificate/ age document.

Dated :

Signature:

Name:

Designation:

(All the parameters should be considered for the age estimation)

h **Body development index method : Optional method**(BDI method is valid upto 18 years)

$$\textbf{BDI} = \frac{\text{Middle breadth x 2 forearm circumference (corrected)}}{\text{Body height x 10}}$$

$$\textbf{Middle breadth} = \frac{\text{Biacromial breadth + Biliospinale breadth}}{2}$$

Forearm circumference (corrected) = Forearm circumference given – Rohrar index (RI) (Corrected)

$$\textbf{Rohrar index} = \frac{\text{Body weight (kg)}}{\text{Body height}^3 \text{ x 10}} = \frac{\text{Kg}}{\text{M}^3 \text{ x 10}}$$

Corrected Rohrar index = Corresponding corrected value to the calculated Rohrar index (Correlate with table 1 : Rohrar index – corrected value)

Biological age = Correspoding age to the BDI index value
(Correlate with table 2 : Mean value of body development index children, wutschrk, 1973)

Table-1: ROHRAR INDEX AND CORRECTED VALUE

RI	Correction	RI	Correction	RI	Correction
0.90	+3.7	1.13	0.0	1.36	-3.7
0.91	+3.5	1.14	0.2	1.37	-3.8
0.92	+3.4	1.15	0.3	1.38	-4.0
0.93	+3.2	1.16	0.5	1.39	-4.2
0.94	+3.1	1.17	0.6	1.40	-4.3
0.95	+2.9	1.18	0.8	1.41	-4.5
0.96	+2.7	1.19	1.0	1.42	-4.7
0.97	+2.6	1.20	1.1	1.43	-4.8
0.98	+2.4	1.21	1.3	1.44	-5.0
0.99	+2.3	1.22	1.5	1.45	-5.1
1.00	+2.1	1.23	1.6	1.46	-5.3
1.01	+1.0	1.24	1.8	1.47	-5.5
1.02	+1.8	1.25	1.9	1.48	-5.6
1.03	+1.6	1.26	2.1	1.49	-5.8
1.04	+1.5	1.27	2.3	1.50	-5.9
1.05	+1.3	1.28	2.4		
1.06	+1.1	1.29	2.6		
1.07	+1.0	1.30	2.7		
1.08	+0.8	1.31	2.9		

Fig. 18.1 Age estimation format from the Ministry of Youth Affairs and Sports, GoI [36]. (Source: Ministry of Youth Affairs and Sports, Government of India, National Code Against Age Fraud in Sports [36])

members from other disciplines may be invited to join the panel according to the requirements of the case.

The age estimation proforma varies for reporting in different cases and in different institutional settings; the following sections are usually part of the proforma (the list is not exhaustive):

1. Informed consent
2. Preliminary details
    2.1. Age Category
    2.2. Case serial number
    2.3. Name
    2.4. Age as stated
    2.5. Availability of any documentation (for example, birth certificate)
    2.6. Sex
    2.7. Address
    2.8. Contact details
    2.9. Parent/guardian/accompanying person name:
    2.10. Relationship:
    2.11. Date and time of examination:
    2.12. Place of examination
    2.13. Marks for identification
    2.14. Thumb impression
    2.15. Signature
3. General physical examination:
    3.1. Height
    3.2. Weight
    3.3. Other relevant details (as per age category)
4. Dental examination

    Charting, radiography, and dental age assessment
5. Radiological examination

    Radiographs are advised according to age category or stated age
6. Gynecological assessment and/or pediatric assessment
7. Psychiatric evaluation (if advised)
8. Any other information
9. Age certificate: an estimated age range considering the opinions of all the experts involved, is signed by panel members. In civil cases, this step is often replaced by verification of age in the documents provided.

18.4 Dental Age Estimation Techniques in India

The two common age estimation methods often used are skeletal maturation and teeth development. These parameters have been revealed to correlate positively with the chronological age. Among the two methods, age estimation using teeth has proved a higher correlation [38].

As teeth are slightly affected by environmental diversities like nutritional and endocrine disturbances and also endure post-mortem destruction [39]. The dental age estimation methods/techniques apply numerous aspects beginning from the appearance of tooth germs to the post-eruption alterations of the teeth [40]. It is found that age estimation of young and adolescent individuals based on stages of tooth development and eruption pattern is of utmost reliability [41].

In forensic age estimation, the choice of a specific age estimation method depends on the age-related dental variables available. Consequently, classifications of the estimation methods are based on the technique used to observe the dental variables or on the dental features inspected in the studied variable. The age-related dental variables are detected clinically utilizing imaging techniques or after tooth extraction. Thus, the method used should be ethical and legal. Therefore, there are many published studies mainly on dental age estimation methods, modifications to the methods, and their validation results on specific Indian populations. As presented in Table 18.3, several population-specific dental age estimation formulas have been developed and validated within Indian cohorts, addressing the need for ethnically and regionally relevant standards rather than relying solely on Western-derived methods.

The topic of "age estimation" has been incorporated into the dental curriculum outlined by the Dental Council of India (DCI) and published in the *Gazette of India* [48]. Based on the inclusion of the topic in the curriculum, it can be implied that dentists, in their capacity, can recommend radiographs for dental observation and age estimation. This can be conducted alone or in conjunction with the medical team with the power invested by the DCI, the supreme regulatory authority that monitors dental practice in India [49].

Table 18.3 Dental age estimation formulas developed and validated in Indian populations

Author	Sample size	M: F	Age range years	Radiograph	Method studied	Inference Indian population	Indian formula
Rai et al. [42]	480	253:227	3–15 years	OPG	Cameriere's formula	Region-specific formulas that account for variations between central/ north and south India.	"Age = 9.402 – 0.879 C + 0.663 No – 0.711s – 0.106sNo"
Acharya [43]	547	199:348	7–25	OPG	Demirjian's	India-specific regression formulas gave better age estimates	"Males = 27.4351 – (0.0097 × S^2) + (0.000089 × S^3) Females = 23.7288 – (0.0088 × S^2) + (0.000085 × S^3)"
Kanchan-Talreja [44]	100		25–77	Intra-oral periapical radiographs	Kvaal's method	The Indian formulae derived produced smaller errors	"All teeth (both Jaws): 123.95–(128.66XUCI BMW)–(93.44XULI ABMW)–(106.06XUP2 BCW)" "All teeth (both Jaws): 182.398–(60.20XUCI AML)–(58.58XULI AMO)–(109.87XLCM)"
Jeevan et al. [45]	240	120:120	16–72	Radiovisiography	Cameriere's	These equations were better able to predict the age at a younger age	"Upper canine age – 96:795 _ 513:561 × 1" "only lower canine age – 88:308 _ 458:137 × 2" "Both upper & lower canines age – 99:190 _ 283:537 × 1 _ 306:902 × 2 t 400:873 × 1 × 2"

Manisha et al. [46]	500	250:250	4–22.1	OPG	Ajit Dinkar formula	Dr. Ajit Dinkar's method is more accurate compared to Acharya's method for Goa Children & adults	"E_ + S = A (E = eruption age; S = calcification stage value in years/months, A = estimated dental age)" "Regression equations for males & females P2M2 P2 M2 P1 Males Y = 0.3905X + 3.7653 0.9887 Females Y = 0.3989X + 3.7604 0.9873 P2 Males Y = 0.3989X + 3.9321 0.9808 Females Y = 0.3836X + 4.4160 0.8875 M2 Males Y = 0.4681X + 4.4805 0.9728 Females Y = 4.4747X + 4.4619 0.9814 (P2 M2) P1 Males Y = 0.4419X + 3.7988 0.9853 Females Y = 0.3794X + 4.2950 0.8731 P2 Males Y = 0.4519X + 4.2053 0.9821 Females Y = 0.4192X + 3.9616 0.9846 M2 Males Y = 0.4547X + 4.2343 0.9844 Females Y = 0.4473X + 3.7890 0.9856 M2 P2 P1 Males Y = 0.4129X + 4.0900 0.9861 Females Y = 0.4179X + 4.0270 0.9868 P2 Males Y = 0.4736X + 4.6756 0.9692 Females Y = 0.4602X + 4.6305 0.9919 M2 Males Y = 0.4120X + 4.3360 0.9733 Females Y = 0.4001X + 4.1509 0.9877"

(continued)

Table 18.3 (continued)

Author	Sample size	M: F	Age range years	Radiograph	Method studied	Inference Indian population	Indian formula
Kiran et al. [47]	250	130:120	7–18	OPG	Demirjian's	Population-specific cubic regression formulas for Bhimavaram town (South India)	"Males: AGE = (7.584933012) + (0.000 × S) + (−0.000395087 × S2) + (1.30357E-05 × S3). Females: AGE = (9.8053) + (0.000 × S) + (−0.0022 × S2) + (2.940E-05 × S3)"

Source: Adapted from Rai et al. (2010), Acharya (2011), Kanchan-Talreja (2011), Jeevan et al. (2011), Manisha et al. (2014), Kiran et al. (2015). See references [42–47]

Case example: Dental age estimation in unidentified human remains

Body of an unidentified female recovered in advanced stages of decomposition from a pond in an urban city in Central India. The body was sent to the designated autopsy centre for post-mortem examination. The cause of death was determined as asphyxia due to ligature strangulation by the autopsy surgeons. The manner of death was still undetermined, as the police continues to investigate. Police have requested a joint age estimation report to create a biological profile of the victim. You were asked to perform dental age estimation, so you went to the mortuary and performed full mouth radiography, using a handheld device. The following radiographs were made by you at the mortuary.

Question: What is the dental age estimated from these radiographs? Describe the population-specific dental age estimation techniques used and the standard error, and provide references for the same. Follow the recommended guidelines for dental age estimation for your report. Include any additional observations made.

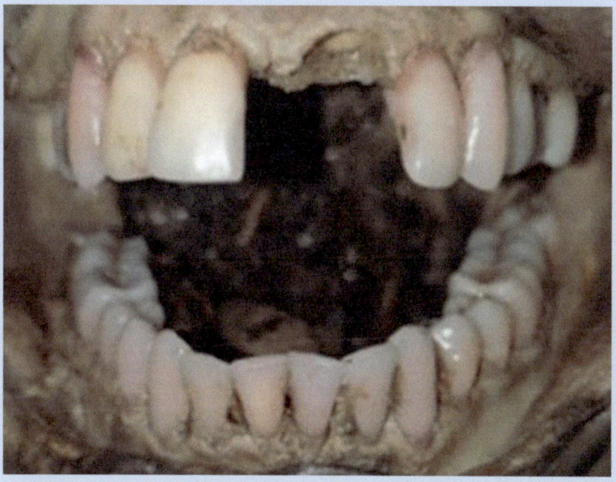

Frontal view

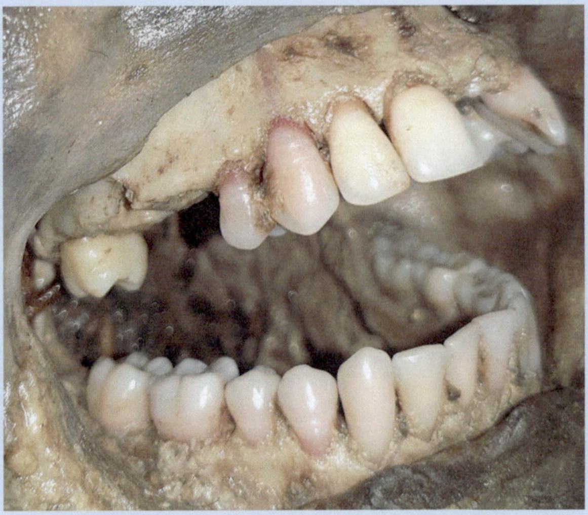

View from the right

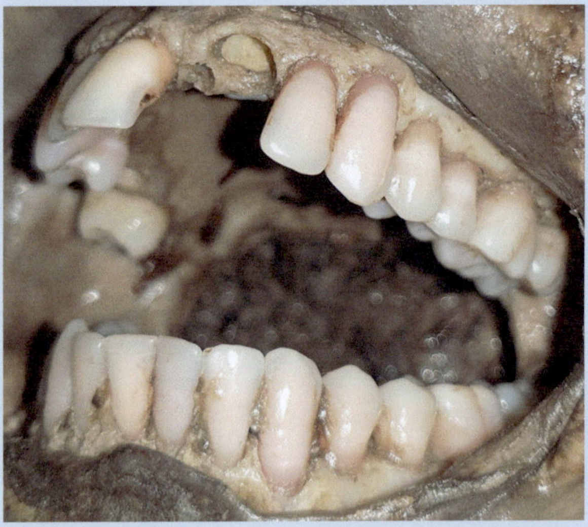

View from the left

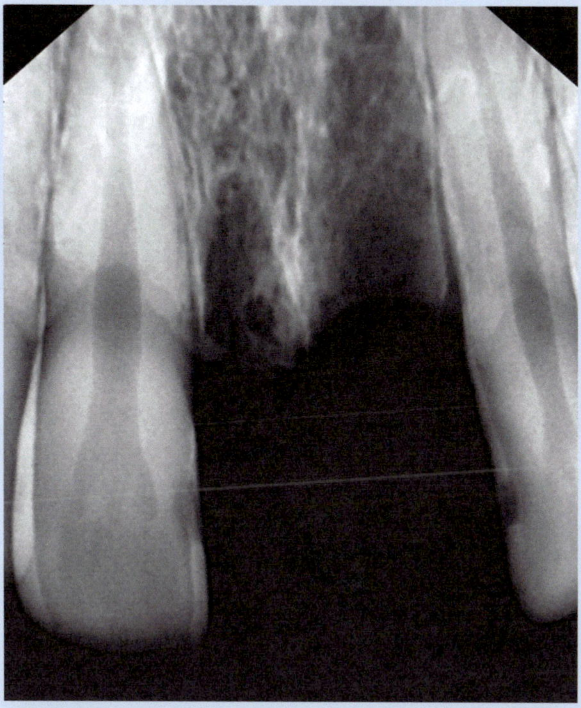

11, present; 21, missing postmortem

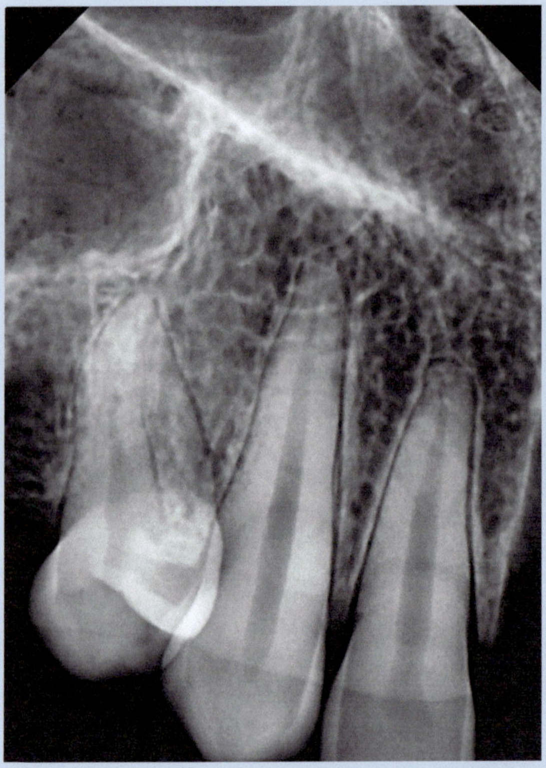

12–14 present; 15, missing antemortem

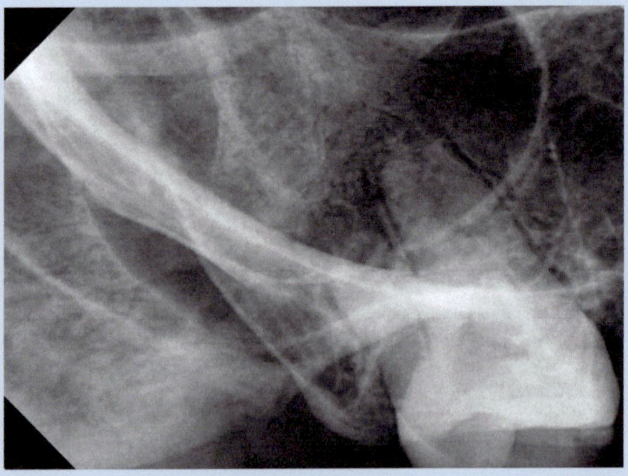

17, present; 16, missing antemortem; 18, missing antemortem

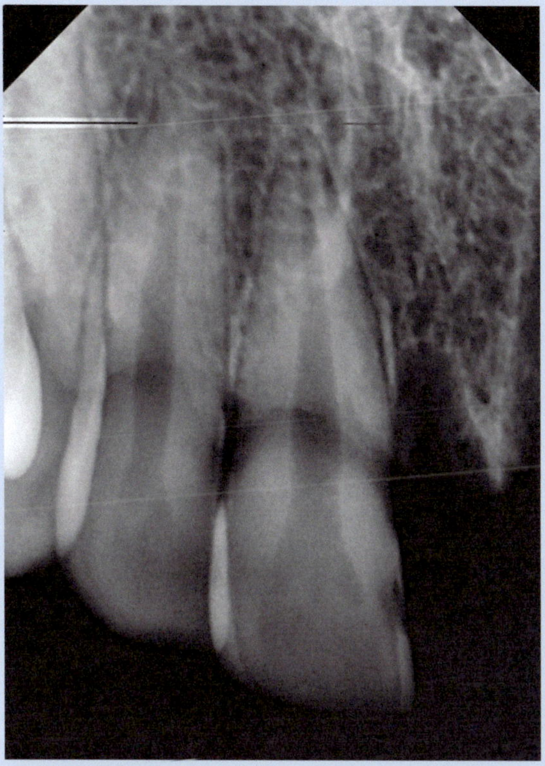

11–12

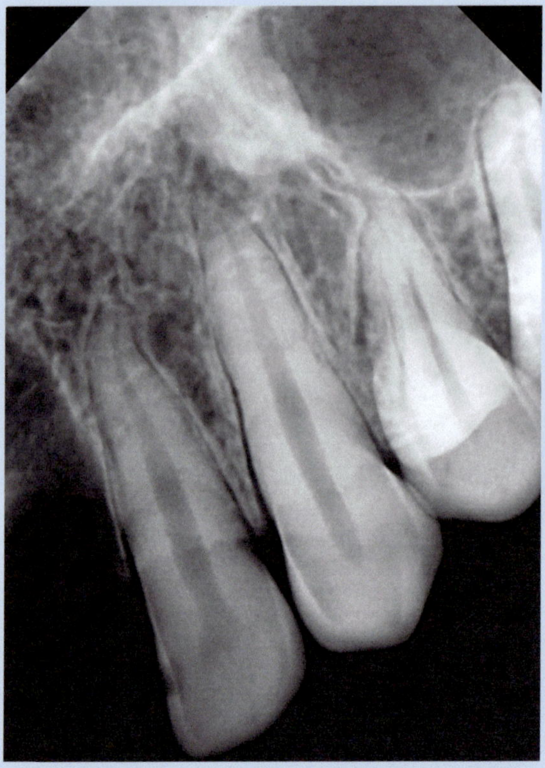

22–24

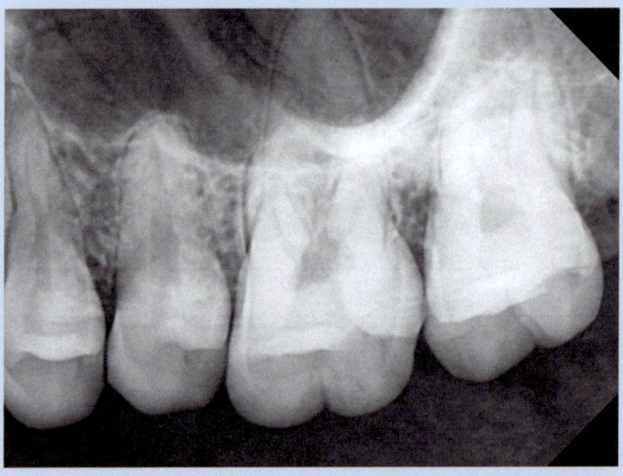

24–27

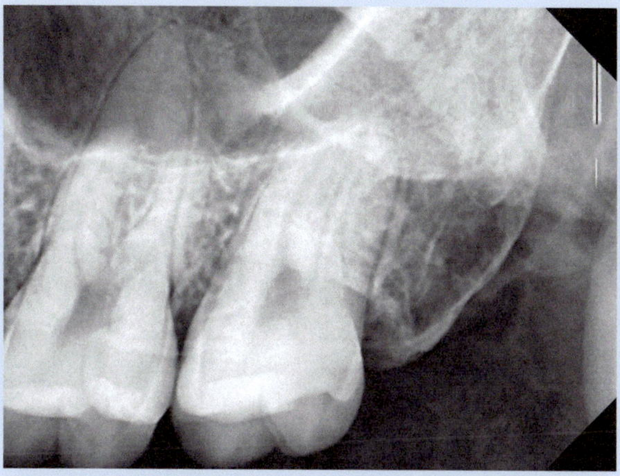

26–27; 28, missing antemortem

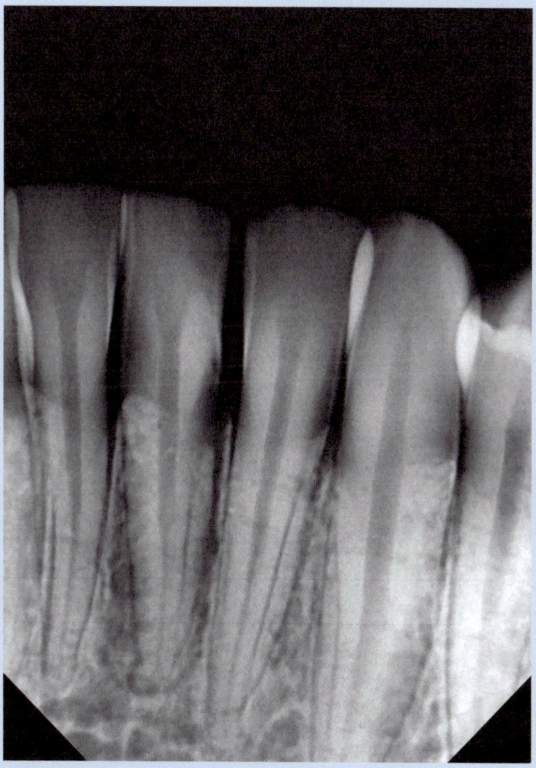

32, 31, 41, 42

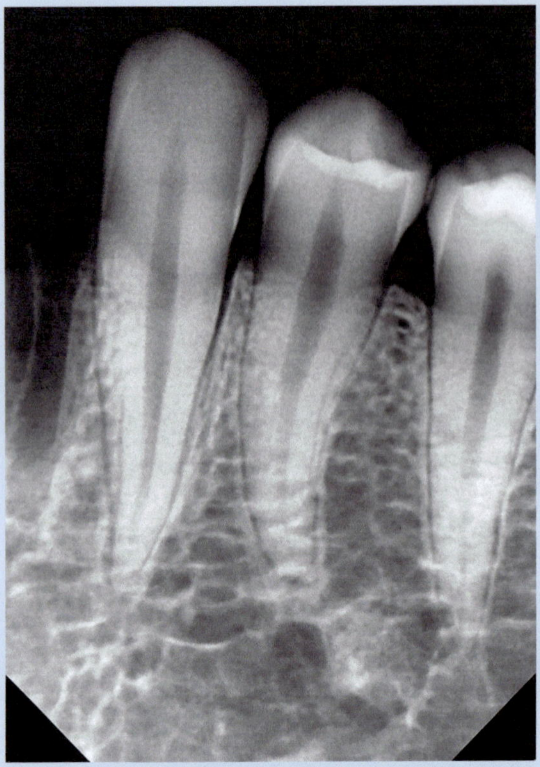

33, 34, 35

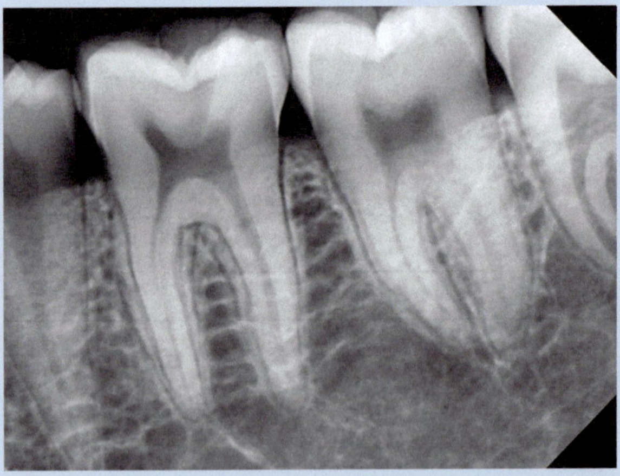

36–37

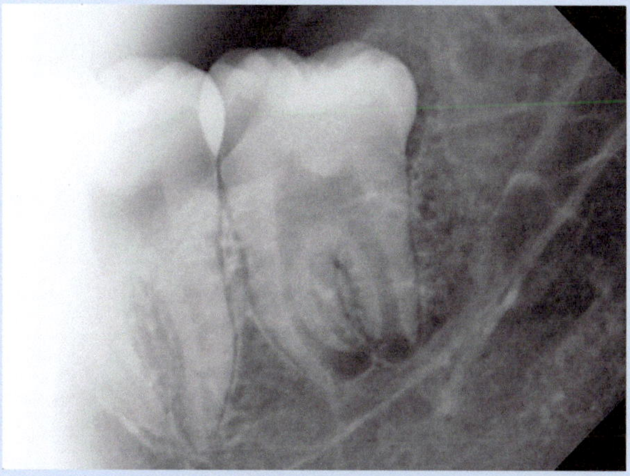

38

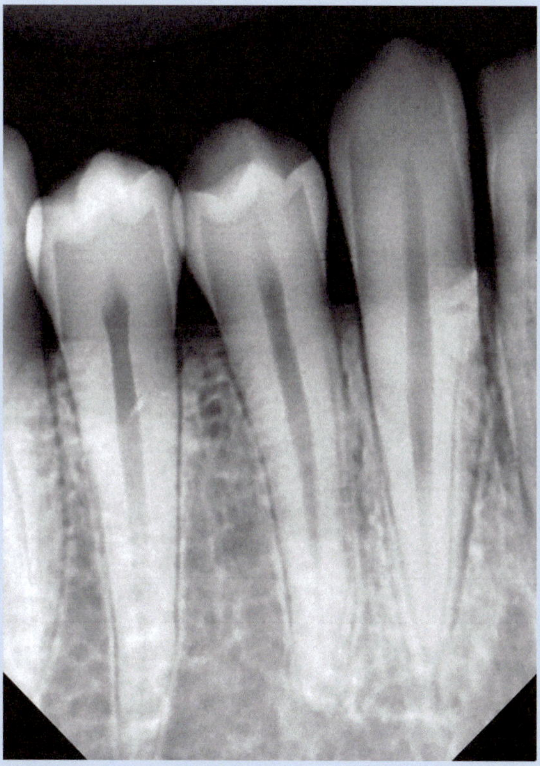

43, 44, 45

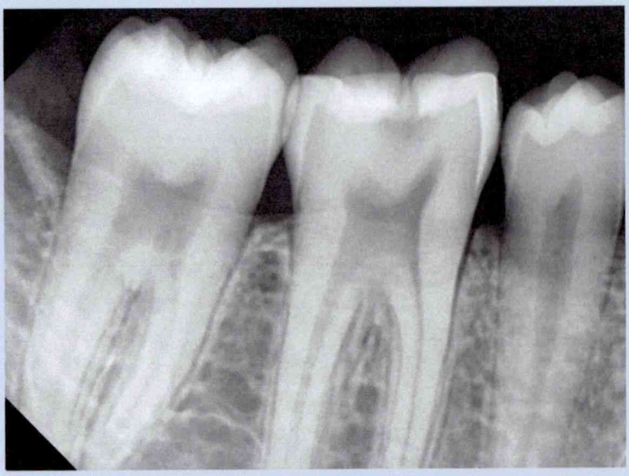

46, 47

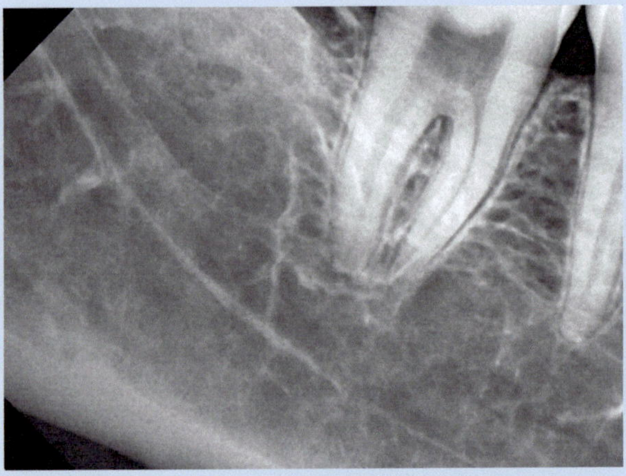

47, present; 48, missing antemortem

Source: Author, HP's own case material, anonymized for publication

This case highlights the importance of dental indicators when skeletal maturity is ambiguous or unavailable, and underscores the need for population-specific standards in age estimation.

18.5 Future of Dental Age Estimation in India

Dentists should be aware of the fact that they can play an important role in age estimation not only for the purpose of criminal investigation but also for helping the Sports Authority of India (SAI) and the Ministry of Youth Affairs and Sports. Both the regulatory bodies mentioned approach dental and medical experts to estimate the age of players involved in age fraud. In their report on "National Code against Age Fraud in Sports," age estimation evaluation includes dental examination and radiographs from orthopantomogram (OPG) and medical examination from hand–wrist radiograph and/or CT scans (SAI, National Code against Age Fraud in Sports, Age Estimation Format) [36]. Likewise, dentist can also extend their help for age estimation during the selection of cricket players. The Board of Control for Cricket in India has adopted bone age tests using hand–wrist radiographs (Tanner Whitehouse—TW3 method) to estimate the age of players in the 16-year-old thresholds [50].

The long-term research objectives are to develop, validate, and facilitate the application of the most accurate methods for age estimation of children and adolescents with a larger population data set. These methods or techniques that are developed should be further validated for accuracy. A dentist interested in age estimation research should try to develop methods that are certain and easily reproducible. To date, there is no such method that can precisely estimate the correct age. The aim and goal of future research, therefore, must be within practical and financial constraints and respect recognized ethical standards. Age estimation studies are of particular significance in India considering poor birth registration practices and issues relating to child rights. There is an imperative need for the protection of the rights of children without birth records and those involved in forged age claims [49].

In the present era of artificial intelligence, even forensic age estimation is being done using machine learning (ML). It is important to understand the advantages and scope of AI over traditional methods and its drawbacks for future studies and perspectives in the Indian scenario. Traditional dental age estimation methods or techniques involve phases as image-preprocessing, segmentation, feature extraction, and classification (categorical) or regression (numerical). The accomplishment of each phase is totally dependent on the compatibility with previous ones. In the classification phase, procedures seek to determine individuals' age groups, whereas the regression phase seeks to pinpoint their precise ages [51].

Deep learning approaches (artificial vision, object detection, recognition, etc.), which have lately succeeded traditional methods, efficiently address numerous issues in diverse scientific fields [52, 53]

The convolutional neural networks can work directly on the input images and generate the required output without requiring the execution of intermediate steps such as segmentation and feature extraction. But the biggest drawback with this latest advancement is that designing and training deep neural networks are complex, time-consuming, and costly affair. Therefore, a study conducted by Isa Atas et al. (2021) adopted the transfer learning approach in the deep learning model proposed for forensic age estimation. This model is intended to accurately predict an individual's forensic age from dental panoramic radiography images in a precise range [54].

In another recent study done by Galibourg A et al. (2021), it was found that machine learning methods used on panoramic radiographs were significantly more accurate than Demerjian's & Willems's method. Further, they concluded ML methods outperform the classic approaches for age estimation based on radiographic dental staging, from childhood up to early adulthood [55].

18.6 Conclusion

The practice of dental age estimation (DAE) plays a pivotal role in the fields of forensic science, law, and public health, particularly in India where age-related issues are often central to both legal and social justice concerns. This chapter has explored the diverse aspects of dental age estimation, focusing on its application in India, the methodologies involved, the specific challenges faced within the Indian context, and the future trajectory of the field.

The practical applications of dental age estimation in India are vast, touching upon a variety of fields such as criminal justice, public health, child protection, and sports. In the field of law, accurate age assessment can aid in resolving cases involving juvenile offenders, victims of sexual abuse, and cases of child trafficking. It can also play a significant role in determining eligibility for various social benefits, including education, healthcare, and pensions.

Given these applications, it is recommended that the Indian government invest in creating standardized protocols for age estimation that are accessible nationwide. This includes the training of forensic professionals, including dentists, in advanced age estimation techniques and the integration of age estimation training into the standard medical and dental curricula. Furthermore, it is crucial to establish nationwide guidelines that can be used across various sectors to ensure consistency and accuracy in age assessment practices.

The future of dental age estimation in India holds great potential, especially with the advent of artificial intelligence (AI) and machine learning (ML). These technologies are already being used in forensic science to enhance the accuracy and efficiency of age estimation techniques. For example, deep learning models that utilize convolutional neural networks (CNN) to directly process panoramic radiographs offer the potential for automating the estimation process, reducing human error, and increasing reproducibility. While these advancements are promising, their application in India remains limited due to resource constraints and the need for specialized training.

Therefore, future research should focus on further developing AI-based methods for dental age estimation, tailored specifically to the Indian demographic. Collaborative research efforts between forensic scientists, dentists, and technologists can lead to the creation of more accurate models that can be widely implemented across the country. Additionally, there is a need to conduct large-scale population-based studies to refine existing methods and create India-specific formulas for dental age estimation, taking into account regional variations in tooth development.

Furthermore, interdisciplinary research is crucial in addressing the ethical and legal challenges associated with dental age estimation. As the use of radiographs and other invasive methods for age estimation raises concerns, it is important to balance the need for accurate age verification with the rights and well-being of individuals, particularly minors. Research into non-invasive methods or advancements in imaging technologies can help mitigate these concerns, offering more ethical and practical solutions for age estimation.

Dental age estimation is a vital tool in forensic science, with significant implications for the legal system, child protection, and public health in India. The key challenges faced in India, such as the lack of reliable birth records, regional disparities in medical infrastructure, and societal pressures on age-related legal processes, highlight the need for standardized, accurate, and easily reproducible methods. While traditional methods of age estimation, such as those based on tooth eruption and skeletal maturity, have proven effective, ongoing advancements in AI and machine learning present exciting new opportunities for improving the accuracy and efficiency of these techniques.

As India continues to address issues such as child rights, age-related fraud, and the need for legal protections for vulnerable populations, the role of dental age estimation will only grow. By investing in research, developing region-specific formulas, and integrating modern technologies into forensic practice, India can enhance its ability to provide fair, just, and timely legal decisions. The future of dental age estimation in India lies in the continued development of interdisciplinary collaborations, technological innovations, and a commitment to improving the accuracy and accessibility of age estimation practices for all.

An important consideration in the Indian context is the lack of uniformity in protocols for age estimation across different states. Despite national guidelines, practices regarding documentation, choice of radiographic indicators, and specialist involvement vary widely. This can impact the standardisation and legal defensibility of age assessments. Furthermore, effective collaboration between disciplines, including pediatricians, radiologists, forensic odontologists, and legal authorities, is essential for ensuring accurate and ethically sound outcomes. Another emerging frontier in age estimation is the integration of artificial intelligence (AI). While promising, its use raises questions of transparency, validation across diverse populations, and the ethical handling of sensitive personal data. As most AI models have been developed and tested on non-Indian datasets, there is a pressing need to develop population-specific training data that reflect the morphological and developmental characteristics of Indian children and adolescents. Incorporating such technological advances into practice will require interdisciplinary research, robust ethical frameworks, and legal scrutiny to ensure fairness and accuracy.

References

1. UNICEF South Asia. Despite significant increase in birth registration, a quarter of the world's children remain unregistered [Internet]. 2019. Available from: https://www.unicef.org/rosa/press-releases/despite-significant-increase-birth-registration-quarter-worlds-children-remain.
2. The Protection of Children from Sexual Offences (Amendment) Act, Ministry of Law and Justice, India. 2019.
3. Nandan P. POCSO Act and Juvenile Justice: an analysis of existing laws and practices in India. Issue 6 Indian JL & Legal Rsch. 2022;4:1.
4. Shreya. Legality of abortion in India: with specific reference to Medical Termination of Pregnancy (Amendment) Act, 2021. Issue 4 Indian JL & Legal Rsch. 2022;4:1.
5. Vijayalakshmi S. The menace of female foeticide and infanticide in India. Editorial Board; 2018. p. 159.
6. Government of India, Press Information Bureau. Features and benefits of Ayushman Bharat Digital Mission [Internet]. 2022 [cited 2024 Dec 3]. Available from: https://pib.gov.in/PressReleasePage.aspx?PRID=1852502.
7. The Juvenile Justice (Care and Protection of Children) Act, 2015 (India) [Internet]. New Delhi: Government of India; 2015 [cited 2024 Dec 3]. Available from: https://www.indiacode.nic.in/handle/123456789/1649?view_type=browse.
8. Government of India, Press Information Bureau. Revised Child Fare Rule becomes applicable for train journey [Internet]. 2016 [cited 2024 Dec 3]. Available from: https://pib.gov.in/newsite/PrintRelease.aspx?relid=138458.
9. Sarkar CC. Right of Children to Free and Compulsory Education Act, 2009 and its implementation. India Infrastructure Report 2012. Routledge India; 2016. p. 33–43.
10. Dadwal L. Juvenility: from criminality to responsibility. Int J Rev Res Soc Sci. 2018;6(4):381–95.
11. Section 369: kidnapping or abducting child under ten years with intent to steal from its person [internet]. Offencein; 2024 [cited 2024 Dec 3]. Available from: https://www.offence.in/section-369-kidnapping-or-abducting-child-under-ten-years-with-intent-to-steal-from-its-person/.
12. Handa RK, Goswami S. The Protection of Children from Sexual Offences Act (POCSO), 2012: The precincts of the law and judicial expositions. J Victimol Victim Justice. 2024;7(2):191–204.
13. National Crime Investigation Bureau. Official website of the National Crime Investigation Bureau [Internet]. [cited 2024 Dec 3]. Available from: https://www.ncib.in/.
14. Virk S, Sekhon YS. Labour Law-Child & Adolescent Labour (Prohibition & Regulation) Act, 1986. Issue 3 Int'l JL Mgmt. & Human. 2020;3:530.
15. Juvenile Justice Committee, Delhi High Court. Official website of the Juvenile Justice Committee, Delhi High Court [Internet]. [cited 2024 Dec 3]. Available from: https://jjcdhc.nic.in/.
16. Government of India. The Criminal Law (Amendment) Act, 2013 [Internet]. 2013 [cited 2024 Dec 3]. Available from: https://prsindia.org/files/bills_acts/bills_parliament/2013/Criminal_Law_(A),_2013.pdf.
17. Anand A. The Juvenile Justice Amendment Bill, 2021: The changes and concerns. Neolexvision Blogs. 2021. https://www.aequivic.in/post/the-juvenile-justice-amendment-bill-2021-the-changes-and-concerns.

18. Government of India. The Majority Act, 1875 [Internet]. 1875 [cited 2024 Dec 3]. Available from: https://www.indiacode.nic.in/bitstream/123456789/15299/1/majorityact.pdf.
19. Umashankar MR. Essential elements for forming a valid contract under the Indian contract Act 1872. Issue 6 Int'l JL Mgmt. & Human. 2020;3:1190.
20. Agarwal P. Prohibition of Child Marriage (Amendment) Act 2006. Jus Corpus LJ. 2021;2.78.
21. Sharma A. The Factory Act, 1948 and social security: concept of factory, manufacturing process, worker and occupier. Issue 2 Indian JL & Legal Rsch. 2023;5:1.
22. Government of India. The Hindu Marriage Act, 1955 [Internet]. 1955 [cited 2024 Dec 3]. Available from: https://www.indiacode.nic.in/bitstream/123456789/1522/1/a1955-57.pdf.
23. Ministry of Road Transport and Highways, Government of India. The Motor Vehicles Act, 1988 [Internet]. [cited 2024 Dec 3]. Available from: https://morth.nic.in/motor-vehicles-act-1988#:~:text=Comprehensive%20Compendium%20Circulars,The%20Motor%20Vehicles%20Act%2C%201988.
24. Borzaga M. Limiting the minimum age: convention 138 and the origin of the ILO's action in the field of child labour. In: Child labour in a Globalized World. Routledge; 2016. p. 39–64.
25. Rana J. Types of Guardians and their rights under Hindu Minority and Guardianship Act, 1956 & Guardians And Wards Act, 1890. Issue 2 Indian JL & Legal Rsch. 2022;4(1)
26. Constitution of India. Article 84: Qualification for Membership of Parliament [Internet]. [cited 2024 Dec 3]. Available from: https://www.constitutionofindia.net/articles/article-84-qualification-for-membership-of-parliament/.
27. Government of India, Department of Public Enterprises. Guidelines on Corporate Governance for Central Public Sector Enterprises [Internet]. [cited 2024 Dec 3]. Available from: https://dpe.gov.in/sites/default/files/R-54%20%28Unsigned%29.pdf.
28. Aggrawal A. Estimation of age in the living–in matters civil and criminal. J Anat. 2008;213(3):342–3.
29. Jayaraman J, Roberts GJ, Wong HM, McDonald F, King NM. Ages of legal importance: implications in relation to birth registration and age assessment practices. Med Sci Law. 2016;56(1):77–82.
30. Government of India, Ministry of Labour and Employment. The Minimum Wages Act, 1948 [Internet]. [cited 2024 Dec 3]. Available from: https://clc.gov.in/clc/sites/default/files/MinimumWagesact.pdf.
31. Government of India, National Commission for Women. The Indian Christian Marriage Act, 1872 [Internet]. 1872 [cited 2024 Dec 3]. Available from: https://ncwapps.nic.in/acts/TheIndianChristianMarriageAct1872-15of1872.pdf.
32. Government of India. The Immoral Traffic (Prevention) Act, 1956 [Internet]. 1956 [cited 2024 Dec 3]. Available from: https://www.indiacode.nic.in/bitstream/123456789/15100/1/immoral_traffic_prevention_act_%28itpa%29_1956.pdf.
33. Chowdhury S. Interpretation of law of succession and inheritance under Hindu Succession Act and Indian Succession Act. Indian JL & Legal Rsch. 2021;3:1.
34. Virat S, Ankur B. The Employee's Compensation Act, 1923 & Code on Social Security. Issue 3 Int'l JL Mgmt. & Human. 2023;6:785.
35. Foster M, Khan AH. Citizenship (Amendment) Act 2019 and international law. Report, Melbourne: Peter McMullin Centre on Statelessness; 2021.
36. Ministry of Youth Affairs and Sports, Government of India. National Code Against Age Fraud in Sports [Internet]. [cited 2024 Dec 3]. Available from: https://yas.nic.in/sports/national-code-against-age-fraud-sports.
37. Kumar K, Saikia N. Determinants of birth registration in India: evidence from NFHS 2015–16. PLoS One. 2021;16(9):e0257014.
38. Makkad RS, Balani A, Chaturvedi SS, et al. Reliability of panoramic radiography in chronological age estimation. J Forensic Dent Sci. 2013;5(2):129–33.
39. Singh S, Venkatatapathy R, Balamurali PD, et al. Digital approach for measuring dentin translucency in forensic age estimation. J Forensic Dent Sci. 2013;5(1):47–51.

40. Periyakaruppan S, Meundi MA, David CM. Accuracy of age estimation in 6-21 year old south Indian population - a comparative analysis of clinical and radiographic methods. J Forensic Odontostomatol. 2018;36(2):10–9. PMID: 30712027; PMCID: PMC6626537.
41. Singh K, Gorea RK, Bharti V. Age estimation from eruption of permanent teeth. JIAFM. 2005;27(4)
42. Rai B, Kaur J, Cingolani M, Ferrante L, Cameriere R. Age estimation in children by measurement of open apices in teeth: an Indian formula. Int J Legal Med. 2010;124(3):237–41. https://doi.org/10.1007/s00414-010-0427-7. Epub 2010 Mar 3.
43. Acharya AB. Age estimation in Indians using Demirjian's 8-teeth method. J Forensic Sci. 2011;56(1):124–7. https://doi.org/10.1111/j.1556-4029.2010.01566.x. Epub 2010 Sep 20.
44. Kanchan-Talreja P, Acharya AB, Naikmasur VG. An assessment of the versatility of Kvaal's method of adult dental age estimation in Indians. Arch Oral Biol. 2012;57(3):277–84. https://doi.org/10.1016/j.archoralbio.2011.08.020. Epub 2011 Sep 17.
45. Jeevan MB, Kale AD, Angadi PV, Hallikerimath S. Age estimation by pulp/tooth area ratio in canines: Cameriere's method assessed in an Indian sample using radiovisiography. Forensic Sci Int. 2011;204(1–3):209.e1–5. https://doi.org/10.1016/j.forsciint.2010.08.017. Epub 2010 Sep 24.
46. Khorate MM, Dinkar AD, Ahmed J. Accuracy of age estimation methods from orthopantomograph in forensic odontology: a comparative study. Forensic Sci Int. 2014;234(184):e1–8. https://doi.org/10.1016/j.forsciint.2013.09.020. Epub 2013 Sep 26.
47. Kiran CS, Reddy RS, Ramesh T, Madhavi NS, Ramya K. Radiographic evaluation of dental age using Demirjian's eight-teeth method and its comparison with Indian formulas in south Indian population. J Forensic Dent Sci. 2015;7(1):44–8. https://doi.org/10.4103/0975-1475.150306. PMID: 25709319; PMCID: PMC4330618.
48. Dental Council of India. Revised BDS Course Regulations; 2007 [Internet]. [cited 2024 Dec 3]. Available from: http://www.dciindia.org.in/Rule_Regulation/Scheme_2006_DCI_Establishment_for_Opening_of_New_Dental_College_Regulations_2006_alongwith_Amendments.pdf.
49. Jayaraman J. Dental age estimation in India: do we have a role beyond publishing scientific evidences? J Forensic Dent Sci. 2018;10:55–7.
50. ESPN Cric info. BCCI adopts new age-verification method [Internet]. [cited 2024 Dec 3]. Available from: http://www.espncricinfo.com/india/content/story/571542.html.
51. Razzak MR, Naz S. Microscopic blood smear segmentation and classification using deep contour-aware CNN and extreme machine learning. In: Proceedings of the IEEE Conference on Computer Vision and Pattern Recognition Workshops; 2017. p. 49–55.
52. Atas I. Human gender prediction based on deep transfer learning from panoramic radiograph images [preprint]. arXiv:2205.09850. 2022.
53. Ozdemir C, Gedik MA, Kaya Y. Age estimation from left-hand radiographs with deep learning methods. Traitement du Signal. 2021;38(6)
54. Ataş İ, Özdemir C, Ataş M, Doğan Y. Forensic dental age estimation using modified deep learning neural network. Balkan J Electr Comput Eng. 2022;11(4):298–305. https://doi.org/10.17694/bajece.1351546.
55. Galibourg A, Cussat-Blanc S, Dumoncel J, Telmon N, Monsarrat P, Maret D. Comparison of different machine learning approaches to predict dental age using Demirjian's staging approach. Int J Legal Med. 2021;135(2):665–75. https://doi.org/10.1007/s00414-020-02489-5.

19 Methods of Skeletal Age Assessment

Anand Marya, Priyanka Kapoor, and Arofi Kurniawan

19.1 Introduction

Skeletal age estimation is an important method used in medicine as well as dentistry. Apart from that, its applications in paediatrics, orthodontics, endocrinology, and forensic science [1]. It defines a person's biological age through the analysis of development and maturation in bones, showing the status of an individual's growth and overall physical development [2]. Sequential age reflects the figure of years from birth, and biological age reflects the category of aging that an independent person has arrived at concerning skeletal aspects. Both of them may vary quite significantly, depending on elements such as general health conditions, nutrition, and genetics [3]. Hence, the approximation of skeletal age creates an important foundation in numerous healthcare settings as it permits a more customised and timely interference, especially through growth spurts.

19.1.1 Importance of Skeletal Age Assessment

Skeletal age assessment is important in fields like orthodontics, where treatment usually relies on growth spurts' timing [4]. Such assessments could be used to make

A. Marya (✉)
Department of Orthodontics, Faculty of Dentistry, University of Puthisastra, Phnom Penh, Cambodia
e-mail: amarya@puthisastra.edu.kh

P. Kapoor
Department of Orthodontics, Faculty of Dentistry, Jamia Millia Islamia, New Delhi, India

A. Kurniawan
Department of Forensic Odontology, Faculty of Dental Medicine Universitas Airlangga, Surabaya, Indonesia

© The Author(s), under exclusive license to Springer Nature Switzerland AG 2026

A. Chowdhry, P. Kapoor (eds.), *Dental Age Assessment*,
https://doi.org/10.1007/978-3-032-08788-1_19

a judgment on whether to use orthodontic appliances or to begin braces in order to treat malocclusions. It would also apply in dental orthopaedics; taking advantage of the peak development time of the patient could enhance the effectiveness of the treatment targeted at skeletal malalignment, such as malalignment of the jaw or crowding of the teeth [5]. Skeletal age evaluation is done quite frequently in paediatric medicine in regard to growth disorders. These include growth hormone deficiencies, premature puberty, and delayed puberty. By determining if the skeletal development in a child is developing normally or not, clinicians are able to make decisions on interventions that might help stimulate or moderate growth. Likewise, the concept of skeletal age can be applied to endocrinology by monitoring patients with hypothyroidism or Turner syndrome, whose main concern is a disturbance in growth of a delayed or abnormal nature [6]. Skeletal age assessment is a method by which, through forensic science, an approximation of the age of unidentified remains is obtained, assisting in narrowing down the identity of unknown individuals. The method is also significant in forensic situations when the determination of age may be necessary to ascertain whether individuals fall into the category of children or adults for certain criminal liabilities or for other legal purposes.

19.1.2 Commonly Used Anatomical Structures for Skeletal Age Assessment

Several anatomical sites can be taken into consideration in order to estimate skeletal age. Each of these regions has a number of advantages in determining an individual's developmental progression. These include the cervical vertebrae, hand-wrist bones, skull, orodental structures, and atlas. Each of the methods is based on specific morphological shifts which have specific ossification patterns that show predictable progressions with time inside an individual [7].

Cervical vertebrae The general morphological and structural changes in cervical vertebrae form the basis for the CVMI, largely done on the pattern change in C2, C3, and C4. Its accuracy in predicting the timing of the pubertal growth spurt, essential for good treatment planning, has made it widely applied in orthodontics. Being the routine use of lateral cephalograms in orthodontics, the CVMI method is not only readily available but also does not involve any additional radiation exposure needs [8].

Hand-wrist bones The hand-wrist radiographic technique is among the oldest and most established methods for the estimation of skeletal maturity. It enables the detailed observation of one's skeletal maturity through the study of patterns of ossification and fusion occurring in the hand and wrist bones. In developing a method to assess skeletal age, schemes such as the Greulich-Pyle or Tanner-Whitehouse systems have been developed, allowing for proper estimates from standard radiographs [7].

Skull It is widely acknowledged that the skull is a crucial component in the field of forensic age estimation and paediatric age determination. One of the earliest indications of growth that may be observed in a child is the development of the sutures and fontanelles of the skull. In forensic investigations that seek to determine the chronological history or evaluate anomalous skull growth, progressive ossification, and suture closure serve as reliable indicators of age [9].

Orodental Structures Dental structures have a unique relationship with skeletal age, as tooth eruption and calcification are closely linked to overall skeletal development. For example, the Demirjian approach uses various stages of tooth development as an effective way to estimate dental age, which typically corresponds with skeletal maturity. The schedule of tooth eruption is pivotal in treatment design and planning for orthodontics and paediatric dentistry [10].

Atlas The atlas (1st cervical vertebra or C1) is another property used in age approximation for its prompt ossification patterns. Age can mainly be derived by noticing morphological changes including size changes over the period. The C1 offers extraordinary insight throughout early childhood; at that time, other skeletal components may not be developed adequately for valid age estimation [11].

19.1.3 Correlation Between Dental Age and Skeletal Age

The main point in estimating skeletal age derives from the relation between dental age and skeletal age. Both of them are biological growth reflectors that often align. However, factors such as nutrition, heredity, or systemic illnesses can lead to variation [12]. Normally children have identical dental and skeletal ages, but a few may encounter delayed or advanced tooth eruption concerning skeletal growth. This combination is crucial in dental departments like orthodontics. In this department, the schedule of tooth eruption concerning skeletal development influences suitable treatment outcomes [13]

19.1.4 Scope of the Chapter

This segment outlines techniques for evaluating age from skeletal structures, concerning clinical as well as forensic purposes. An extended overview will be narrated of how skeletal age evaluation is done and implemented, including procedures like the CVMI, skull-based research, hand-wrist radiographs, dental structures, and atlas ossification. To provide information related to biological age, the current chapter is going to talk about morphological age-related switches such as mental foramen position, bone density variation, and the constriction of the gonial angle. However, changes will be consented to dental developments, further prioritizing the significance of skeletal age evaluation from both a forensic perspective and a clinical perspective.

19.2 Cervical Vertebral Maturation Index (CVMI)

The Cervical Vertebral Maturation Index is an accepted method for estimating skeletal age, mainly in orthodontics including growth-related factors. Different from traditional radiographs like taking of the hand-wrist area, the method of CVMI causes changes in the morphology of C2, C3, and C4 in the lateral cephalogram [8]. Clinicians can estimate the skeletal age of any given patient by observing the shape, size, and development of these vertebrae, which also have high correlations with pubertal growth (Table 19.1). This information helps very much in treatment planning, particularly the timing of interventions: orthodontic braces, correction, and growth modulation treatments [14].

The CVMI method offers, for other skeletal age assessment methods using Tanner-Whitehouse or Greulich-Pyle—which both need specific radiographs of the hand-wrist area—an effective, completely non-invasive alternative. One of the clear advantages is the use of routine lateral cephalograms, already generally taken on orthodontic patients. The changes in the shape and size of the vertebrae mark a very good indicator of when the growth spurt occurs, enabling the clinician to plan the best possible treatment strategy [15].

19.2.1 Stages of CVMI

The cervical vertebral maturation method categorises skeletal development into six separate stages. Each of these stages differs from the others due to morphological changes in vertebrae C2, C3, and C2, respectively. The main characteristics that define these stages are changes in the height and shape of the vertebral bodies and the development of concavities in the inferior margins of the vertebrae. Accurate prediction of a patient's pubertal growth spurt is important in orthodontics to maximise the effectiveness of growth-related treatments. This is a widely used six-stage model for this motive [16].

Advantages of CVMI include estimation of remaining growth in the lateral cephalogram which is a routine orthodontic record and hence no additional radiograph like a hand-wrist is required. Disadvantages include that serial radiographs are not possible due to radiation exposure, subjective evaluation of growth is based on the shapes of vertebrae, and in case a lead band is worn in the neck while taking a radiograph, the vertebrae are not visible. It may be useful in forensic anthropology for age determination, along with other techniques like dental or skull-based assessments [17].

Limitations These include individual variation in vertebral shapes and sizes due to genetic, nutritional, and environmental factors [18]; subjectivity in stage

Table 19.1 Diagrammatic representation of cervical staging of 2nd, 3rd, and 4th vertebrae and their interpretation, as identified in a lateral cephalogram

Cervical Stage (CS)	Growth status in relation to stage	Interpretation of stage
CS 1	At least 2 years from the beginning of peak mandibular growth Growth remaining: 80–100%	Lower borders of 2nd, 3rd, and 4th vertebrae straight Shape is a wedge with taper of the superior border from posterior to anterior
CS 2	1 year from the beginning of peak mandibular growth. Growth remaining: 65–85%	2nd and 3rd vertebrae interior border shows concavities 4th vertebrae inferior border is flat Shape of 3rd and 4th vertebrae roughly rectangular
CS 3	Peak mandibular growth already commenced and probable completion within 1 year Growth remaining: 25–65%	2nd and 3rd vertebrae interior border shows distinct concavities 4th vertebrae inferior border concavity begins Shape of 3rd and 4th vertebrae rectangular
CS 4	Completion of peak mandibular growth immediate or within the past 1 year Growth remaining: 10– 25%	2nd, 3rd, and 4th vertebrae interior border show distinct concavities Shape of 3rd and 4th vertebrae roughly square
CS 5	Completion of peak mandibular growth one year ago Growth remaining: 5–10%	2nd, 3rd, and 4th vertebrae interior border concavities accentuated Shape of 3rd and 4th vertebrae roughly square
CS 6	Completion of peak mandibular growth 2 years ago Growth remaining little/no growth	2nd, 3rd, and 4th vertebrae interior border concavities deep Shape of 3rd and 4th vertebrae roughly rectangular vertically

Adapted from (Hegde *et al.*, [19])

identification due to variability in assessment between observers [20]; is most effective for tracking growth during puberty but not useful after skeletal growth is complete [21].

19.2.2 MP3 (Middle Phalanx of the Third Finger)

The timing of the spurt of pubertal growth seems important for clinical orthodontic decision-making due to the utilization of somatic growth rate for the correction of skeletal discrepancies [22] described the ossification stages of MP3 (middle phalanx of the third finger) with respect to pubertal growth.

Advantages include a closer estimation of skeletal growth status based on a radiograph of a single finger; hence, the possibility of evaluation in IOPA would require less radiation exposure, even if serial radiographs are taken. Disadvantages include a subjective evaluation of growth based on the shapes of the metaphysis and epiphysis.

19.3 Hand-Wrist Skeletal Age Assessment

Hand-wrist skeletal age assessment is a traditional and widely used method for estimating biological age. It has proven especially useful in paediatric endocrinology, orthodontics, and growth-related research, where understanding skeletal maturation is crucial for diagnosing growth disorders, predicting growth potential, and deciding the optimal timing for interventions like orthodontic treatment. By monitoring the growth stages of hand and wrist bones, clinicians can record how far the development has progressed during puberty including the expected growth in the future [23].

The hand-wrist area contains numerous bones that reveal expected patterns of epiphyseal and ossification fusion, making it an outstanding site for estimating skeletal age. Throughout the years, multiple standardised procedures have been established, with the Greulich-Pyle and Tanner-Whitehouse methods being the most frequently utilised. These approaches evaluate the stage of bone ossification including the completion of growth plates to evaluate age, which can then be collated to a patient's sequential age to point out any growth divergence [7].

19.3.1 Ossification and Growth Centres

Ossification of the hand and wrist region's bones follows a systematic path from birth to adolescence, making them important markers of skeletal development. This area contains 19 bones, phalanges or finger bones, metacarpals or hand bones, and carpals or wrist bones, including the distal ends of the ulna and radius or forearm bones. These bones pass through well-defined stages of growth, beginning with the formation of ossification centres in infancy besides culminating in late adolescence with the fusing of growth plates [24].

19.3.2 Tanner-Whitehouse and Greulich-Pyle Methods

Two of the popular methods for evaluating skeletal age using hand-wrist radiographs are the Greulich-Pyle method and Tanner-Whitehouse (TW2) method. These approaches give systematic techniques to interpret radiographs by collating the maturation of specific bones to optimum growth charts, allowing precise evaluation of skeletal age.

19.3.2.1 Tanner-Whitehouse Method (TW2)

The Tanner-Whitehouse method (TW2) is an all-inclusive, bone-specific record system used to evaluate skeletal age. It assesses the developmental stages of twenty bones in the wrist and hand, and the ulna, radius, carpals, phalanges, and metacarpals. Every bone has a score depending on the degree of ossification including epiphyseal fusion found in the radiograph. These solo scores are then counted to create a maturity score, and that determines the skeletal age [25].

Procedure After taking the radiographs of the wrist and hand, the bones are assessed depending on their ossification stage, size, and shape. Every bone is scored based on its level of maturity, starting from initial ossification to full epiphyseal fusion. These scores are then counted to form an overall maturity score, collated against standard age charts.

Accuracy The TW2 method is well known for its better accuracy because of its all-inclusive, bone-specific scoring system. In paediatric and growth assessments, where precise skeletal age evaluation is important for the diagnosis of growth-related problems and treatment planning, this technique is quite helpful.

Applications This technique is mainly applied in clinical situations that need precision, like evaluating a child with an abnormal growth pattern. This technique is used in research to record the effect of growth-related treatments.

19.3.2.2 Greulich-Pyle Method

The Greulich-Pyle technique removes the complexities from skeletal age evaluation by collating a hand-wrist radiograph to reference images from the Greulich-Pyle Atlas and radiographs showing different stages of bone maturation. The child's radiograph is coordinated to the closest matching image in the atlas to evaluate their skeletal age [26].

Procedure By comparing the patients' hand-wrist radiographs to standardised images from the Greulich-Pyle Atlas, clinicians evaluate the patient's situation by highlighting compatibilities in bone ossification including fusion. To specify bone age, an image that most closely fits the child's radiograph is chosen from the atlas.

Efficiency The Greulich-Pyle technique is quick and needs less effort in comparison to TW2 method, and it has become a common option in time-dependent clinical environments. Despite that, its accuracy is less because it depends on visual comparison and not a detailed scoring process.

Limitations The Greulich-Pyle method is quick and quite convenient. However, it is not as accurate as the TW2 approach. This is applicable when the patient's bone growth varies much from the reference images of the atlas.

19.3.3 Limitations

The hand-wrist technique is broadly known as the gold standard technique for skeletal age evaluation, but this technique has some limitations and needs to be contemplated for accurate results and application.

Radiation exposure By the time hand-wrist radiographs show lower radiation levels in comparison with other imaging methods, they still expose the child to radiation. This is a particular concern in paediatric cases, where repeated imaging may be required during critical growth phases, raising potential health risks over time [27].

Genetic and environmental variability Bone development in the hand and wrist is shaped by several factors, including genetics, nutrition, and overall health. These individual differences can result in discrepancies between skeletal age and chronological age. For example, children with growth disorders may experience delayed ossification, while those with conditions like precocious puberty might show accelerated bone maturation [28].

Gender differences Significant gender differences exist in the timing of ossification and epiphyseal fusion, with females generally maturing earlier than males. Most skeletal age assessment methods are designed to account for these variations, but neglecting to consider gender in clinical practice can result in inaccurate skeletal age estimates [29].

Timing of growth spurts Hand-wrist radiographs are most effective for evaluating skeletal maturity during childhood and adolescence, especially during periods of rapid growth. However, after epiphyseal fusion occurs, usually by late adolescence, this method loses its utility. In adults, alternative skeletal assessment techniques, such as those based on cervical vertebrae or dental structures, are often more suitable [18].

19.4 Skull-Based Age Assessment

Skull-based age assessment is essential for estimating skeletal age, particularly in forensic anthropology, archaeology, and paediatric medicine. As one of the first structures to ossify, the skull offers critical insights into early and late stages of skeletal development. Its maturation and growth follow consonant patterns, which can be analysed to approximate biological age, mainly in young children and infants. In adults and adolescents, age gauges such as the changes in bone density, cranial morphology, and timing of suture closure provide important details for age evaluation [30].

In the field of forensic anthropology, the assessment of skull-based age is valuable for evaluating the age of skeletal residue, as skull features frequently remain preserved over time. By inspecting sutures, fontanelles, including other age-related changes, a forensic scientist can evaluate the age at death with a high accuracy rate. In clinical scenarios, orthodontists and paediatricians use skull-based estimation to monitor regular growth patterns or recognise developmental abnormalities [31].

19.4.1 Sutures and Fontanelles

The skull includes several bones associated with cranial sutures, which are joints made of fibres that support growth in the initial stages of development. The soft, membranous spaces identified as fontanelles in between the cranial bones permit the skull to grow fast in the starting few years of life. These fontanelles' and sutures' predictable closure deliver useful measures for assessing skeletal maturity [32].

19.4.1.1 Fontanelle Closure

Fontanelles play an important role in initial skull development, allowing the skull bones to increase as the brain grows. During childbirth, there are multiple primary fontanelles: the anterior, mastoid, sphenoidal, and posterior fontanelles. The posterior and anterior fontanelles are mainly useful for evaluating age in infants due to their larger size along with consistent closure timelines [33].

Posterior fontanelle closure Normally, the posterior fontanelle is found in the meeting place of the parietal and occipital bones, the smallest of the two main fontanelles. It closes by 2 to 3 months of age. Its closure in the early stage is a sign of normal skull development and also acts as an important indicator for evaluating the skeletal age of young infants [34].

Anterior fontanelle closure Normally, the anterior fontanelle is found at the meeting point of the parietal and frontal bones, it is large and quite noticeable. It closes between 18 and 24 months, providing continued skull growth through an important phase of brain development. A significant premature closure or delay may show developmental issues like craniosynostosis or other growth abnormalities, making it an important topic of paediatric assessments [35].

In clinical and forensic contexts, the area of fontanelle closure is frequently used to evaluate an infant's age. Early or delayed closure can indicate underlying health issues, on the other hand, normal closure times indicate a reliable reference point for evaluating skeletal maturity during infancy.

19.4.1.2 Suture Closure

The cranial sutures are evident as fibrous joints between the skull bones, where the cranial bones become mature and fuse as the child grows. In the initial life stage, these sutures—the squamosal, coronal, lambdoid, and sagittal—remain open to allow brain growth. Adulthood and adolescence see the continuance of suture fusion, and that happens in the expected order. Suture closure is a significant benchmark of skeletal age, mainly in adults and adolescents [36].

Coronal suture The second or third decade of life is normally when the coronal suture, which joins the parietal and frontal bones horizontally, starts to fuse. Adolescence can see the first signs of ossification. However, full fusion doesn't happen till later in adulthood, at the ages of 40–50 [37].

Sagittal suture In early adulthood or late adolescence, the sagittal suture runs between the parietal bones beside the midline of the skull, from beginning to close. The ages of 30–40 are the time to complete fusion, though this period might vary, mostly based on things such as general health and heredity [38].

Lambdoid suture One of the last sutures to completely close is the lambdoid suture, it is situated between the parietal and occipital bones closer to the rear of the skull. It may stay partially open in middle age, but most of the people experiencing complete closure in the age of 50–60 [39].

In the Department of Forensic Anthropology, closure of suture serves as a dependable indicator for evaluating age at death, mainly in adults. The degree of suture fusion is normally evaluated through direct examination of skeletal remains or radiographs, helping to estimate the individual's age. In living individuals, abnormal suture closure patterns can signal developmental disorders or congenital conditions like craniosynostosis, where early fusion of sutures results in abnormal skull shape and restricted growth.

19.4.2 Age-Related Changes in the Skull

As a person ages, various changes occur in the skull that can be used to estimate biological age. While these changes are most noticeable during infancy and adolescence, they continue to offer important clues throughout adulthood. Two key factors in skull-based age estimation are the thickness of the cranial bones and the enlargement of the paranasal sinuses. These features develop predictably over time, making them valuable in assessing age.

19.4.2.1 Cranial Bone Thickness

As a person ages, especially during childhood and adolescence, the cranial bones become thicker. In infants and young children, these bones are relatively thin and flexible to accommodate the rapid growth of the brain. As individuals near skeletal maturity, the bones of the cranium thicken and strengthen, providing increased protection for the brain. In adulthood, the thickening process continues, though it significantly slows down once the growth plates close [32].

Infants and Children In young children, the cranial bones are quite thin, enabling flexibility for deformation during childbirth and accommodating rapid growth in infancy. As the child develops, the bones gradually thicken, and by adolescence, they achieve a more mature thickness.

Adolescents During adolescence, the skull attains its adult size, and the bones experience substantial thickening. This thickening coincides with the fusion of cranial sutures, signalling the conclusion of rapid cranial growth.

Adults In adulthood, cranial bone thickness continues to increase, albeit at a slower pace. Over time, the bones become denser, which can be observed through radiographic imaging. Bone density scans of the skull may highlight age-related changes, offering insights into an individual's age.

19.4.2.2 Expansion of the Paranasal Sinuses

The paranasal sinuses, consisting of the frontal, maxillary, ethmoidal, and sphenoidal sinuses, expand considerably during childhood and adolescence. Their development follows a predictable pattern, making them valuable markers for estimating age, especially in children and adolescents [40].

Infants At birth, the paranasal sinuses are not fully developed, with only the maxillary and ethmoidal sinuses showing initial signs of formation. During infancy and early childhood, these sinuses remain relatively small.

Children In the initial time of childhood, the sphenoidal and frontal sinuses begin to develop. On the other hand, ethmoidal and maxillary sinuses proceed to grow. During the ages of 6–8, these sinuses are more distinguishable on radiographs, but they are still smaller in comparison with those in adults.

Adolescents The paranasal sinuses quickly enlarge in adolescence to correspond with the pubertal growth rush. The sinuses become mature in size by the end of the phase. It can be seen on radiographic imaging. Skeletal age by this time can be evaluated from the shape and size of the sinuses.

Adults During adulthood, paranasal sinuses maintain their size, but their extent of pneumatization (air cavity formation) and shape can differ regarding individual health factors. Sinus expansion is a reliable factor for evaluating skeletal age, mainly during the growth period.

19.5 Orodental Structures in Skeletal Age Assessment

Orodental structures deliver a reliable and mostly used method for evaluating skeletal age, and dental development is parallel to overall skeletal maturation. The procedure of tooth eruption followed by calcification, and resorption follows a particular timeline, offering important insights into someone's biological age. Dentists, orthodontists, and forensic anthropologists frequently use dental indicators to estimate age, especially in paediatric patients and young adults. This approach proves particularly useful when other skeletal age markers are unavailable or when radiographic imaging of skeletal structures is limited [41].

Dental age estimation relies on several key factors, including the sequence of tooth eruption, stages of tooth calcification, and the degree of tooth resorption. Since these factors progress in a predictable pattern, clinicians can estimate a person's biological age with a fair degree of accuracy. In addition, comparing skeletal age with dental age helps identify growth discrepancies and detect conditions like precocious or delayed puberty [42]. It can depend on tooth eruption sequence, *Tooth Calcification and Resorption, as taken separately in other chapters.*

19.5.1 Dental Age Versus Skeletal Age

Skeletal and dental ages are usually aligned, yet discrepancies may occur. However, dental development normally parallels skeletal growth. There are cases in which the timing between the two varies. Clinicians need to interpret these differences carefully to avoid inaccurate diagnoses or badly timed treatments.

19.5.1.1 Correlation Between Dental and Skeletal Age

In healthy adolescents and children, skeletal and dental development is likely to follow similar timelines. Moreover, various factors, including genetics, environmental influences, and hormones, can result in deviations. For example, a child having delayed tooth eruption can show signs of delayed skeletal growth, and early tooth development may correlate with an accelerated growth phase [43].

Studies recommend that dental age can be a more reliable indicator than skeletal age sometimes, mainly in children having growth-related conditions [44, 45]. In scenarios where nutritional deficiencies or chronic illness impact skeletal growth, dental development might still progress normally, creating a better gauge of biological age [46].

19.5.1.2 Discrepancies Between Dental and Skeletal Age

Lagging dental age Conditions like hypothyroidism, growth hormone deficiency, or poor nutrition can lead to dental development lagging behind skeletal growth, resulting in delayed tooth eruption and root calcification. Clinicians need to identify whether this delay is because of is simply a normal variation or a medical condition [47].

Advanced dental age Contrarily, conditions like hyperthyroidism or precocious puberty can cause teeth to develop faster than the skeleton, resulting in early tooth eruption. This can cause challenges for orthodontists, and skeletal growth may still be happening, requiring heedful consideration to avoid premature growth plate closure at the time of treatment [48].

19.5.1.3 Clinical and Forensic Applications

In clinical orthodontic practice, appreciating the connection between skeletal and dental ages is important for better treatment planning. It is important to time interventions to conflict with periods of active growth, mainly when addressing major skeletal abnormalities such as jaw discrepancies or malocclusions. In situations where skeletal remains are not enough, dental age is frequently utilised in forensic science to assess the age of the unidentified person. The eruption of third molars is quite helpful in evaluating a teen or young adult's age [49].

19.6 Atlas-Based Skeletal Age Assessment

The first cervical vertebra, referred to atlas or C1, is the main point of atlas-based skeletal age evaluation. C1 creates a junction between the spine and head, which is important for both permitting head movement and supporting the skull. The atlas is a helpful marker for evaluating skeletal age, mainly in adolescents and children, because of its early distinct developmental stages and ossification. The atlas gives an alternative to standard methods for evaluating skeletal maturity, such as dental examinations or hand-wrist radiography. This is useful in scenarios where other skeletal identification points are not accessible [50].

With its two lateral masses attached by posterior and anterior arches, the C1 has a unique shape. Due to its distinct growth pattern along with the lack of a vertebral body, C1 is a trustworthy identification point of skeletal development. Adolescence and childhood bring about prominent structural changes, and recording these changes shows us a lot about an individual's biological age [51].

19.6.1 Ossification Centres in the Atlas

C1 develops through an expected sequence, starting with primary ossification formation early in infancy. Recording the progression of these centres permits clinicians to evaluate skeletal maturity.

19.6.1.1 Primary Ossification Centres

Primary ossification centres are present in the atlas' lateral masses, predominantly composed of cartilage at birth. The foundation of the vertebra is formed by these sites, which ossify first. Around the 7th or 8th week of fetal development, the lateral masses begin to ossify as well as continue to expand throughout infancy [52].

Lateral masses The lateral masses act as the atlas' primary structural supports and are the early regions to ossify. These regions help form the axis or portions of the atlas that attach to the skull base and the second cervical vertebra (C2) [53].

Posterior arch ossification When a child reaches 3 years, the posterior arch of the C1 starts to ossify, attaching the lateral masses. This posterior arch formation creates a ring-like shape of C1 and is a key milestone in early skeletal maturity [54].

19.6.1.2 Posterior Arch Fusion

In the age between ages 3 and 8, the fusion of the posterior arch in C1 occurs, and it can differ depending on individual growth patterns. The fusion of this arch is an important benchmark in cervical spine development and is frequently used to evaluate skeletal age in young children. If fusion doesn't take place within the presumed age range, it may indicate conditions affecting bone growth or developmental delays [55].

Fusion timeline The fusion typically takes place between the ages of 3 and 5. Before-time fusion may suggest faster-than-average skeletal development, and delayed fusion may suggest slower maturation [56].

19.6.1.3 The Dens (Odontoid Process) and the C2 Vertebra

Apart from the C1, another important element in evaluating skeletal maturity is the maturation of the dens, or odontoid process, on the axis (C2 vertebra). The head can rotate due to the dens, a bony protrusion that slides into the C1. It fused with the axis's body at a later age (normally around 12) than the C1 ossification [57].

Dens ossification Although the dens begin to ossify immediately after birth, they don't completely fuse with the C2 until adolescence. This fusion shed further light on skeletal age, mainly in adolescence.

Clinical significance Observing the timing of ossification along with fusion in both the C1 and C2 helps diagnose growth disorders. Delays in fusion can represent conditions like other issues affecting the cervical spine or developmental dysplasia.

19.6.2 Atlas Morphology and Growth

The growth and shape of the atlas vertebra or C1 are key points in determining skeletal age. As children grow, the C1 changes in structure and size, with the height of the length of the vertebral arch and the vertebral body acting as crucial markers of the development of the skeleton. Radiographic imaging can be used to collect these measurements, showing a non-invasive method of assessing a child's growth.

19.6.2.1 Growth Patterns in the Atlas

Throughout adolescence and early childhood, the C1 changes, increasing in both width and height. By using radiographic images, a growth pattern can be tracked, showing valuable indicators of skeletal maturity [58].

Height of the vertebral body While the child grows, the atlas height increases. Measuring the atlas' height developmental progress can be monitored. The height represents both overall and ossification growth, creating it a trustworthy marker of skeletal age [59].

Length of the vertebral arch during childhood, the posterior arch of the C1 also grows and normally completes its fusion by the age of 8. Incomplete fusion or delayed growth of the arch may indicate growth issues or developmental delays [60].

19.6.2.2 The Ratio of Height to Length

The ratio of the vertebral body's height to the vertebral arch's length is an important criterion for evaluating atlas growth. This ratio changes as a person grows and offers a reliable gauge of bone development [61].

Height-to-length ratio The C1 has a shorter vertebral body in young children. Following this ratio can help in determining the child's stage of skeletal development, and as they grow older, their height develops faster than their length [61].

Predictive value Comprehensive knowledge of skeletal age can be gained by combining this ratio with additional indicators, such as posterior arch fusion. Another method like hand-wrist radiography, is impractical, or additional confirmation of bone maturity is required; this method can be helpful [62].

19.6.2.3 Clinical Applications

The changes and growth in the atlas have important clinical uses, mostly in paediatric orthodontics. By analysing the atlas's development, healthcare providers can detect spinal growth abnormalities, diagnose congenital issues affecting the cervical spine, and track the effectiveness of growth-related treatments.

Paediatric assessments In children who may have growth delays, examining the growth and ossification of the atlas can help confirm diagnoses and guide treatment plans. Early identification of abnormal atlas development allows for timely interventions that support healthy skeletal growth [18].

19.6.2.4 Forensic Applications

The C1 vertebra is a helpful instrument in forensic science for evaluating the age of skeletal remains. Mainly in cases when the deceased was a teenager, or child, or infant, the degree of fusion and ossification in the atlas provides specific hints related to the age of the deceased.

Age estimation in remains Forensic anthropologists can identify the age of a deceased person by seeing the ossification centres and fusion patterns in C1. This can be very useful in evaluating unexplained remains, typically if other skeletal signs are absent or not accessible [63].

19.7 Scoring

19.7.1 Tanner-Whitehouse Method (TW2)

The Tanner-Whitehouse (TW2) approach is a comprehensive framework for estimating skeletal age that focuses on hand and wrist bones. This method was created by J.M. Tanner and R.H. Whitehouse, including their associates, and rates 20 bones according to their developmental stage. Clinicians can then evaluate skeletal age by comparing these values to traditional growth charts. In a clinical scenario, the TW2 method is normally employed to diagnose developmental problems along with determining the optimal timing of therapies in fields like orthodontics and endocrinology [25].

19.7.1.1 Bone-Specific Scoring System

The Tanner-Whitehouse Method evaluates the following twenty bones from the hand-wrist region:

- *Radius and ulna*
- *Eight carpal bones*: capitate, hamate, triquetral, lunate, scaphoid, trapezium, trapezoid, pisiform
- *Five metacarpals*

- *Six Phalanges*: proximal, middle, and distal phalanges from the first, third, and fifth digits

Early expansion, ossification, the creation of secondary ossification centres, and finally the fusion of the growth plates are the special developmental stages that each bone goes through. Every bone is given a maturity score, keeping a record of these stages with higher scores indicating a more advanced development [64].

19.7.1.2 Stages of Ossification

The form and size of the growth plates, the presence or absence of secondary ossification centres, and the degree of fusion are some of the points used to assess each bone. After that, a score is created with the help of this data, which goes towards evaluating the total skeletal maturity score [18].

19.7.1.3 Total Maturity Score and Skeletal Age

The maturity score is matched with skeletal age with the help of standardised reference charts, followed by the results are compared after the scores for all 20 bones have been generated. These charts reflect whether an individual's growth is advanced, delayed, or normal by comparing their chronological and skeletal ages.

Skeletal age determination The reference data offers age ranges for numerous scores after considering population-specific and gender growth patterns and is compared to the total maturity score.

Clinical applications For the treatment of growth abnormalities like early puberty, growth hormone shortages, and Turner syndrome, the TW2 method is useful. It's also often utilised in orthodontics to find out what time to start treatments which change the way the skeleton or the jaw grows [65].

19.7.1.4 TW2 Variants: TW3 Method

The TW3 method is the result of updates made to the TW2 method to increase its accuracy over time. This updated version has fresh information on patterns of bone maturation. The new method provides better accurate age evaluation for modern populations, and growth patterns may have slightly changed in comparison to earlier data sets, even though the variations between TW2 and TW3 are rather tiny [44].

19.7.1.5 Advantages and Limitations of the TW2 Method

Advantages

Precision: The TW2 method is quite accurate because of its bone-specific approach.

Validated system: It has been highly validated by various populations and is widely received in research and clinical settings.

Comprehensive assessment: By analysing 20 different bones, it gives a thorough estimation of skeletal age.

Limitations

Time-consuming: The TW2 method may be labour-intensive because it involves scoring a large number of bones, making it more time-consuming compared to simpler methods of skeletal age estimation.

Complexity: The TW2 method can only be applied in particular clinical situations by specialists, who have specialised training in explaining the numerous stages of bone formation.

19.7.2 Fishman Skeletal Maturity Indicators (SMI)

Compared to more intricate methods like the TW2 method, the Fishman Skeletal Maturity Indicators (SMI) method created by Dr. Leonard Fishman provides a higher straightforward means of estimating skeletal age. It concentrates on four essential hand and wrist regions: the radius, finger epiphyses, thumb, and ulna. By grouping skeletal development into specific maturity stages, the Fishman method offers a quicker and reliable way to estimate skeletal age, which is especially helpful in orthodontics and clinical settings where fast decisions are needed for treatment planning [66] (Table 19.2).

19.8 Enumerating Age-Related Changes

Skeletal age can be determined by looking at the predictable changes that people's skeletons go through as they age. These changes are essential for specialists tracking growth, biological maturity, and developmental anomalies in both forensic and medical contexts. The mandible, bone density, and certain anatomical landmarks such as the gonial angle and the position of the mental foramen are important skeletal regions that show these age-related changes. These characteristics offer important insights into how the skeleton develops during childhood, adulthood, and old age [68].

19.8.1 Gonial Angle

An accurate indicator of skeletal age is the gonial angle, which is created between the mandible (lower jaw) and the upward branch of the jaw, or back edge of the ramus. This angle is helpful in areas like orthodontics, craniofacial growth research, and forensic science since it changes dramatically in size and shape as a person ages. These modifications show how the jawbone and the muscles attached to it have changed throughout time [69] (Table 19.3, Fig. 19.1).

19.8.2 Bone Density

Bone density, also known as bone mineral density (BMD), is a key indicator of skeletal health and development. It gradually increases throughout childhood and adolescence as bones undergo ossification and mineralization, reaching its highest levels during early adulthood. Bone density begins to decline after this peak, which often occurs in the late 20 s, as a result of hormonal changes, aging, diseases like osteoporosis, and diet. Skeletal age including general bone health can be estimated by measuring bone density, mainly in weight-bearing bones and the mandible [75].

Table 19.2 Fishman Skeletal Maturity Indicators (SMI) stages and interpretation

Stages	Growth status	Key indicators	Clinical implications
1	Prepubertal	The proximal phalanx of the third finger shows equal width of the epiphysis and diaphysis.	Significant growth potential remains. Early orthodontic or growth interventions not yet indicated.
2	Prepubertal	The middle phalanx of the third finger shows equal width of the epiphysis and diaphysis.	Growth potential remains high. Still too early for growth-modifying treatments.
3	Prepubertal	The middle phalanx of the fifth finger shows equal width of the epiphysis and diaphysis.	Growth is ongoing, but rapid growth spurts have not started.
4	Pubertal growth spurt	Appearance of the adductor sesamoid of the thumb.	Ideal phase to begin growth-modifying orthodontic treatments (e.g., jaw alignment).
5	Pubertal growth spurt	Capping of the epiphysis of the distal phalanx on the third finger.	Continued skeletal growth. Orthodontic interventions highly effective at this stage.
6	Pubertal growth peak	Capping of the epiphysis on the middle phalanx of the third finger.	Peak growth; critical period for treatment adjustments to capitalise on rapid growth.
7	End of growth spurt	Capping of the epiphyses of the middle phalanx on the fifth finger.	Nearing completion of skeletal growth; less growth-modifying potential remains.
8	Post-puberty	Fusion between the epiphysis and diaphysis of the distal phalanx on the third finger.	Orthodontic treatments focus on final adjustments rather than growth modification.
9	Post-puberty	Fusion between the epiphysis and diaphysis of the proximal phalanx of the third finger.	Growth largely complete; interventions focus on stabilizing results.
10	Post-puberty	Fusion between the epiphysis and diaphysis of the middle phalanx on the third finger.	Final skeletal development: orthodontic treatment focuses on retention and maintenance.
11	Post-puberty	Fusion of the epiphysis and diaphysis seen in the radius.	Skeletal maturity is complete; no further growth-modifying interventions possible.

Adapted from Mohammed et al. [67]

19.8.2.1 Bone Density During Growth

As bones develop and stiffen during childhood and adolescence, they gradually get denser. Growth hormones and the mechanical stress incurred from physical activity are the driving forces behind this process. The late teens and early twenties are considered the years of full skeletal maturity, as this is when bone density usually reaches its maximum. Bone density is a consistent indicator of the skeleton's developmental stage during this growth phase [76].

Radiographic assessment Bone density can be measured using techniques like dual-energy X-ray absorptiometry (DEXA) and other imaging methods. In children and adolescents, an increase in bone density in areas such as the mandible, spine, and femur indicates healthy skeletal development [77].

19.8.2.2 Peak Bone Density and Decline

Bone density reaches its highest point in early adulthood, typically in the late twenties, when bone formation outpaces bone resorption. After this peak, bone density begins to decline, especially in women after menopause, due to a drop in estrogen levels, which accelerates bone breakdown. Men also experience a gradual decline in bone density, though it occurs at a slower rate compared to women [78].

Osteoporosis and aging As bone density decreases with age, conditions like osteoporosis can develop, particularly in postmenopausal women. Osteoporosis makes bones fragile and more prone to fractures. This loss of density can also be seen in radiographic images of bones such as the mandible, where the cortical bone thins [79].

Table 19.3 Gonial angle development across different life stages

Life stage	Gonial angle	Description	Clinical relevance
Children	>130 degrees	The large angle is due to the vertical growth of the mandible and weaker muscles. It indicates that the mandible is still growing.	Indicates active growth of the jaw; used in orthodontics to track skeletal development.
Adolescence	Gradually narrows as growth continues	As children transition into adolescence, the gonial angle decreases with continued jaw development and muscle strengthening.	Reflects skeletal maturation and the ongoing remodelling of the mandible.
Adults	110–120 degrees	The angle narrows further, reflecting full skeletal maturity and muscle development.	Used in forensic science to estimate age and assess skeletal maturity.
Elderly	May widen again	Due to tooth loss and bone resorption, particularly in the alveolar bone, the gonial angle may increase slightly in old age.	Relevant in geriatric care and forensic anthropology as it indicates bone resorption and changes in mandible structure.

Adapted from [70–74]

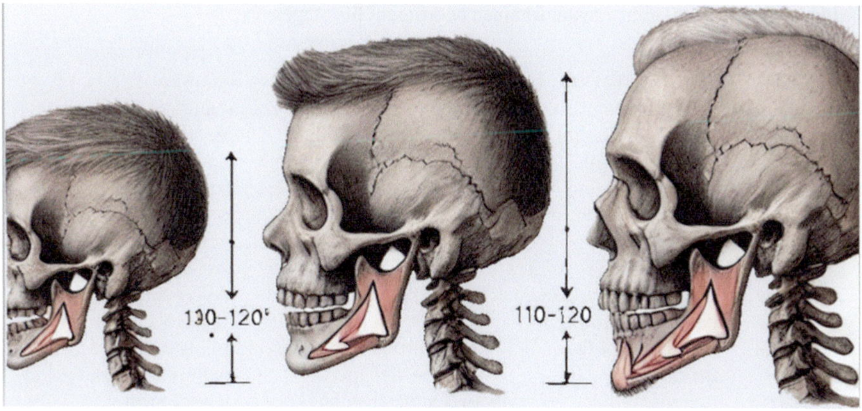

Fig. 19.1 Gonial angle

Bone density and orthodontics In orthodontic treatment planning, bone density is an important factor. Denser bones provide more resistance to tooth movement, which affects how forces are applied during treatment. This is crucial when considering treatments like braces or jaw modifications [80].

19.8.2.3 Bone Density in Age Estimation

Bone density is also a valuable tool in forensic anthropology and gerontology for estimating age, especially in older adults. The gradual decrease in bone density, particularly in areas like the mandible, spine, and femur, is a clear marker of aging. By assessing these changes, experts can estimate an individual's age at death or evaluate their overall bone health [81].

Mandibular bone density The mandible shows noticeable age-related changes in bone density. As a person ages, the bone in the mandible, especially around the tooth sockets (the alveolar process), becomes less dense. Radiographs can show thinning of the cortical bone and increased porosity, both of which are signs of aging [82].

19.8.3 Position of the Mental Foramen

The mental foramen is a small opening on the front surface of the mandible, through which the mental nerve and blood vessels pass. Its position changes throughout life, reflecting the growth and development of the mandible. This shifting position makes the mental foramen a helpful marker for estimating skeletal age, particularly in children and adolescents [83, 84] (Table 19.4).

Table 19.4 Position of the mental foramen at different life stages

Life stage	Mental foramen	Description	Clinical/forensic relevance
Children	Relatively high on the mandible, near the alveolar margin Reflects ongoing vertical and horizontal growth of the mandible.	Distance between the alveolar crest and the mental foramen is shorter.	Important for planning paediatric dental treatments such as extractions and implants, as the location impacts surgical planning.
During growth (adolescent)	Shifts downward and backward, settling in the middle of the mandible	The foramen moves as the mandible grows and the alveolar process develops. Usually settles midway between the alveolar margin and the lower mandible edge.	X-rays can track the foramen's position to estimate skeletal age and monitor mandibular development.
Adult	Mid-height of the mandible, between first and second premolars	In adults, the foramen stabilises in this position. Loss of teeth may cause bone resorption, making the foramen appear higher over time.	Useful in forensic anthropology for age estimation, as its position changes with skeletal maturity and bone loss.

Adapted from [85–89]

19.9 Correlation with Dental Age

Skeletal age and dental age are two related but distinct markers of biological development. Dental age refers to the stages of tooth development, such as eruption, calcification, and root formation. In contrast, skeletal age is determined by the maturation of bones, often assessed through radiographic images of areas like the hand and wrist. Even though these two measurements often show a close developmental trajectory, there are times when nutritional, genetic, and environmental effects cause them to diverge. Each exam is helpful separately, and combining them yields a complete picture of a person's developmental level [90].

In specialities such as orthodontics, paediatric endocrinology, and forensic science, the relationship between dental and skeletal age is crucial. In these domains, appropriate age estimation and treatment options depend on a thorough understanding of an individual's growth and development. A discernible difference in the ages of the skeleton and teeth may point to underlying medical conditions or developmental abnormalities; therefore, it's critical to take both into account when diagnosing and treating a patient [91].

19.9.1 Synchronization of Growth Spurts

Skeletal growth and dental development generally reach their zenith throughout adolescence, especially during the pubertal growth spurt. This synchronisation is essential, particularly in orthodontics, for determining age and scheduling treatments. Clinicians can decide when to intervene with growth-dependent treatments, such as those that attempt to guide tooth eruption or alter jaw alignment, by knowing how dental and skeletal ages correlate with puberty [92].

19.9.1.1 Pubertal Growth Spurt and Its Impact on Skeletal and Dental Development

The pubertal growth spurt, which usually happens between the ages of 12 and 16 for boys and between 10 and 14 for girls, is a time of extremely rapid physical development. Height and facial shape alter significantly during this phase due to a notable acceleration of bone growth, especially in the long bones and the jaw. Concurrently, there is an advancement in dental growth as permanent teeth, particularly second molars and third molars (wisdom teeth), erupt. In order to pinpoint critical growth phases and schedule orthodontic treatments that take advantage of these times of active development, it is imperative to comprehend the relationship between these two processes [93].

Skeletal growth during puberty Bones grow swiftly in length and density during this era of rapid growth, especially in places like the spine, mandible, and limbs. Significant structural alterations take place, as evidenced by X-rays, which show the increased ossification of long bones and the narrowing of the gonial angle [94].

Dental development during puberty Dental growth occurs simultaneously, and by mid-adolescence, the majority of permanent teeth erupt. By now, third molar growth is well underway, and second molars have typically fully erupted. Because the development of the skeleton and the teeth occurs at the same time, adolescence is essential for determining biological age [95].

19.9.1.2 Relationship Between Skeletal and Dental Development in Adolescence

The close relationship between skeletal and dental growth during adolescence is well-established, especially in orthodontic studies. Research shows that the timing of peak mandibular growth often coincides with the final stages of dental development, particularly the eruption of second molars. This alignment is key for determining when to start treatments like braces or orthopaedic appliances, which are most effective when timed with the active growth of the jaw and facial bones [96].

Skeletal and dental growth spurts Studies reveal that the peak in mandibular growth occurs around the same time that the permanent teeth, including the second molars, complete their eruption. This makes the pubertal growth spurt an ideal time for certain orthodontic treatments. For instance, functional appliances used to correct jaw discrepancies work best when applied during this period, as the jaw is most responsive to change [97].

Clinical implications Orthodontists rely on both skeletal and dental maturity to guide treatment plans, particularly those involving jaw growth modifications or tooth realignment. For example, if a patient's dental age suggests the second molars are about to erupt but skeletal maturity indicates the growth spurt is nearing its end, the orthodontist may need to accelerate treatment to take full advantage of the remaining growth period [98].

19.9.1.3 Individual Variations in Growth Timing

While dental and skeletal development often progress together during adolescence, the timing can vary significantly from person to person. Factors such as genetics, nutrition, and hormone levels can cause differences in growth rates, sometimes leading to discrepancies between dental and skeletal maturation. Because of this variety, doctors need to use a thorough, multidisciplinary approach in order to appropriately diagnose patients and develop treatment plans. For example, early or delayed growth spurts can be caused by disorders such as growth hormone shortages or precocious puberty, which can impact skeletal and dental development [99].

Genetic factors When skeletal growth spurts and dental eruption occur is mostly determined by genetics. It may be more difficult to synchronise treatments like orthodontic interventions for some people due to early or delayed development. Children who have a family history of premature skeletal maturation, for instance, may also have faster dental growth and need treatment earlier than is usual for their age group [100].

Hormonal influences Growth time can also be impacted by hormonal abnormalities, such as those brought on by thyroid issues or shortages in growth hormone. When a child has delayed puberty, their skeletal growth may slow down while their teeth continue to grow, resulting in an age discrepancy between their skeleton and teeth. On the other hand, premature puberty can cause skeletal and dental development to speed up, resulting in more advanced growth than is typical for the individual's age [101].

19.9.1.4 Multidisciplinary Approach to Age Assessment

In order to produce precise diagnoses and treatment strategies, a multidisciplinary approach to age assessment is frequently required due to the possibility of differences between skeletal and dental development. In order to evaluate tooth development and bone maturation, this method may combine a number of radiographic techniques. Clinicians can more clearly identify any growth mismatch and modify their therapy by comparing these two signs.

Combining assessments For instance, in orthodontics, utilising panoramic X-rays to evaluate dental development and lateral cephalograms to assess skeletal age using the Cervical Vertebral Maturation Index provides a more comprehensive view of a patient's growth. For treatments like braces, maxillary expansion, or functional appliances that rely on continued bone growth, this dual strategy is crucial.

Forensic applications In forensic anthropology, comparing dental and skeletal age can be valuable in estimating the age of unidentified remains. By analysing bone ossification and the eruption or wear of teeth, forensic experts can narrow down the age range of a deceased individual, even when only partial remains are available. This combination of indicators helps create a more accurate age estimate.

19.10 Conclusion

In disciplines including paediatrics, orthodontics, forensic science, and endocrinology, skeletal age estimation is important. The chapter covers several techniques for estimating skeletal maturity and offers crucial insights into biological development. These techniques include hand-wrist radiography, dental age appraisal, CVMI, and skull-based assessments. These methods are based on age-related changes in the skeleton that may be seen, like dental development, suture closures, and ossification patterns. Forensic investigators and physicians can diagnose developmental abnormalities, arrange treatments, and estimate age more precisely when they have a thorough understanding of these techniques for skeletal maturity.

Skeletal and dental development in childhood and adolescence follow regular timetables that correspond with significant growth periods, like the pubertal growth spurt. Nonetheless, disparities in dental and skeletal age can result from dietary, hormonal, or genetic variables, which is why a multidisciplinary approach is crucial. In clinical settings, particularly in orthodontics, techniques like the Tanner-Whitehouse method (TW2) and Fishman Skeletal Maturity Indicators (SMI) are widely employed to optimise treatment time. These techniques provide systematic and reliable means to estimate skeletal age.The significance of integrating several age assessment techniques for a thorough comprehension of a person's biological development is emphasised in this chapter. Professionals can obtain more precise assessments and customise interventions to the individual's growth trajectory by merging skeletal and dental exams. Skeletal age evaluation is still an essential component in assessing human growth, guaranteeing good treatment outcomes, and estimating age, whether in clinical settings or forensic investigations.

References

1. Sinha A. Comparison and estimation of dental age and skeletal age by radiographic methods with chronological age in children of 8–9 Years. Rajiv Gandhi University of Health Sciences (India); 2020.
2. Boldsen JL, et al. Paleodemography: from archaeology and skeletal age estimation to life in the past. Am J Biol Anthropol. 2022;178:115–50.

3. Ruchira S, Shweta J. “Hand anthropometry - a valuable parameter for grip strength and hand functional assessment”. Asian Journal of Pharmaceutical and Clinical Research, 2023;16(10):pp. 121–4, https://doi.org/10.22159/ajpcr.2023.v16i10.48934.
4. Kahaki SM, et al. Deep convolutional neural network designed for age assessment based on orthopantomography data. Neural Comput Appl. 2020;32:9357–68.
5. Zhou C, et al. Expert consen sus on pediatric orthodontic therapies of malocclusions in children. Int J Oral Sci. 2024;16(1):32.
6. Spadoni GL, Cianfarani S. Bone age assessment in the workup of children with endocrine disorders. Horm Res Paediatr. 2010;73(1):2–5.
7. Manzoor Mughal A, et al. Bone age assessment methods: a critical review. Pak J Med Sci. 2014;30(1):211–5.
8. McNamara JA Jr, Franchi L. The cervical vertebral maturation method: a user’s guide. Angle Orthod. 2018;88(2):133–43.
9. Geoffroy M, et al. Paediatric skull growth models: a systematic review of applications to normal skulls and craniosynostoses. J Stomatol Oral Maxillofac Surg. 2022;123(5):e533–43.
10. Brotons A, et al. Concordances and correlations between chronological, dental and bone ages: a retrospective study in French individuals. Forensic Sci Int. 2022;331:111150.
11. Sarakinova O, et al. Skeletal age determination by using maturational stages of cervical vertebrae. Acta Morphol. 2017;14(1):63–9.
12. Gelbrich B, et al. Comparison of three methods to estimate dental age in children. Clin Oral Investig. 2020;24:2469–75.
13. Huo B, et al. Timing of early correction of mandibular hypoplasia in skeletal class II malocclusion: a review. J Clin Pediatr Dentist. 2023;47(6)
14. Utter MS. The ability of machine learning to predict skeletal maturation using the cervical vertebrae maturation (CVM) method on traced lateral cephalograms. The University of Iowa; 2021.
15. Knoefel M-U. Age-related morphological changes in fifth cervical verterbrae. 1999.
16. Henriques dos Santos MF, et al. Developmental steps of the human cervical spine: parameters for evaluation of skeletal maturation stages. Anat Sci Int. 2010;85:105–14.
17. Różyło-Kalinowska I, et al. Relationship between dental age according to Demirjian and cervical vertebrae maturity in Polish children. Eur J Orthod. 2011;33(1):75–83.
18. Cavallo F, et al. Evaluation of bone age in children: a mini-review. Front Pediatr. 2021;9:580314.
19. Hegde P, Shetty S, Gupta L. Role and Importance of forensic odontology in identification. Int Interdiscip J Sci Res. 2014;1:64–9.
20. Dzemidzic V, et al. Computer based assessment of cervical vertebral maturation stages using digital lateral cephalograms. Acta Inform Med. 2015;23(6):364–8.
21. Cericato GO, et al. Validity of the assessment method of skeletal maturation by cervical vertebrae: a systematic review and meta-analysis. Dentomaxillofac Radiol. 2015;44(4):20140270.
22. Hägg U, Taranger J. Maturation indicators and the pubertal growth spurt. Am J Orthod. 1982;82(4):299–309.
23. Hägg U, Taranger J. Skeletal stages of the hand and wrist as indicators of the pubertal growth spurt. Acta Odontologica Scandinavica. 1980;38(3):187–200.
24. Flores-Mir C, et al. Use of skeletal maturation based on hand-wrist radiographic analysis as a predictor of facial growth: a systematic review. Angle Orthod. 2004;74(1):118–24.
25. Malina RM, et al. Tanner–Whitehouse skeletal ages in male youth soccer players: TW2 or TW3? Sports Med. 2018;48:991–1008.
26. Widek T, et al. Bone age estimation with the Greulich-Pyle atlas using 3T MR images of hand and wrist. Forensic Sci Int. 2021;319:110654.
27. Ludlow JB. Hand-wrist, knee, and foot-ankle dosimetry and image quality measurements of a novel extremity imaging unit providing CBCT and 2D imaging options. Med Phys. 2018;45(11):4955–63.
28. Weaver CM, Fuchs RK. Skeletal growth and development. In: Basic and applied bone biology. Elsevier; 2014. p. 245–60.

29. Algee-Hewitt BF. Age estimation in modern forensic anthropology. In: Forensic anthropology: an introduction. CRC Press; 2013. p. 181–230.
30. Mesejo P, et al. A survey on artificial intelligence techniques for biomedical image analysis in skeleton-based forensic human identification. Appl Sci. 2020;10(14):4703.
31. Aldrees AM, et al. Orthodontic treatment and referral patterns: a survey of pediatric dentists, general practitioners, and orthodontists. Saudi Dent J. 2015;27(1):30–9.
32. Lipsett BJ, et al. Anatomy, head and neck, fontanelles. StatPearls Publishing; 2019.
33. Adeyemo A, Omotade O. Variation in fontanelle size with gestational age. Early Human Develop. 1999;54(3):207–14.
34. Kiviranta AM, Rusbridge C, Lappalainen AK, Junnila JJT, Jokinen TS. Persistent fontanelles in Chihuahuas. Part I. Distribution and clinical relevance. J Vet Intern Med. 2021;35(4):1834–47.
35. McKinney AM, McKinney AM. Normal variations and developmental anatomy of the calvarial sutures and fontanelles above the skull base. In: Atlas of normal imaging variations of the brain, skull, and craniocervical vasculature. Springer; 2017. p. 815–58.
36. White HE, et al. The intertwined evolution and development of sutures and cranial morphology. Front Cell Develop Biol. 2021;9:653579.
37. Atkinson ME. Development and growth of the skull and age changes. In: Anatomy for dental students. Oxford University Press.
38. Sandoval JI, De Jesus O. Scaphocephaly. In: StatPearls [Internet]. StatPearls Publishing; 2023.
39. Cirpan S, et al. The morphological grading and comparison of sutural patency among cranial sutures in dry human skulls. J Craniofac Surg. 2017;28(8):2155–8.
40. Lee S, et al. Pediatric paranasal sinuses-Development, growth, pathology, & functional endoscopic sinus surgery. Clin Anat. 2022;35(6):745–61.
41. Nilendu D. Optical properties of oro-dental tissues in forensic dentistry: implications for identification and age estimation. Arch Biol Life Sci. 2024;1(1):1–6.
42. Priyadarshini C, et al. Dental age estimation methods-a review. LAP Lambert Academic Publ; 2015.
43. Choukroune C. Tooth eruption disorders associated with systemic and genetic diseases: clinical guide. J Dentofac Anom Orthod. 2017;20(4):402.
44. Franklin D. Forensic age estimation in human skeletal remains: current concepts and future directions. Legal Med. 2010;12(1):1–7.
45. Cunha E, et al. The problem of aging human remains and living individuals: a review. Forensic Sci Int. 2009;193(1–3):1–13.
46. Schmeling A, et al. Forensic age estimation in unaccompanied minors and young living adults. In: Forensic medicine-from old problems to new challenges. Rijeka: InTech; 2011. p. 77–120.
47. Garn SM, et al. Endocrine factors in dental development. J Dent Res. 1965;44(1):243–58.
48. Tabakcilar D, et al. Dental age in precocious and delayed puberty periods. Eur J Dent. 2021;15(3):539–45.
49. Ubelaker DH, Khosrowshahi H. Estimation of age in forensic anthropology: historical perspective and recent methodological advances. Forensic Sci Res. 2019;4(1):1–9.
50. Hashim HA, et al. Assessment of skeletal age using hand-wrist radiographs following Bjork System. J Int Soc Prev Community Dent. 2018;8(6):482–7.
51. Prasad C, et al. Objective evaluation of cervical vertebral bone age' its reliability in comparison with hand-wrist bone age: by TW3 method. J Contemp Dental Pract. 2013;14(5):806–13.
52. Chaturvedi A, et al. Malformed vertebrae: a clinical and imaging review. Insights Imaging. 2018;9:343–55.
53. Cramer GD. The cervical region. In: Clinical anatomy of the spine, spinal cord, and ANS. Elsevier; 2013. p. 135–209.
54. Menezes AH. Craniocervical developmental anatomy and its implications. Child's Nerv Syst. 2008;24:1109–22.
55. Wang JC, et al. Growth and development of the pediatric cervical spine documented radiographically. J Bone Joint Surg Am. 2001;83(8):1212–8.

56. Torriani M, Lourenço JLG. Agenesis of the posterior arch of the atlas. Revista do Hospital das Clínicas. 2002;57:73–6.
57. Ishak B, et al. The retroverted dens: a review of its anatomy, terminology, and clinical significance. World Neurosurgery. 2020;137:304–9.
58. Faria AV, et al. Atlas-based analysis of neurodevelopment from infancy to adulthood using diffusion tensor imaging and applications for automated abnormality detection. Neuroimage. 2010;52(2):415–28.
59. Zhang A, et al. Racial differences in growth patterns of children assessed on the basis of bone age. Radiology. 2009;250(1):228–35.
60. Ghanem I, et al. Pediatric cervical spine instability. J Child Orthop. 2008;2(2):71–84.
61. Sone T, et al. Age-related changes in vertebral height ratios and vertebral fracture. Osteoporos Int. 1997;7(2):113–8.
62. Priya E. Methods of skeletal age estimation used by forensic anthropologists in adults: a review. Foresic Res Criminol Int J. 2017;4(2):41.
63. Langley NR, et al. Age estimation methods. In: Forensic anthropology. CRC Press; 2017. p. 193–212.
64. Sousa ESP, et al. Skeletal age assessed by TW2 using 20-bone, carpal and RUS score systems: intra-observer and inter-observer agreement among male pubertal soccer players. PLoS One. 2022;17(8):e0271386.
65. Satoh M. Bone age: assessment methods and clinical applications. Clin Pediatr Endocrinol. 2015;24(4):143–52.
66. Jamir T, et al. Skeletal and dental age assessment methods: a review. J Pharm Negat Results. 2023;14:1603–10.
67. Mohammed RB, et al. The reliability of Fishman method of skeletal maturation for age estimation in children of South Indian population. J Nat Sci Biol Med. 2014;5(2):297–302.
68. Garvin HM, et al. Developments in forensic anthropology: age-at-death estimation. In: A companion to forensic anthropology. Wiley; 2012. p. 202–23.
69. Mehta H, et al. Gender determination using mandibular ramus and gonial angle on OPG. J Indian Acad Oral Med Radiol. 2020;32(2):154–8.
70. Jensen E, Palling M. The gonial angle: a survey. Am J Orthod. 1954;40(2):120–33.
71. Bajracharya M, et al. Gonial angle by lateral cephalogram in orthodontic patients of a tertiary care hospital: a descriptive cross-sectional study. JNMA J Nepal Med Assoc. 2021;59(237):482–5.
72. Vidarsdottir US. Changes in the form of the facial skeleton during growth: a comparative morphometric study of modern humans and Neanderthals. London: University of London, University College London; 1999.
73. Sikaria S, et al. Gonial angle in forensic anthropology to determine age and gender: a population-specific analysis. Cureus. 2024;16(6)
74. Yanıkoğlu N, Yılmaz B. Radiological evaluation of changes in the gonial angle after teeth extraction and wearing of dentures: a 3-year longitudinal study. Oral Surg Oral Med Oral Pathol Oral Radiol Endodontol. 2008;105(6):e55–60.
75. Darelid, A., Bone density, bone geometry and bone development in young men. 2015.
76. Huang TH, Ables GP. Dietary restrictions, bone density, and bone quality. Ann New York Acad Sci. 2016;1363(1):26–39.
77. Gulsahi A, et al. Assessment of bone density differences between conventional and bone-condensing techniques using dual energy x-ray absorptiometry and radiography. Oral Surg Oral Med Oral Pathol Oral Radiol Endodontol. 2007;104(5):692–8.
78. Kleerekoper M. Assessment of bone density and bone strength. In: Treatment of the postmenopausal woman. Elsevier; 2007. p. 331–6.
79. Eastell R, et al. Postmenopausal osteoporosis. Nat Rev Dis Prim. 2016;2(1):1–16.
80. Chang H-W, et al. Effects of orthodontic tooth movement on alveolar bone density. Clin Oral Investig. 2012;16:679–88.
81. Bethard JD, et al. Bone mineral density adult age estimation in forensic anthropology: a test of the DXAGE application. J Forensic Sci. 2019;64(4):1125–8.

82. Jonasson G, et al. Skeletal bone mineral density in relation to thickness, bone mass, and structure of the mandibular alveolar process in dentate men and women. Eur J Oral Sci. 2007;115(2):117–23.
83. Hasan T. Mental foramen morphology: a must know in clinical dentistry. J Pak Dent Assoc. 2012;21(03)
84. Almutairi M, et al. Mental foramen as an indicator of patient's gender, panoramic study in Qassim province, Saudi Arabia. J Dent Health Oral Disord Ther. 2022;13(3):69–72.
85. Cellina M, et al. Anatomy of the mental foramen: relationship among different metrical parameters for accurate localization. Appl Sci. 2023;13(16):9235.
86. Lim M, et al. Age-related changes in the location of the mandibular and mental foramen in children with Mongoloid skeletal pattern. Eur Arch Paediatr Dentist. 2015;16:397–407.
87. Begum S, Gupta S. Methods of age estimation. Dentomed Publication House.
88. Udhaya K, et al. The morphometric analysis of the mental foramen in adult dry human mandibles: a study on the South Indian population. J Clin Diagn Res. 2013;7(8):1547–51.
89. Shaaban A, El-Shall O. Study of age and gender related variations in position of mental foramen of some Egyptians using digital panoramic radiography. Ain Shams J Forensic Med Clin Toxicol. 2017;29(2):36–47.
90. Macha M, et al. Estimation of correlation between chronological age, skeletal age and dental age in children- a cross-sectional study. J Clin Diagn Res. 2017;11(9):Zc01–zc04.
91. Jourieh A, et al. The correlation between dental stages and skeletal maturity stages. Biomed Res Int. 2021;2021:9986498.
92. Flores-Mir C, et al. Association between growth stunting with dental development and skeletal maturation stage. Angle Orthod. 2005;75(6):935–40.
93. Soliman A, et al. Advances in pubertal growth and factors influencing it: can we increase pubertal growth? Indian J Endocrinol Metabol. 2014;18(Suppl 1):S53–62.
94. Sanders JO, et al. The uniform pattern of growth and skeletal maturation during the human adolescent growth spurt. Sci Rep. 2017;7(1):16705.
95. Rai V, et al. Dental and skeletal maturity-a biological indicator of chronologic age. J Clin Diagn Res: JCDR. 2014;8(9):ZC60.
96. Ghafari JG, et al. Monitoring growth during orthodontic treatment. In: Seminars in orthodontics. Elsevier; 1995.
97. Franchi L, et al. Long-term skeletal and dental effects and treatment timing for functional appliances in Class II malocclusion. Angle Orthod. 2013;83(2):334–40.
98. Kirschneck C, Proff P. Age assessment in orthodontics and general dentistry. Quintessence Int. 2018;49(4)
99. Rapaport R, Bowlby DA. Clinical aspects of growth and growth disorders. In: Pescovitz OH, Eugster EA, editors. Pediatric endocrinology: mechanisms, manifestations, and management. Philadelphia: Lippincott Williams&Willkins; 2004. p. 172–90.
100. Suri L, Gagari E, Vastardis H. Delayed tooth eruption: pathogenesis, diagnosis, and treatment. A literature review. Am J Orthod Dentofacial Orthop. 2004;126(4):432–45
101. Dattani M, Preece M. Growth hormone deficiency and related disorders: insights into causation, diagnosis, and treatment. The Lancet. 2004;363(9425):1977–87.

Mind Maps and Illustrative Dental Age Assessment

20

Aman Chowdhry, Priyanka Kapoor, and Pooja Chakraborty

20.1 Introduction to Dental Age Estimation Mind Map

A *mind map* is a useful tool for organizing and displaying complicated information in a flexible yet ordered way. It offers a succinct and straightforward method of arranging and presenting different aspects of a subject, which facilitates comprehension and memory. Mind maps are multisensory tools used in medical and dental science that help medical students integrate, organize, visualize, and then retain and recall information for extended periods of time [1–4].

The mind map presented in this chapter will aid in the smoothening of the complex process of dental age estimation (DAE) into easily understood parts, including estimating techniques, important developmental milestones, and the importance of each stage in diverse clinical contexts. Practitioners can quickly access and use pertinent information in real-world situations with the help of a well-structured mind map.

A. Chowdhry (✉)
Oral Pathology & Microbiology, Faculty of Dentistry, Jamia Millia Islamia, New Delhi, India
e-mail: achowdhry@jmi.ac.in

P. Kapoor
Orthodontics, Faculty of Dentistry, Jamia Millia Islamia, New Delhi, India
e-mail: pkapoor@jmi.ac.in

P. Chakraborty
Forensic Biology Expert, Chandigarh Police, Chandigarh, India

© The Author(s), under exclusive license to Springer Nature Switzerland AG 2026

A. Chowdhry, P. Kapoor (eds.), *Dental Age Assessment*,
https://doi.org/10.1007/978-3-032-08788-1_20

20.2 Reasons to Classify and Segregate Dental Age Estimation Methods

The ability of mind maps to cohesively convey both conceptual and procedural information is what makes them significant in DAE. When learned or explained in linear formats, the variety of techniques used in DAE—such as radiographic analysis, tooth eruption stages, and mineralization patterns—can be daunting. One can demonstrate the connections between these techniques and give a visual depiction of how they affect dental age by making a mind map. This promotes active recall and problem-solving skills while also helping researchers, physicians, and students better understand the full extent of DAE.

- *Need for this mind map*: A mind map can assist in streamlining and organizing the decision-making process, even though the vast array of DAE techniques poses a challenge. The mind map can be a useful tool for choosing the best approach in any particular circumstance by outlining approaches according to population-specific demands, practicality, accuracy, and resource requirements. It simplifies intricate comparisons, clarifies the areas in which each approach is most effective, and helps the practitioner make well-informed, fact-based judgments.
- *Components of a mind map*: Parts of a mind map [5] in a DAE context:
  (a) The central theme in this instance is "Age estimation" for kids, teens, and adults.
  (b) The branching theme includes several DAE techniques.
  (c) Visual representation is denoted by colors, patterns, and shapes that distinguish the many themes and concepts depicted.
  (d) Connections between branches (such as DAE techniques) are emphasized to show how concepts are built upon and linked to one another.
- *Novelty*: To the best of our knowledge, there isn't a current, user-friendly mind map. For a more thorough and organized understanding of the subject, we divided the use of DAE techniques into three categories: children, adolescents, and adults.

20.3 The Mind Map (Fig. 20.1)

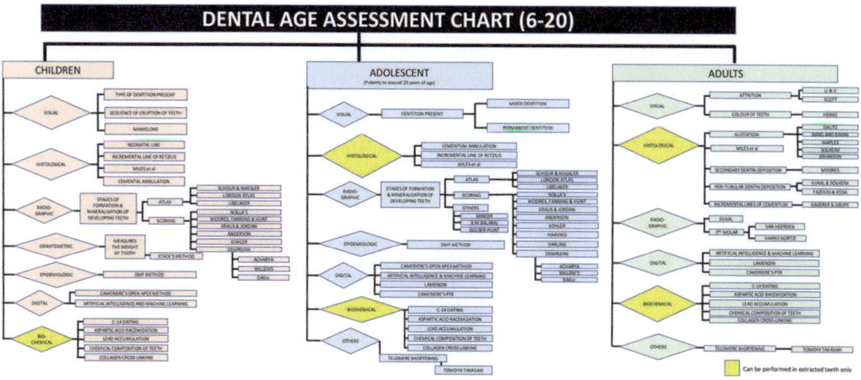

Fig. 20.1 After a careful appraisal of the literature [6–20] and drawing from personal research experience in DAE, a condensed mind map showing many DAE techniques compiled and structured into a classification scheme. This Mind map will surely improve the conceptual comprehension of the readers

20.4 Application of Dental Age Estimation Mind Map in Forensic Setup

By using of mind map for DAE, both professionals and students can easily navigate a tool that will enhance their understanding in this field. This mind map in the current chapter will help with decision-making and increase precision and productivity in all of its fieldwork applications. Such a mind map can be useful in the following ways:

(a) Arranges the main ideas and methods of DAE.
(b) Provides a comprehensive overview of DAE techniques.
(c) Fast reference for professionals
(d) Support forensic investigations and provide prompt on-site references
(e) Encouraging inter-disciplinary communication
(f) Training and student educational tool
(g) Research and development
(h) Tracking developmental trends
(i) Ethical and legal aspects
(j) Visualizing several DAE techniques for various age groups

20.5 Summary and Conclusions

In clinical and educational contexts, using a mind map to illustrate DAE procedures offers a number of benefits. By graphically structuring intricate, multi-step procedures, it first improves clarity and makes the material easier to understand. A mind map can be a great teaching tool that ensures practitioners have a thorough understanding of the area by displaying the many DAE approaches and their applicability across different specializations. Furthermore, it promotes improved memory and retention of important ideas, which is essential in clinical practice when prompt, precise choices are required. In the end, this mind map improves patient outcomes across several disciplines by streamlining the learning process and facilitating the more efficient use of DAE approaches.

References

1. Shrivastava SR, Shrivastava PS. From chaos to clarity: use of mind maps as a tool to ensure better learning among medical students. Indian J Community Med. 2024;49(1):233–6.
2. Edwards S, Cooper N. Mind mapping as a teaching resource. Clin Teach. 2010;7(4):236–9.
3. Tattersall C, Powell J, Stroud J, Pringle J. Mind mapping in qualitative research. Nurs Times. 2011;107(18):20–2.
4. Ordu Y, Caliskan N. The impact of a web-based mind map learning technique on students' nursing knowledge of the nursing process. Int J Nurs Knowl. 2023;34(2):108–15.
5. Williams B. What is a mind map: 7 key elements explained [Internet]. Insight7 - AI Tool For Interview Analysis & Market Research. 2024 [cited 2025 Jun 11]. Available from: https://insight7.io/what-is-a-mind-map-7-key-elements-explained/.
6. Vila-Blanco N, Varas-Quintana P, Tomás I, Carreira MJ. A systematic overview of dental methods for age assessment in living individuals: from traditional to artificial intelligence-based approaches. Int J Legal Med. 2023;137(4):1117–46.
7. AlQahtani SJ, Hector MP, Liversidge HM. Accuracy of dental age estimation charts: Schour and Massler, Ubelaker and the London Atlas. Am J Phys Anthropol. 2014;154(1):70–8.
8. Demirjian A, Goldstein H, Tanner JM. A new system of dental age assessment. Hum Biol. 1973;45(2):211–27.
9. Kvaal SI, Kolltveit KM, Thomsen IO, Solheim T. Age estimation of adults from dental radiographs. Forensic Sci Int. 1995;74(3):175–85.
10. Willems G, Van Olmen A, Spiessens B, Carels C. Dental age estimation in Belgian children: Demirjian's technique revisited. J Forensic Sci. 2001;46(4):893–5.
11. Chowdhry A, Kapoor P, Bablani PD. Oral pathologist in development of the subject of forensic odontology-the road ahead. J Indo Pacific Acad Forensic Odontol. 2020;9(2):113–6.
12. Haavikko K. Tooth formation age estimated on a few selected teeth. A simple method for clinical use. Proc Finn Dent Soc Suom Hammaslaakariseuran Toim. 1974;70(1):15–9.
13. Chowdhry A, Kapoor P, Bhargava D, Bagga DK, Mehta A. Comparison of Demirjian's comprehensive chart with the London atlas of tooth development in children and adolescents: a pilot study. Forensic Sci Res. 2023;8(4):332–7.
14. Kapoor P, Jain V. Comprehensive chart for Dental Age Estimation (DAEcc8) based on Demirjian 8-teeth method: simplified for operator ease. J Forensic Leg Med. 2018;59:45–9.
15. Jain V, Kapoor P, Miglani R. Demirjian approach of dental age estimation: abridged for operator ease. J Forensic Dent Sci. 2016;8(3):177.
16. Cameriere R, Ferrante L, Belcastro MG, Bonfiglioli B, Rastelli E, Cingolani M. Age estimation by pulp/tooth ratio in canines by peri-apical X-rays. J Forensic Sci. 2007;52(1):166–70.
17. Kashyap VK, Koteswara Rao NR. A modified Gustafson method of age estimation from teeth. Forensic Sci Int. 1990;47(3):237–47.
18. Gustafson G, Malmö DO. Age determinations on teeth. J Am Dent Assoc. 1950;41(1):45–54.
19. Moorrees CF, Fanning EA, Hunt EE. Age variation of formation stages for ten permanent teeth. J Dent Res. 1963;42:1490–502.
20. Cameriere R, Ferrante L, Cingolani M. Age estimation in children by measurement of open apices in teeth. Int J Legal Med. 2006;120(1):49–52.

MIX
Papier aus verantwortungsvollen Quellen
Paper from responsible sources
FSC® C105338
FSC
www.fsc.org

If you have any concerns about our products,
you can contact us on
ProductSafety@springernature.com

In case Publisher is established outside the EU,
the EU authorized representative is:
Springer Nature Customer Service Center GmbH
Europaplatz 3, 69115 Heidelberg, Germany

Printed by Libri Plureos GmbH
in Hamburg, Germany